Infected Total Joint Arthr

Rihard Trebše

Editor

Infected Total Joint Arthroplasty

The Algorithmic Approach

Springer

Editor
Rihard Trebše
Orthopedic Hospital Valdoltra
Ankaran
Slovenia

ISBN 978-1-4471-2481-8   ISBN 978-1-4471-2482-5   (eBook)
DOI 10.1007/978-1-4471-2482-5
Springer London Heidelberg New York Dordrecht

Library of Congress Control Number: 2012952504

Printed on acid-free paper

Springer is part of Springer Science+Business Media (www.springer.com)

Foreword

The authors of this book are outstanding experts on implant-associated complications. This has qualified them to write a well-structured and singularly interesting contribution on the subject.

To begin with, the history of implants is reviewed and the biomaterials used for them are described. This leads on to a special section devoted to the influence of wear particles on the local and systemic immune system emphasizing that for metal-on-metal articulations, for example, the effects on the entire body need to be considered over and above local responses like corrosion particles and lymphocyte infiltration. These are, no doubt, less dramatic with ceramic-on-ceramic articulations than with cross-link articulations. However, the ultimate effects of the cross-link particles generated are, for instance, not yet predictable.

The differential diagnosis of septic and aseptic complications and the entire battery of microbiologic tests are given extensive attention. All diagnostic approaches including histology, cytology, microbiologic sampling, and microbial spectra as well as newest state-of-the-art modalities like molecular biology tests are described and discussed at great length. Based on these diagnostic tests, the most recent insights into antibiotic medication, dosage, and adverse events are addressed. Interactions between bacteria and biomaterials and those between implant materials and peri-implant tissues in both septic and aseptic complications are also reviewed and more sophisticated diagnostic modalities like imaging techniques including isotope studies are described.

All of these subjects make the reader aware of the complexity of the problem and the potential of diagnostic studies. In a similar approach, potential treatments are described and an easily comprehensible algorithm associating diagnosis and treatment is defined. This should guarantee optimal function achieved with the most effective therapeutic modalities in terms of permanent infection control. The use of bone grafts and bone substitutes in one- or two-stage procedures for infected hip implants is also addressed.

Arranged in clearly structured sections, this book thus offers helpful guidelines for diagnosing and treating implant-associated problems. The different aspects of the problem are given equal weight so that the reader can expect a well laid out, wide-range and – more important still – user-friendly practical guide to decision-making.

Karl Zweimuller

Contents

Part I

Chapter 1
Introduction

Rihard Trebše

Keywords Processes • Errors • Controlling

With the advent of low-friction total hip replacements in the 1960s, total joint replacements (TJR) have become predictable and reliable procedures. Although infections have been present throughout the history of TJR the major focus of development, in the field was concentrated on improvements in the design and the materials of implants. Despite the fact that prosthetic joint infections (PJI) have been, since the early days of the alloarthroplasty era, a main area concern for both orthopedic surgeons and patients the prevention and treatment of such infections was never the primary focus of scientific research. era (Fig. 1.1).

Surgeons had (and still have) the tendency to hide the problem or to inadvertently misdiagnose the condition until the development of purulent discharge that can not be ignored or misinterpreted. Difficult and disappointing treatment as well as frequent and frustrating communication with the affected patients and their relatives, led to the tendency for the treating surgeon to provide treatment even if he was not actually interested in it and did not have the appropriate experience to administer it, not to mention, the team, and knowledge (and general support).

As a result the problem was traditionally solved radically by removal of the implant and radical debridement accompanied by the predictable control of sepsis even in cases of suboptimal antibiotic support. Although the infection was brought under control, the patient was frequently left with no joint and limited function. The issue and the timing of reimplantation become a matter for discussion between the treating surgeon and the patient based on historical practice in the hospital.

Over time, this issue has improved but not sufficiently. Making matters more difficult, the condition is generally treated by low volume surgeons who, because of

R. Trebše, Ph.D., M.D.
Department for Bone Infections and Adult Reconstructions,
Orthopaedic Hospital Valdoltra,
Jadranska cesta 31, Ankaran SI-6286, Slovenia
e-mail: rihard.trebse@ob-valdoltra.si

R. Trebše (ed.), *Infected Total Joint Arthroplasty*,
DOI 10.1007/978-1-4471-2482-5_1, © Springer-Verlag London 2012

Fig. 1.1 Pain (By Dr.
Silvester Fonda, Orthopedic
Hospital, Valdoltra, Slovenia)

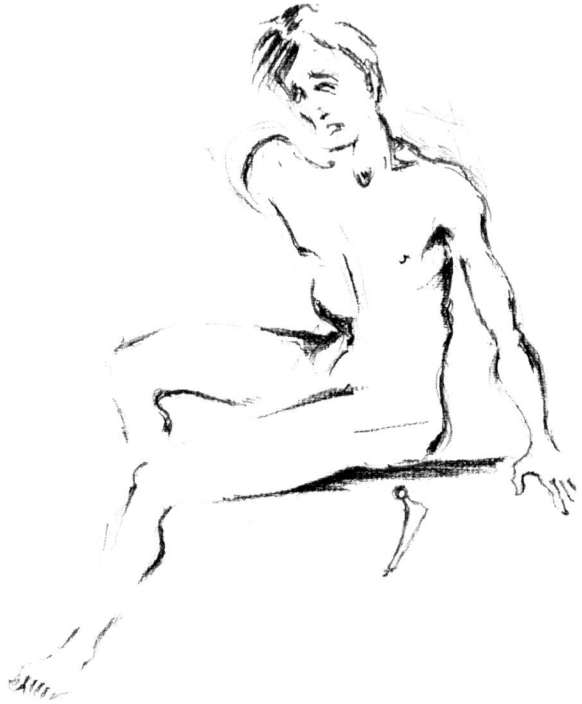

their limited experience and knowledge, tend to cause proportionately more complications in joint replacement procedures, as the incidence of infection is highly correlated to the surgical volume of both surgeon and hospital.

There are nearly no randomized studies in this field, and strong unequivocal evidence is being gathered very slowly. Only a few centers have adopted any consistency in terms of diagnostic and therapeutic processes involved. Comparisons are thus very difficult.

During the period of rapid industrialization, the process of industrial quality control developed with the aim to identify mistakes and remove defective products to decrease costs and to improve performances and customers' satisfaction. The consistent analyses of defective products provided a basis for introducing corrective measures to improve quality. The introduction and implementation of standards (such as ISO) was relatively slow and costly, but the improvements have been substantial.

Contemporary industrial standards are based on preventive measures. The institutions adopt strictly defined measures including meticulous analysis of the incoming products (subjects), activities, and potential risks, which can affect the quality of the product or the service.

In medicine, we lag far behind industry in this respect. All doctors occasionally make terrible mistakes [1, 2], but it is the lack of institutionalized preventive processes and measures that allow the repetition of errors and malfeasance within a hospital. The complexity of biological processes in medicine has provided excuse for avoiding the standardization of our procedures. One of the first radical improvements in process control in medicine was achieved by anesthesiologists who in the 1990s implemented regulations in their working processes, which resulted in dramatic improvements of the safety of their work [3, 4]. The medical community found it difficult to accept the implementation of these processes, but the results have been outstanding and in the end were appreciated by all those involved.

In recent years, changes have been under way to implement standards in hospitals similar to those implemented by industry decades ago. Some hospitals have succeeded controlling many processes, particularly those not directly involving medicine, but the standardization of the pure medical field is still relatively undeveloped in large part because of the variety views that doctors have on what is correct, appropriate, and acceptable and what is not.

There have always been studies in medicine that enabled us to accumulate a great deal of knowledge, and yet the appropriate and widespread implementation of that knowledge within real clinical setting has not been successful. In recent years, due to the increased expectations of patients and insurance providers, there has been a movement to institute quality control even in the difficult and variable field of clinical work in order to improve results and reduce mistakes. By making use of precise definitions of processes that govern treatment, identifying and focusing on potential risks, analyzing of protocol deviations, medicine, similarly to industry, can augment the safety of the patients and improve treatment outcomes. The downside is increased administration and work burden for medical personnel, especially doctors.

Total joint arthroplasty surgery has just exited the exponential growth period and is entering a steady phase. In the developing world, and to a certain extent even in the West, projections still show considerable growth in this important orthopedic field. The problem of PJI, which causes much suffering, distress, and considerable costa, is thus becoming even more pressing.

The concept of this book is to objectively present the basic knowledge regarding microprocesses that are involved in the evolution of a PJI, to present the current clinical evidence regarding established treatment options, and, based on this presentation to comprehensively define appropriate procedures for diagnostic evaluation and patient allocation to defined treatment options and finally to describe the specific treatment protocols involved.

It is our goal to contribute to the efforts to establish standards of treatment for PJI. Only when we are able to set a standpoint it will it be possible to study the variations that will eventually lead to substantial improvements in treatment.

References

1. Brennan TA, et al. Incidence of adverse events and negligence in hospitalized patients: results of Harvard Medical Practice study I. N Eng J Med. 1991;324:370–6.
2. Localio AR, et al. Relation between malpractice claims and adverse events due to negligence: results of Harvard Medical Practice Study III. N Eng J Med. 1991;325:245–51.
3. Cooper JB, et al. Preventable anesthesia mishaps: a study of human factors. Anesthesiology. 1978;49:399–406.
4. Pierce EC, et al. The 34th Rovenstine Lecture: 40 years behind the mask – safety revisited. Anesthesiology. 1996;84:965–75.

Chapter 2
Joint Replacement: Historical Overview

Rihard Trebše and Anže Mihelič

Abstract Joint diseases have troubled people since the ancient times. Many devoted surgeons have introduced numerous surgical techniques and important progress was made in the development of materials and implant designs. Prosthetic joint infections were the main reason for poor success of the early implants.

Keywords Artificial joints • History • Development • Surgeons

Joint diseases, their wear in particular, and bone fractures have troubled people since the ancient times, as proved by numerous excavations from different time periods [1–3]. Even Hippocrates in his texts considered sprains and fractures separately. From the ancient times until present days, many different and innovative attempts of bone disease treatments have been invented with many successes as well as terrible failures [4].

The history of artificial joints and internal fixation of fractures is already very long and infections, were present from the very beginnings. Already the first documented artificial joint had to be removed because of this complication. Historically, infections were the most common cause of failure and very frequently fatal. They represented the main obstacle in the widespread development of bone surgery [5].

In London in 1822 Anthony White (1782–1849) from Westminster Hospital performed the first excision joint arthroplasty [6]. The first surgical principles and techniques for bone fracture treatment developed in the eighteenth and nineteenth century. The first fixation plate was made by Hansmann from Hamburg in 1886. In the early times very cumbersome instruments were used for fracture stabilization, and usually, highly unstable osteosynthesis followed open reduction of the fracture [7].

Artificial joints appeared during this period, too. They were fully unsuccessful in almost all cases, mainly due to septic complications. Professor Themistocles Glück

R. Trebše, Ph.D., M.D. (✉) • A. Mihelič, M.D.
Department for bone infections and adult reconstructions,
Orthopaedic Hospital Valdoltra,
Jadranska cesta 31, Ankaran SI-6286, Slovenia
e-mail: rihard.trebse@ob-valdoltra.si; anze.mihelic@ob-valdoltra.si

R. Trebše (ed.), *Infected Total Joint Arthroplasty*,
DOI 10.1007/978-1-4471-2482-5_2, © Springer-Verlag London 2012

7

Fig. 2.1 The explanted Judet
acrylic hemi hip arthroplasty
51 years after implantation

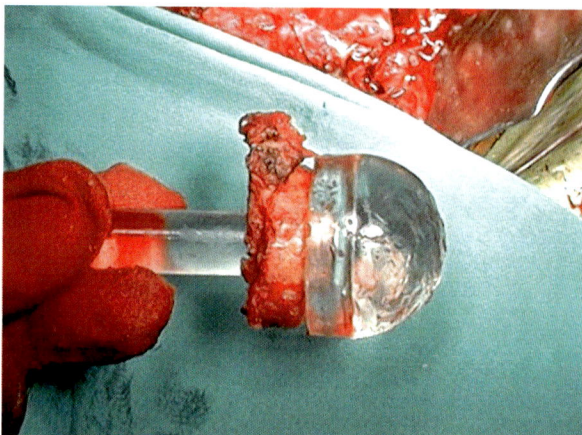

(1853–1942) from Berlin implanted the first artificial knee in 1890 and manufactured and implanted the first artificial hip in 1891 as well. The ivory head was fixed to the bone with a nickel plate and screws [8]. He is also credited for introducing the term arthroplasty in 1902. In 1893 the French surgeon Pean implanted the first artificial shoulder joint. The implant, made of natural, biological materials, lasted for 2 years which is almost incredible [9].

Before Charnley's "low-friction arthroplasty," hip implants were predominating, and most of the development was also concerning the hips. Typically the implants were used as an interposition arthroplasty and made from various materials with unpredictable results. The pioneer of these surgical procedures was renowned American surgeon of Norwegian origins, Marius Smith Petersen (1886–1953). With the introduction of Vitallium® interposition implant (Co-Cr-Mo alloy), he achieved the first predictable and lasting results of this type of surgery [10].

In this period surgeons experimented with real bone-joint replacements from various materials. The acrylic implant from brothers Robert (1901–1980) and Jean (1905–1995) Judet from Paris achieved the greatest popularity. It was introduced in 1948. This implant holds the current world record in the implant in vivo durability – 51 years [11] (Fig. 2.1).

Artificial knees were developed in the same period but they were less successful if compared to hip implants. The reason for the inferior results was probably not in the implants but resulted from inadequate surgical technique. Contemporary principles of mechanical axis balance and the importance of joint stability evolved only in the mid-1980s. Following the example of Smith-Petersen, Boyd introduced Vitallium (Co-Cr alloy) femoral coating. Similar implants for femoral and tibial part were tested also by others, including Smith Petersen, but without success [12]. In 1957 Walldius published his comparison of hinge knee endoprostheses and resection arthroplasties (Fig. 2.2). Good results of the hinged knee implant opened a new era of total knee replacements, which prevailed for the next 30 years, in some centers almost to the present days. The study was a landmark for another reason. It was

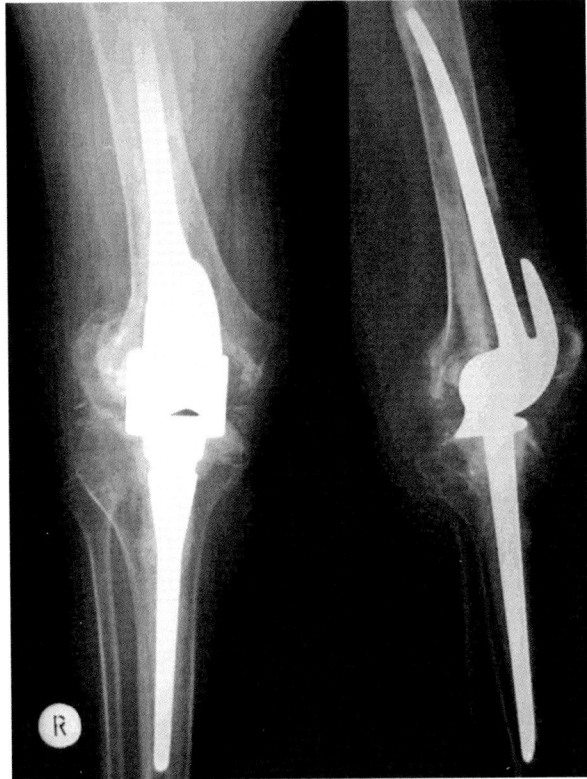

the first one with pain as the indication for the implantation of an artificial joint [13].
Until then, limited range of movements was virtually the only appropriate
indication.

Following the example of J. Charnleya, in Wrightington Hospital Gunston was
the first to used polyethylene against metal in his knee replacement which represented
the predecessor of the contemporary condylar type of knee replacements [14].
Gunston devoted considerable attention to the kinematics of the knee but neglected
efficient fixation, which made his implant unsuccessful.

Only in 1974, following the example of Freeman's implants (Fig. 2.3), Insall
introduced the first successful total condylar knee replacement and developed a
surgical technique that was indispensable for this type of knee replacement to function effectively [15].

In the same fashion, implants for other joints were developed. These are, however, much less frequently used today, although the incidence is increasing,
especially for the shoulders.

Further development of the implants was based on the introduction of new materials, different ways of fixation, advances in implant design, properties and coatings,
and new, less invasive surgical techniques [16]. Today the list of materials used for
production of artificial joints is very extensive.

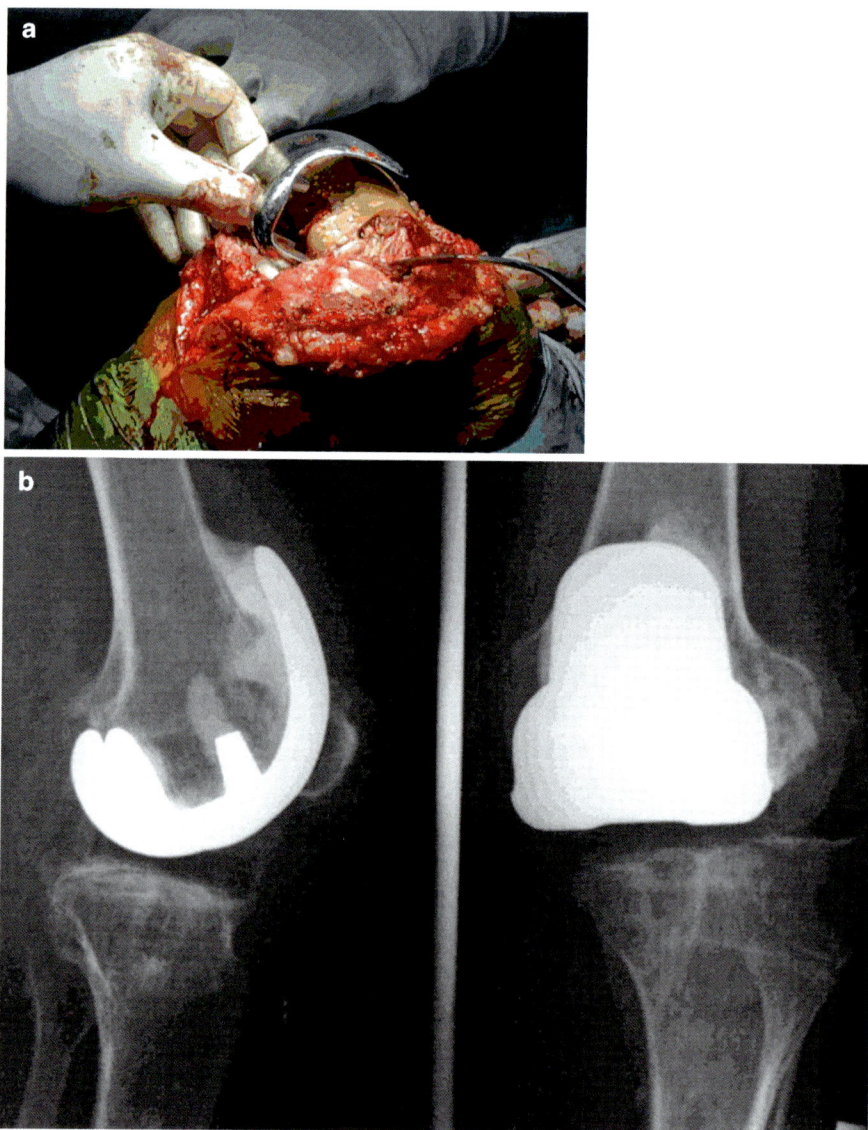

Fig. 2.3 (a) Revision of a Freeman total knee arthroplasty 20 years after implantation that failed due to instability. (b) X-ray of the same knee before explanation

References

1. Rogers J, Watt I, Dieppe P. Arthritis in Saxon and mediaeval skeletons. Br Med J. 1981;283:1668–70.
2. Thould AK, Thould BT. Arthritis in Roman Britain. Br Med J. 1983;287:1909–11.

3. Trinkaus E. Pathology and the posture of the La Chapelle-aux-Saints Neandertal. Am J Phys Anthropol. 1985;67:19–41.
4. MacLennan WJ. History of arthritis and bone rarefaction: evidence from paleopathology onwards. Scot Med J. 1999;44:18–20.
5. Gomez PF, Morcuende JA. Early attempts at hip arthroplasty 1700s to 1950s. Iowa Orthop J. 2005;25:25–9.
6. Anon. Anthony White (obituary). Lancet. 1849;1:324.
7. Broos PL, Sermon A. From unstable internal fixation to biological osteosynthesis. A historical overview of operative fracture treatment. Acta Chir Belg. 2004;104:396–400.
8. Rang M. Anthology of orthopaedics. Edinburgh/London/New York: Churchill Livingstone; 1966.
9. Rockwood CA, Matsen F, Wirth M. The shoulder. 3rd ed. Philadelphia: Saunders; 2004.
10. Smith-Petersen M. Evolution of mould arthroplasty of the hip joint. J Bone Joint Surg Br. 1948;30:59.
11. Kovač S, Pišot V, Trebše R, Rotter A. Fifty-one years survival of a Judet polymethylmethacrylate hip prosthesis. J Arthroplasty. 2004;19:664–7.
12. Klenerman L, editor. The evolution of orthopaedic surgery. London: The Royal Society of Medicine Press Limited; 2002.
13. Walldius B. Arthroplasty of the knee joint using an endoprosthesis. Acta Orthop Scand Suppl. 1957;24:1–112.
14. Gunston FH. Polycentric knee arthroplasty. Prosthetic simulation of normal knee movements. J Bone Joint Surg Br. 1971;53:272–7.
15. Insall J, Scott WN, Ranawat CS. The total condylar knee prosthesis. A report of two hundred and twenty cases. J Bone Joint Surg Am. 1979;61(2):173–80.
16. Konttinen YT, Milošev I, Trebše R, Rantanen P, Linden R, Tiainen V, Virtanen S. Metals for joint replacement. In: Ravel PA, editor. Joint replacement technology. New developments. Cambridge: Woodhead Publishing; 2008.

Chapter 3
Biomaterials in Artificial Joint Replacements

Rihard Trebše

Abstract Prosthetic joint infection is by definition a disease determined by the presence of a foreign body. Since the materials used for joint implants vary considerably, it is important to have a basic knowledge of the characteristics of the materials used in joint replacement technologies. An overview of the biomaterials and their characteristics is presented in this chapter, focusing on the features important for infection development. Orthopedic metals, ceramics, and polymers are described in some detail as well as novel approaches to functionalize the surfaces to prevent bacterial colonization and subsequent infection.

Keywords Metals • Polymers • Corrosion • Mechanical proprieties

3.1 Introduction

Biomaterials are substances used for medical applications in the human body. Their use is increasing rapidly. In the developed world nearly every aged person was carrying some sort of device during the life span. The biomaterial market is valued as more than $300 billion US Dollars and increasing by 20 % per year [4].

Biomaterials have many limitations. They must satisfy biofunctionality and biocompatibility requirements. The real and potential hazards must be acceptable and in line with the purpose. The production and handling are strongly regulated with special emphasis on the proprieties, production, testing requirements, toxicity, sterilization, traceability, and others. The core standards that regulate biomaterials have been published in EN ISO 10993 series, which includes many criteria.

According to their chemical composition, biomaterials can be classified as metals, ceramics, polymers, composites, and substances from biological origin. According to the host reaction, the biomaterials are:

R. Trebše, M.D., Ph.D.
Department for Bone Infections and Adult Reconstructions,
Orthopaedic Hospital Valdoltra,
Jadranska cesta 31, Ankaran SI-6286, Slovenia
e-mail: rihard.trebse@ob-valdoltra.si

R. Trebše (ed.), *Infected Total Joint Arthroplasty*,
DOI 10.1007/978-1-4471-2482-5_3, © Springer-Verlag London 2012

Biotolerant, like bone cement. These biomaterials are in the body usually covered with a fibrous membrane.

Bioinert, which can in certain conditions form direct chemical bonds with tissues, like Ti and Al oxides.

Bioactive, which directly incorporate in the bones hydroxyapatite or bioglass.

Bioresorbable, which undergo partial (Ca phosphate) or full (polyglycolides) resorption.

According to surface reactivity biomaterials can be divided as:

1. Almost inert – smooth surface
2. Almost inert – porous surface
3. Those having chemically reactive surfaces
4. Bioresorbable materials

Metallic joint implants belong to group one or two depending on the surface finish. Mostly they become covered with a fibrous membrane that represents a result of the foreign body reaction to metal. The material is in this case considered biotolerant. Metals can be bioinert, too. Especially titanium and its oxides can make bonds to bone in appropriate conditions. Surface reactive materials directly bind to bone. The examples are bioglasses and hydroxyapatite.

In bone surgery [8] the most important biomaterials are metals, ceramics polymers, and, to a smaller extent, other materials. Among the metals, surgical steel, Co and Cr alloys, commercially pure titanium (CPT), Ti alloys, aluminium, and tantalum alloys prevail. Silver, and other noble metals are rarely adopted.

The features that are important for their applications include biocompatibility, elasticity, toughness, fatigue resistance, corrosion resistance [21], and allergic diathesis.

3.2   Metals for Joint Replacements

Surgical steel (AISI 316 L) is an alloy of steel, carbon, and at least 11 % of chrome. Chrome on the surface forms the durable passive oxide layer that protects the surface against corrosion. Although the corrosion resistance of surgical steel is high, other materials like cobalt or titanium alloys perform better in this term. Being relatively sensitive to pit and crevice corrosion steel should not have a porous coating. Anticorrosive properties of steel may be further improved by the addition of nickel and molybdenum. Nickel also stabilizes the austenitic organization of the material which is responsible for nonmagnetic nature of the material that allows for magnetic resonance imaging. Stainless steel is in use already for a long time, and today it is mainly used for the implants that are intended to be subsequently removed, although the organism tolerates well the metal ions that are slowly released from the material. Good fatigue resistance of $350/400$ MPa/10^7 walking cycles makes it lasting indefinitely. Adverse conditions with improper design, material defects, and corrosion resulted in occasional failure (Fig. 23.5). With the elastic modulus of 200 GPa, it is approximately ten times stiffer than bone. Fixation of steel with bone cement,

Fig. 3.1 Bone ongrowth on
CPT Allofit cementless cup
removed for infection

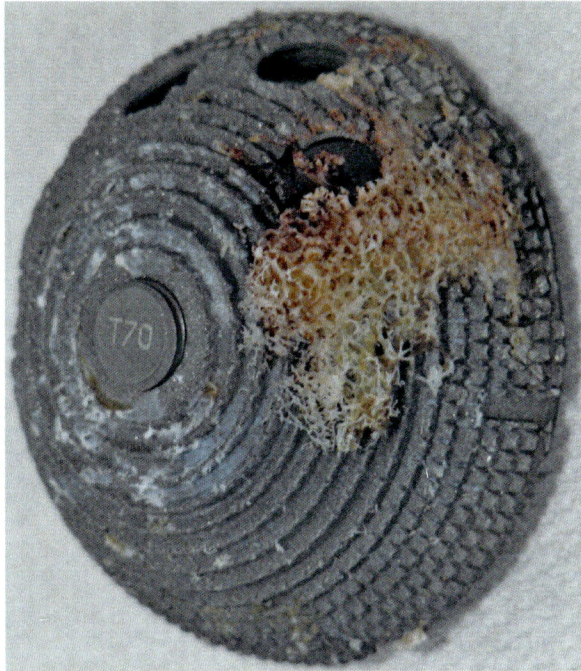

which serves for stress distribution, reduces the stress-shielding effect due to much lower elastic modulus of bone cement.

Co and Cr alloys (like CoCr29Mo5, F-75) usually contain 30–60 % Co and 20–30 % Cr, and the rest is mainly Mo and sometimes Ni. They are the most frequently used materials for arthroplasty components for fixation with cement. Fixation with cement is necessary due to its low elastic modulus of 200–300 GPa (10–15 times stiffer than diaphyseal bone). As in surgical steel, cement serves for stress distribution and reduction of stress-shielding effect. Due to the formation of a passive layer of Cr oxides [21], on their surface these alloys are very resistant to corrosion. High resistance of these alloys also to galvanic corrosion makes it possible to combine Co and Ti alloy components.

Titanium (commercially pure titanium) and its alloys (mainly $TiAl_6V_4$, rarely $TiZr_{13}Nb_{13}$ and others) have better corrosion resistance than steel- or cobalt-based alloys. Ti oxide that forms on the surface provides the passive protection layer against corrosion. In case this passive surface is abraded; the surface is spontaneously repassivated. Ti oxides accumulated around the implant in abrasion conditions stain the tissues black (metallosis). Aluminium has been associated with osteomalacia and dementia. Ti alloys contain aluminium that is uniformly distributed and does not accumulate on surface. There are no reports of dementia or osteomalacia linked to the use of aluminum containing Ti alloys. Excellent corrosion resistance allows the use of porous surface (pore size, e.g., 50–400 μm, pore interconnectivity, e.g., 75–150 μm), which facilitates biological ingrowth (Fig. 3.1).

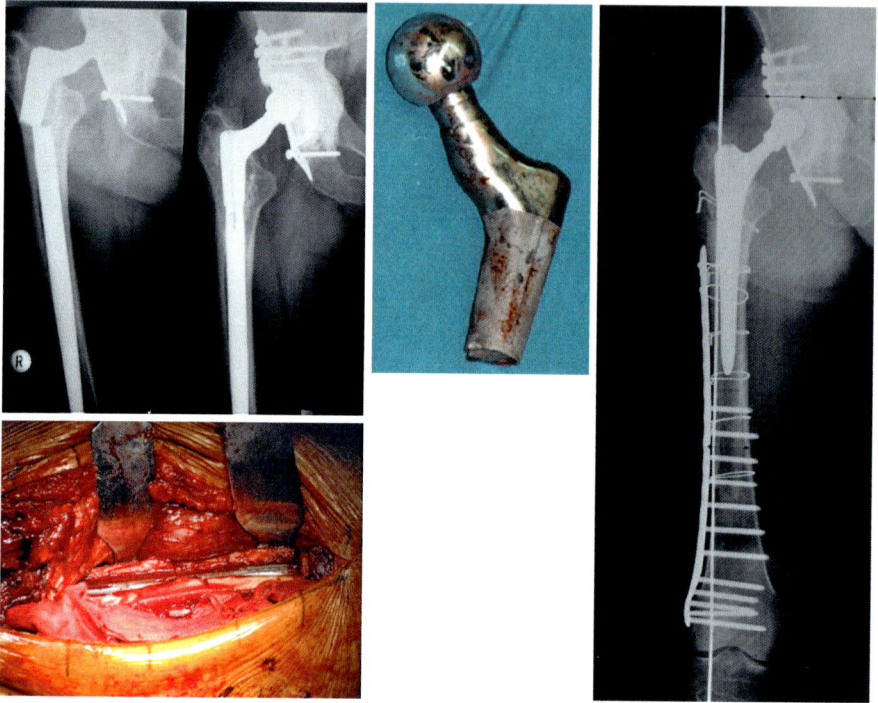

Fig. 3.2 Revision Ti alloy cementless stem failed due to crevice corrosion. Radiography showing the implant after breakage and after revision through a transfemoral approach

Ti and its alloys are the most frequently used material for cementless application because of their lower elastic modulus (110 GPa) that matches more closely that of the bone, high fatigue resistance (500–650 MPa at 10^7 cycles), and osteoconductive proprieties. These alloys are very tough, corrosion resistant, and biocompatible. They are not applicable for cemented applications in circumstances where micromotions are considerable, because of the deleterious tribocorrosive phenomena that may happen in these occasions [8, 9].

3.2.1 Corrosion and Infections

Gradual degradation of metals that occurs in electrolytic solutions like body fluids due to the electrolytic attack represents corrosion. All metals are subject to corrosion, although to a different extent. Different types of corrosion occur in vivo. Crevice corrosion occurs between two closely approximated metal surfaces (like head-neck taper junction) with fluid in between. The lack of oxygen in this microenvironment impairs the protective passive oxide surface layer, accelerating the corrosion process (Fig. 3.2). Pitting corrosion is guided by the same principles. Galvanic corrosion results from different electrochemical potentials between two metals [21]. Corrosion products alter the chemical environment around the joint implants and may have negative influence on the local innate and adaptive immune capability. The possible consequence is the increased incidence of infections in metal-on-metal (MOM) [9] total hip arthroplasty where corrosion of metal micro-and nanoscale debris with extremely large total surface area produces increased amounts of toxic corrosion products (Chap. 13).

3.3 Polymers

Among the polymers by far, the most successfully and frequently encountered in total joint replacement is polyethylene (PE). Teflon [3] and polyacetal [20] were used as well, but rather unsuccessfully. Ziegler in Natta received a Nobel Prize award in the 1963 for the invention of the polymerization of ethylene [17]. There are many types of PE on the market. In the recent past the most employed was the ultra-high molecular weight PE (UHMWPE), with acceptable tribological features. Wear with particulate debris formation, resulting in development of osteolyses and resultant loosening, presented an important drawback [22].

UHMWPE is formed from simple carbon backbone chain with hydrogen atoms attached. It is a homopolymer of ethylene gas (C_2H_4) with large number of units and an average molecular weight of $3.5–6 \times 10^6$ g/mol. As the length of the molecule increases, branching and complexity increase as well. Higher density is associated with lower wear. Its mechanical characteristics (impact resistance, ductility, and toughness), wear resistance, and oxidative degradation resistance make it an excellent material for use in joint replacements.

Native UHMWPE is supplied in the form of a resin. Today two resins known as GUR (*G*ranular, *U*HMWPE, *R*hurchemie) 1020 and 1050 predominate, but others are in use as well (GUR 1120 and 1150). If the first number of the code is 1, it indicates that the PE is designated for orthopedic devices. The second specifies the presence (1) or absence (0) of Ca stearate, the third (2 or 5) stands for molecular weight either 2×10^6 g/mol or 5×10^6 g/mol, and the fourth digit (0) is internal Hoechst (the company that used to produce PE) code [11].

GUR resins are successors of the resin that was used by Sir J. Charnley in the 1960s. With the implementation of PE cup and surgical steel (EN 58J) stem, Charnley set the fundamentals for the modern joint arthroplasty era [1]. The survivorship of this implant was hardly surpassed.

Advanced PE treated with gamma or beta irradiation to increase cross-linking and consecutive wear resistance are mostly in use today. Already in the 1970s Oonishi introduced irradiated polyethylene cups to reduce particulate wear debris and subsequent osteolyses. Contemporary heat-treated cross-linked PE (XLPE) was introduced late in the 1990s [13]. To produce XLPE, standard UHMWPE (GUR 1020 or 1050) is irradiated with beta or gamma rays. The irradiation splits the long PE chains, generating free radicals that combine among themselves and produce cross-linking covalent bonds between long PE molecules. The resulting material is more wear resistant but very prone to oxidation due to residual free radicals locked within the material. To improve oxidative stability various postir-radiation processes are applied, including annealing or remelting. With anneal-ing the irradiated PE is heated below the melting point. The number of free radicals is greatly reduced, but they are not fully annihilated. The advantage of the annealed material is that the mechanical proprieties are retained, but oxida-tive stability is not perfect. Remelted material has no residual free radicals because all of them combine among themselves, but the mechanical proprieties are considerably reduced. The remelted XLPE is more brittle [15]. Novel strate-gies are being developed to eliminate free radicals but retaining the mechanical proprieties. Vitamin E doping of the resin and sequential annealing are among the most promising [15]. In general XLPE has shown excellent results with only a few concerns [15].

3.4   Ceramics

Ceramics have been introduced in the hip arthroplasty surgery in the early 1970s [2]. The material has been gradually improved after the introduction of ISO 6474 standard [7], especially the structural density that has nowadays reached near theoretical values with 3.98 g/cm^3 and the grain size below 2 μm. The improvements have been achieved in the level of impurities and surface finish. Currently third-generation alumina is produced using modern technologies such as clean room processing, hot isostatic pressing subsequent to sintering, laser engraving instead of mechanical engraving, proof testing, and total quality management [23].

There are two types of ceramics, alumina (Al_2O_3) and zirconia (Zr_2O_3). Contemporary alumina ceramics have shown excellent wear resistance and excel-lent survivorship curves with the only major drawback being ceramic components fractures [16]. The incidence of this complication is decreasing, and the reported rate was 0.16 % in 2006 [14]. Especially in Asian population in some recent papers, authors reported that the fracture incidence reached even >3 % [5, 15]. Zirconia ceramics has been abandoned because of high failure rates related to the in vivo phase transformation issue and consequent high wear. Recently composite high-performance ceramic material (Biolox Delta® – zirconia toughened alumina [ZTA]) has been introduced with improved mechanical proprieties and fracture resistance (ISO 6474-2). It is composted from high-purity alumina (80 %) and reinforcing elements like zirconia (17 %) strontium aluminate (3 %) and some other minor con-stituents like Cr and Yt. Chromium is included to increase hardness (it is also responsible for the pink color), and small amount of Yttrium (Y_2O_3), to partly stabi-lize zirconia [10].

3.5 Antibacterial Coatings

Conventional systemic drug delivery has many shortcomings like potential systemic toxicity and the need for hospitalization and monitoring of serum drug levels, not to mention other problems discussed in detail in Appendix A. Local delivery of antibiotics and other bioactive molecules maximizes their effect where needed the most and concomitantly reduces the potential for side effects and other application-related disadvantages.

The presence of an implant decreases the minimal infecting dose of *Staphylococcus aureus* up 100,000-fold [24]. If bacterial adhesion is faster than host tissue regeneration, host defenses are unable to remove bacteria from the surface, and a device-related infection occurs and persists under the protection of biofilm layer. Preventing bacterial adhesion is thus crucial to prevent implant-associated infection because mature biofilm is difficult to destroy and remove both for the immune system and antibiotics.

It is known for a long time that different types of surfaces have different affinity for bacterial attachment. The variability is mainly resulting from different hydrophobicity, electrical charge, surface chemistry, and porosity. The differences were however not substantial. The trend today is to functionalize the surfaces of the implants to retain the potential for biological fixation but to implement strong bacterial repellent functionalization as well. Recently inorganic and organic–inorganic composite coatings were developed to functionalize the surfaces of the implants to have a potential for delivery of drugs to combat infections.

The coatings of interest include polymeric coatings, inorganic coatings, and recently nanoceramics. Polymeric coatings have some disadvantages like limited chemical stability, local inflammatory reaction, and uncontrolled drug-release kinetics. Consequently inorganic coatings like bioceramics and bioactive glasses become interesting. The most sophisticated, recently introduced surface delivery systems are nanoceramics. Surface nanostructuring provides improved cellular adhesion, surface osteoblast proliferation, and differentiation with increasing biomineralization. By combining biopolymers and bioactive ceramics that can mimic bone structure, scientists developed composite coatings that can carry different functional biomolecules for local delivery [19].

Antibiotic impregnation of the coatings capable of binding to different surfaces, coatings with antimicrobialy active metals like silver and copper, and nitric oxide (NO)-releasing materials are among the most promising [19]. Nanostructured HA coatings including silver nanoparticles in combination with biocompatible polymers and TiO_2 nanotubes have proven efficient in some studies. Coatings with NO-loaded silica and gold nanoparticles have shown antimicrobial activity with controlled release of NO.

Nanostructured coatings have already shown great promise for the development of novel biomedical coatings and implants. Nanofilms, nanocoatings, and nanostructured surfaces are being widely exploited for biomedical applications [12]. The advantages are reduced inflammation and controlled drug-release kinetics. The most promising nano-surface modifications are TiO_2 nanotubes [18], which can be loaded with different substances like (gentamycin) and have controllable drug-releasing kinetics by controlling the size of the tubes. Nanodiamonds (ND) are the new promising materials because of their biocompatibility and low toxicity for many cell types. The ND drug-loaded microfilms (2–8 nm) embedded in a polymer matrix can release drugs for months. Another possibility for local antibiotic release is HA-based nanostructured bioactive inorganic coating and silica-based sol-gels, being biocompatible and bioactive with controlled release potential [19].

Nanotechnology carries its inherent known and unknown risks that need to be addressed before wide implementation of this technology on implants [6] intended for human wide-scale use. Further research should evaluate in detail the effect of nanostructures on healthy tissues.

References

1. Berry DJ, Hamsen WS. The Charnley: the Mayo Clinic. In: Finerman GAM et al., editors. Total hip arthroplasty outcomes. New York: Churchill/Livingstone; 1998.
2. Boutin P, Christel P, Dorlot J-M, Meunier A, de Roquancourt A, Blanquaert D, Herman S, Sedel L, Witvoet J. The use of dense alumina-alumina ceramic combination in total hip replacement. J Biomed Mater Res. 1988;22:1203–32.
3. Charnley J. Low friction principle. In low friction arthroplasty of the hip: theory and practice. Berlin: Springer; 1979.
4. Chu PK, Liu X. Preface. In: Chu PK, Liu X, editors. Biomaterials fabrication and processing handbook. Boca Raton: CRC Press/Taylor & Francis Group; 2008.
5. Hasegawa M, Sudo A, Hirata H, Uchida A. Ceramic acetabular liner fracture in total hip arthroplasty with a ceramic sandwich cup. J Arthroplasty. 2003;18:658–61.
6. Hoet PHM, Bruske-Hohlfeld I, Salata OV. Nanoparticles- known and unknown health risks. J Bionanotechnol. 2004;2:12–27.
7. International Standard ISO 6474 standard, second edition 1994-02-01. Implants for surgery – ceramic materials based on high purity alumina.
8. Konttinen YT, Milošev I, Trebše R, Rantanen P, Linden R, Tiainen V-M, Virtanen S. Metals for joint replacement. In: Ravel P, editor. Joint replacement technology: new developments. Cambridge: Woodhead Publishing Limited; 2009.
9. Kovač S, Trebše R, Milošev I, Mihalič R, Levašič V. Incidence of inflammation of the THP with metal on metal articulation. 9th EFORT Congress, Nice, France; 29 May–1 June 2008. p. 1449.
10. Kuntz M, Masson B, Pandorf T. Current state of the art of the composite material Biolox delta. In: Menndels L, editor. Strength of materials. New York: Nova Science; 2009.
11. Kurtz SM, Muratoglu OK, Evans M, Edidin AA. Advances in the processing, sterilization, and crosslinking of ultra-high molecular weight polyethylene for total joint arthroplasty. Biomaterials. 1999;20:1659–88.
12. Liu H, Webster TJ. Nanomedicine for implants: a review of studies and necessary experimental tools. Biomaterials. 2007;28:354–69.
13. McKellop H, Shen FW, Lu B, Campbell P, Salovey R. Development of an extremely wear-resistant ultra high molecular weight polyethylene for total hip replacements. J Orthop Res. 1999;17:157–67.
14. Mehmood S, Jinnah RH, Pandit H. Review on ceramic-on-ceramic total hip arthroplasty. J Surg Orthop Adv. 2008;17:45–50.
15. Milosev I, Trebše R, Kovac S. Materials development and latest results of various bearings. In: Aoi T, Toshida A, editors. Hip replacements, approaches, complications and effectiveness. New York: Nova Science Publishers Inc; 2009.

16. Milošev I, Kovač S, Trebše R, Levašič V, Pišot V. Comparison of 10-year survivorship of a hip prosthesis using conventional polyethylene, metal-on-metal or ceramic-on-ceramic bearings. J Bone Joint Surg Am. 2012;94:1756–65.

17. Morawetz H. Polymeres. The origins and growth of a science. New York: Wiley; 1985.

18. Popat KC, Eltgroth M, LaTempa TJ, Grimes CA, Desai TA. Decreased *Staphylococcus epidermis* adhesion and increased osteoblast functionality on antibiotic-loaded titania nanotubes. Biomaterials. 2007;28:4880–8.

19. Simchi A, Tamjid E, Pihbin F, Boccacini AR. Recent progress in inorganic and composite coatings with bactericidal capability for orthopaedic applications. Nanomedicine. 2011; 7:22–39.

20. Trebše R, Milosev I, Kovac S, Mikek M, Pisot V. The isoelastic total hip replacement: a fourteen to seventeen years follow-up study. Acta Orthop. 2005;76:169–76.

21. Virtanen S, Milošev I, Gomez-Barrena E, Trebše R, Salo J, Konttinen YT. Special modes of corrosion under physiological and simulated physiological conditions. Acta Biomater. 2008;4:468–76.

22. Willert H. Reactions of articular capsule to wear products of artificial joint prostheses. J Biomed Mater Res. 1977;11:157–64.

23. Willmann G. Ceramic femoral head retrieval data. Clin Orthop Relat Res. 2000;379:22–8.

24. Zimmerli W. Prosthetic-joint-associated infections. Best Pract Res Clin Rheumatol. 2006;20:1045–63.

Chapter 4
The Definition of Prosthetic Joint Infections (PJI)

Rihard Trebše and Andrej Trampuž

Abstract It seems simple to define what a PJI is. The problem is that definitions vary depending on the author involved. It has become accepted that the PJI diagnosis is confirmed when there is purulence around the joint, there is a communication between the skin and the implant, and when causative agent(s) are isolated in multiple samples. In this chapter each of these criteria is discussed in some detail to help in diagnosing PJI as unambiguously as possible.

Keywords Definitions • Pseudotumor • Diagnostic criteria • Metallosis

4.1 The Definition of PJI

Before proceeding to the details of the procedures that are necessary in the evaluation of a PJI, it is useful to define the pathologic process in a way that is clear and can serve as a basis for determination of diagnostic and treatment decisions (Table 4.1).

Generally speaking, living microorganisms on or around an artificial joint are the necessary condition for PJI. Occasionally they can be difficult to isolate and identify. For clinical purposes a symptomatic artificial joint is infected if at least one or more of the following conditions is fulfilled [1–3]:

1. There is a sinus tract (fistula) communicating with the implant.
2. There is purulence around the joint (see boxes).
3. Microorganisms are isolated from the liquids or tissues around the joint implant or from the implant itself.

R. Trebše, M.D., Ph.D. (✉)
Department for Bone Infections and Adult Reconstructions,
Orthopaedic Hospital Valdoltra,
Jadranska cesta 31, Ankaran SI-6286, Slovenia
e-mail: rihard.trebse@ob-valdoltra.si

A. Trampuž, M.D.
Division of Infectious Diseases & Septic Unit, University Hospital of Lausanne,
Rue du Bugnon 46, Lausanne CH-1011, Switzerland
e-mail: andrej.trampuz@chuv.ch

R. Trebše (ed.), *Infected Total Joint Arthroplasty*,
DOI 10.1007/978-1-4471-2482-5_4, © Springer-Verlag London 2012

Table 4.1 Overview of diagnostic criteria for PJI

Sinus tract (fistula)
Acute inflammation in tissue histology
≥1 to ≥10 neutrophils/high-power field
Leukocytes in synovial fluid[a]
Knee and hip arthroplasty: ≥1.7 × 10⁹/L leukocytes and/or ≥65 % neutrophils
Purulence[b]
Puss around an artificial joint
Microbial growth
Positive culture from sinovial fluid aspiration
Growth of the same organism in 2 or more periprosthetic tissue samples from 3 or more collected
Sonication fluid (>50 CFU/mL)

[a] Not validated in the Early postoperative (3 months) and in case of inflammatory joint diseases
[b] Except in the cases with "pseudopus" which is sterile and caused by a foreign body reaction. (see box)

4.1.1 Sinus Tract Communicating with the Implant

In all instances where there is a communication between the implant and the skin, we can diagnose infection even if we are not able to find the causing agent. It is however difficult to exactly define when early wound-healing problem with drainage trough stitches or drain hole becomes a fistula. Persistent drainage ten or more days after surgery may be defined as a fistula which needs assessment and revision. In the case of a superficial infection, the subcutaneous sinus tract is not communicating with the joint. Fistulography is helpful to determine the extension of the communicating sinus. If fistulography does not confirm the communication with an artificial joint, it does not necessarily mean that the communication does not exist. In superficial infections sinus excision during revision usually results in complete healing.

4.1.2 Purulence Around the Joint

Purulence around the joint can be diagnosed: macroscopically, in high-grade processes, by tissue histology and/or pseudosynovial fluid cytology. Acute inflammation in tissue histology is defined when there are ≥1 to ≥10 neutrophils/high-power field (refer to Chap. 16). Pseudosynovial fluid can be obtained preoperatively by joint aspiration or during the surgery if preoperative aspiration was dry [4]. In case of intraoperative aspiration and assessment, it is necessary that the laboratory is prepared to provide the values as soon as possible still during the surgery to help with the decisions on how to proceed with the operation. The cutoff value for diagnosing infection by counting leucocytes in pseudosynovial fluids [2, 5]:

Knee and hip: ≥1.7 × 10⁹/L leukocytes, ≥65 % neutrophils. In the case of a metal-on-metal (MOM) articulation (Figs. 4.1 and 4.2) or in any case where there is attrition between two hard implant parts (Figs. 4.3 and 4.4), like screw rubbing against a plate or if the prosthesis or a metal part of the joint implant has worn through the plastic, the interpretation of puss around the joint must be very cautious. The resultant metallosis may be associated with a so-called pseudotumor or pseudoinfection. The process is frequently associated with production of massive granulomas (Fig. 4.5a, b), and the pseudosynovial fluid may macroscopically look exactly like pus, but it is mostly sterile [6].

The exact cause of the phenomenon is not yet fully understood, but it is thought to be either an allergic or a toxic reaction to metal particles formed by the abrasive process. Although it may be found in any metal to metal or ceramic to metal attrition case [7], it is most frequently encountered in failed resurfacing arthroplasties with unacceptable component position and a resultant poor tribology [8]. Recently it has been proposed that the purulent reaction is due to corrosion of metal particle debris. Fagocitosed metal particles are prone to corrosion within the lysosomes and release ions that are toxic for the cell. Ions and alarmins are released from the lysed cell. High ion concentration drive the influx of water and alarmins stimulate the innate immune system and the inflammation process with the consequent inflammatory cell accumulation.

4.1.3   Isolation of Microorganisms from the Artificial Joint

Joint aspiration (Fig. 4.6) is the most frequently employed diagnostic procedure for evaluation of PJI. There is a lot of evidence confirming that joint aspiration for culture and synovial fluid cell count and differential are strongly recommended in the evaluation of PJI [2, 9, 10]. Any growth from the sample obtained by joint aspiration is enough for the diagnosis of infection because its specificity is high. It is however wise to confirm the presence of the same organism during surgery by tissue cultures or implant sonication. Aspiration is not enough to rule out infection in cases where clinical history, patient examination, and other diagnostic modalities indicate infection because of its variable sensitivity that ranges from 11 to 100 % [11, 12], but it is in general around 70 %, as shown recently by Meermans in a meta-analysis [13]. Limited sensitivity is explicable by the biofilm growth pattern of the bacteria. Only a small share is released into a planktonic form and can be obtained by aspiration [14]. Intraoperative tissue biopsies are recognized as a gold standard for diagnosing PJI. Two or more out of three or more samples growing the same bacteria with the same antibiogram are considered diagnostic [15]. For high-virulence organisms such as Staphylococcus aureus, one positive culture suffices. Recently sonication [1] of the explanted material is gradually replacing the tissue biopsies as the gold standard for etiologic diagnosis of PJI. The diagnostic threshold was set at 50 CFU/mL of sonicate fluid. Lower counts are being considered for low-grade infections, especially with Propionibacterium acnes isolates.

It must be emphasized to avoid swabs, especially swabs from sinus tract exudates. There is always something growing from these samples, but only rarely the organism is the same as within the infected joint [3, 16].

Fig. 4.1 McKee–Farrar early MOM
total hip arthroplasty

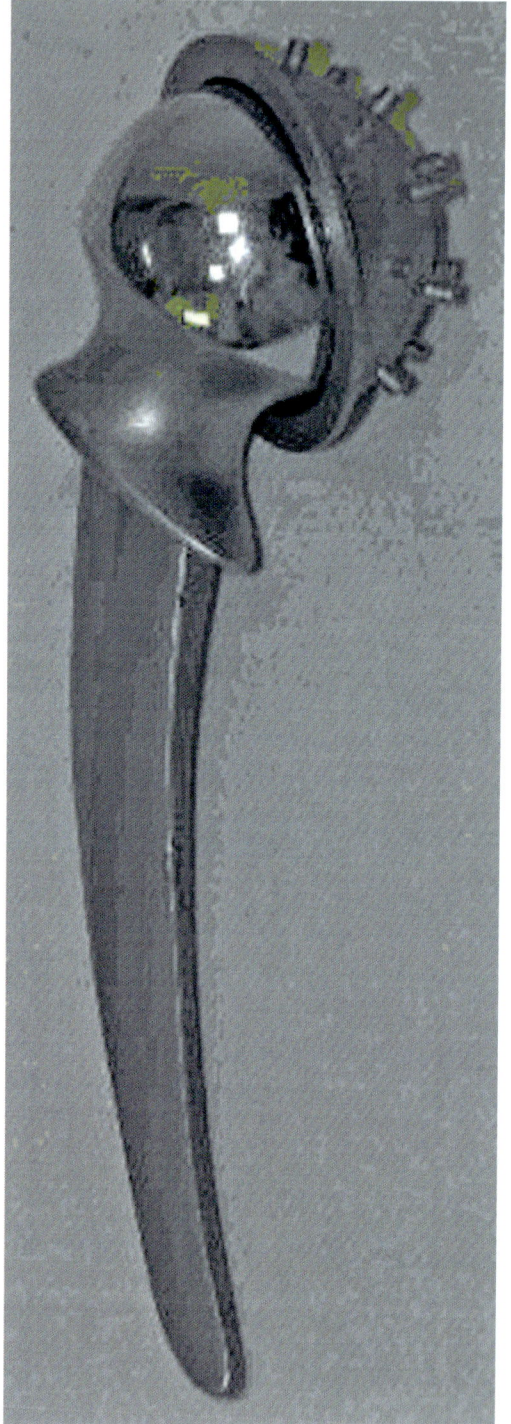

Fig. 4.2 Contemporary
MOM resurfacing THA

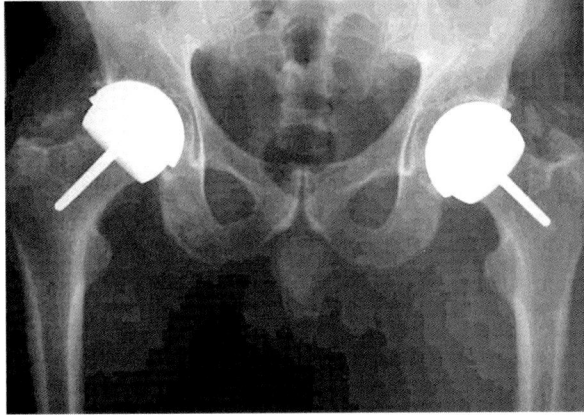

Fig. 4.3 Worn metal surface
from a MOM THA

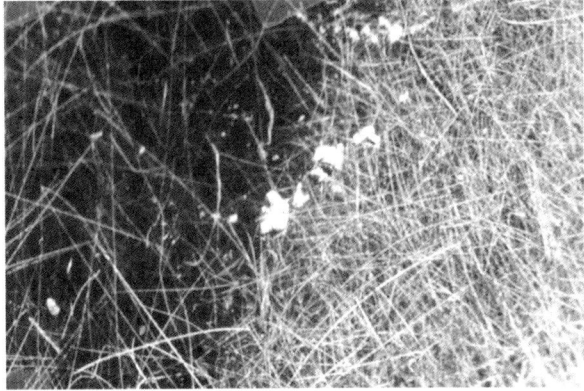

Fig. 4.4 Ceramic particle
third-body wear of the metal
head after previous ceramic
on ceramic bearing fracture

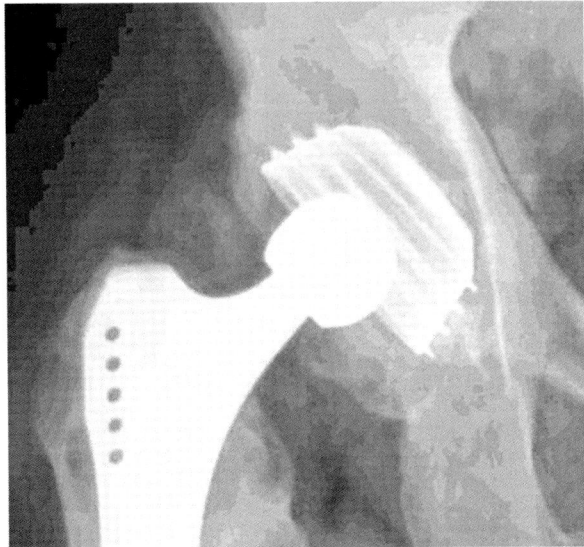

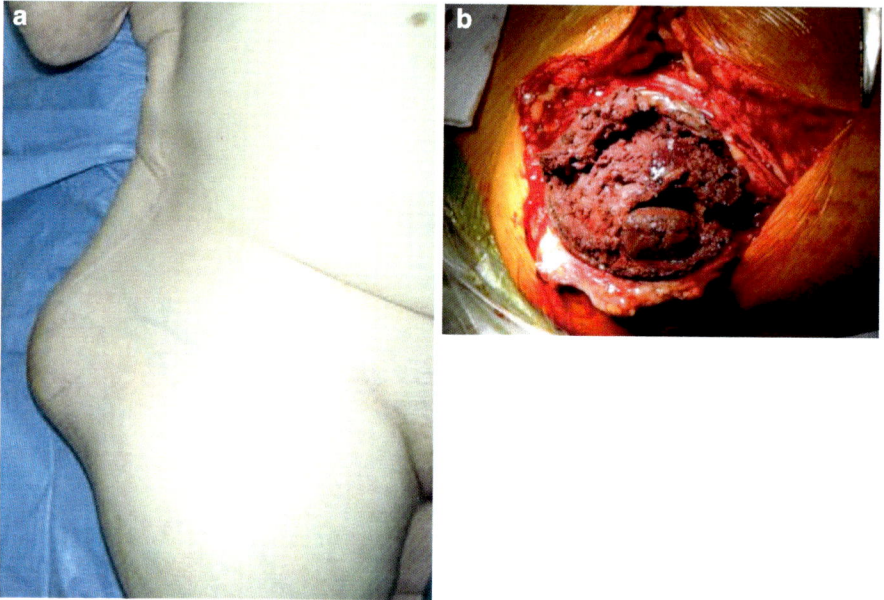

Fig. 4.5 (**a**, **b**) Giant granuloma in MOM THA

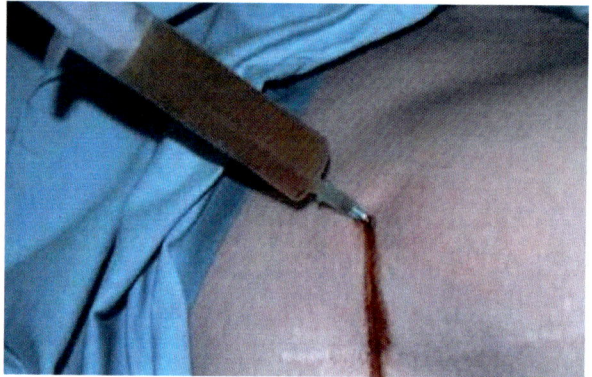

Fig. 4.6 Pus-like
pseudosynovial fluid

Puss by definition is a collection of whitish-yellow, sometimes greenish, blue
(pyocyanin), or bloody, generally viscous protein-rich inflammatory exudate
formed within the tissues consisting of polymorphonuclear (PMN) leukocytes,
necrotic liquefied tissues, microorganisms, and tissue fluids. It accumulates
around the source of infection.

Pseudopus can be similar, but it is not caused by an infection. Many joint aspirates
of MOM bearings look like puss, but microscopic examination of fresh joint aspirates and cyt ological sediment assessment of stained aspirate smears show a different picture. Macroscopically they may be milky, yellow, grayish, chocolate brown,

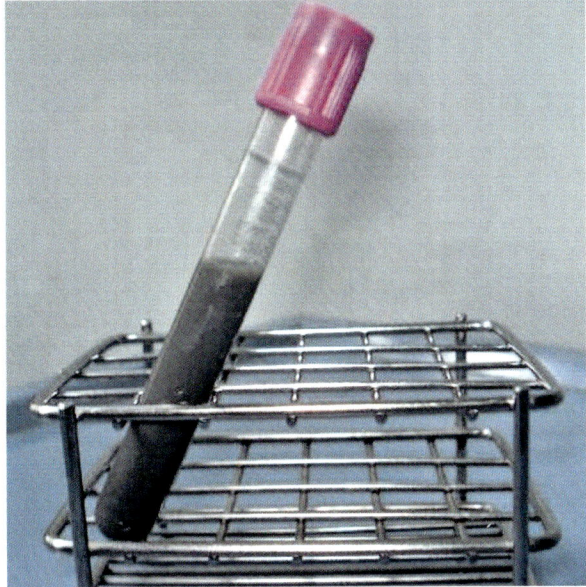

Fig. 4.7 Grayish pseudopus obtained from MOM THA

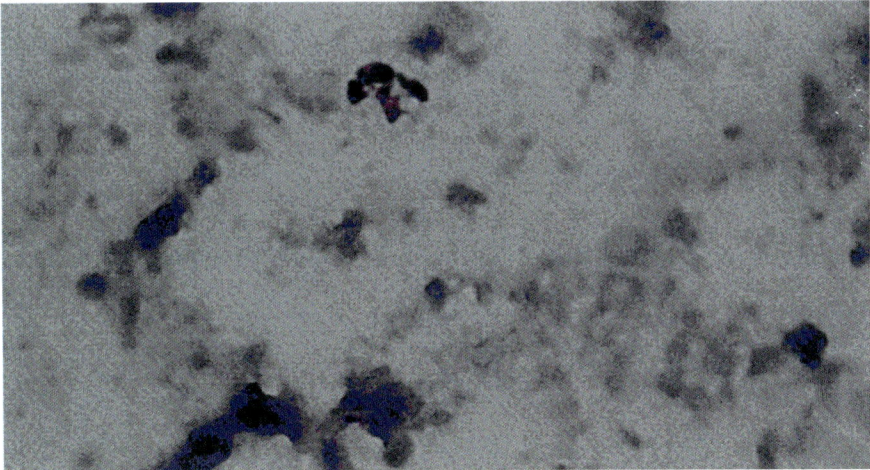

Fig. 4.8 Microscopy of pseudopus with PE and metal particles

brown grayish, metallic grey (Fig. 4.7), or even black and bloody. Sometimes the aspirate is filled with metal debris visible by naked eye.

The cytological examination is difficult to interpret. The leukocyte count is sometimes difficult to perform because of various particles and artifacts present in the sample (joint tissue and prosthesis remnant). Leucocytes are few, almost always below the cutoff value for PJI. For differential cell count examination, the joint aspirate cytological sediment smear is stained according Pappenheim. In the MOM smears we can find lymphocytes, PMN (3–85 %), which are almost all vacuolized or lysed, and monocytes-macrophages (3–27 %) with phagocytized deep violet-stained metal particles. Occasionally in some samples with gross metallosis, eosinophils appear in 3–13 %. Besides violet-stained metal particles all around the smear, PE particles are also present in some samples. They appear as transparent, slightly blue-stained plaques (Fig. 4.8).

References

1. Trampuz A, Piper KE, Jacobson MJ, Hanssen AD, Unni KK, Osmon DR, Mandrekar JN, Cockerill FR, Steckelberg JM, Greenleaf JF, Patel R. Sonication of removed hip and knee prostheses for diagnosis of infection. N Engl J Med. 2007;357:654–63.
2. AAOS (American academy of orthopedic surgeons). The diagnosis of periprosthetic joint infections in the hip or knee. Guideline and evidence report. 1st ed. AAOS, Rosmont. 2010. http://www.aaos.org/research/guidelines/guide.asp
3. Del Pozzo JL, Patel R. Infections associated with prosthetic joints. N Eng J Med. 2009; 361:787–94.
4. Mihalič R, Trebše R, Terčič D, Trampuž A. Synovial fluid cell count for rapid and accurate intraoperative diagnosis of prosthetic joint infection. In: 10th EFORT Congress, Vienna. 2009.
5. Trampuž A, Hanssen AD, Osmon DR, Mandrekar J, Steckelberg JM, Patel R. Synovial fluid leukocyte count and differential for the diagnosis of prosthetic knee infection. Am J Med. 2004;117:556–62.
6. Canadian Hip Resurfacing Study Group. A survey on the prevalence of pseudotumors with metal-on-metal hip resurfacing in Canadian academic centers. J Bone Joint Surg. 2011;93 Suppl 2:118–21.
7. Milošev I, Trebše R, Simon K, Andrej C, Venčeslav P. Results and retrieval analysis in Sikomet metal-on-metal total hip arthroplasty at a mean follow-up of seven years. J Bone Joint Surg Am. 2006;88:1173–82.
8. Glyn-Jones S, Roques A, Taylor A, Kwon YM, McLardy-Smith P, Gill HS, Walter W, Tuke M, Murray D. The in vivo linear and volumetric wear of hip resurfacing implants revised for pseudotumor. J Bone Joint Surg. 2011;93:2180–8.
9. Bauer TW, Parvizi J, Kobayashi N, Krebs V. Diagnosis of periprosthetic infection. J Bone Joint Surg. 2006;88:869–82.
10. Trampuž A, Hanssen AD, Osmon DR, Mandrekar J, Steckelberg JM, Patel R. Synovial fluid leukocyte count and differential for diagnosis of prosthetic knee infection. Am J Med. 2006;117:556–62.
11. Bernard L, Lubbeke A, Stern R, Bru JP, Feron JM, Peyramond D, Denormandie P, Arvieux C, Chirouze C, Perronne C, Hoffmeyer P. Value of preoperative investigations in diagnosing prosthetic joint infection: retrospective cohort study and literature review. Scand J Infect Dis. 2004; 36:410–6.
12. Ali F, Wilkinson JM, Cooper JR, Kerry RM, Hamer AJ, Norman P, Stockley I. Accuracy of joint aspiration for the preoperative diagnosis of infection in total hip arthroplasty. J Arthroplasty. 2006;21:221–6.
13. Meermans G, Haddad FS. Is there a role for tissue biopsy in the diagnosis of periprosthetic infection? Clin Ortop. 2010;468:1410–7.
14. Costerton JW. Biofilm theory can guide the treatment of device-related orthopaedic infections. Clin Orthop Relat Res. 2005;437:7–11.
15. Tunney MM, Patrick S, Gorman SP. Improved detection of infection in hip replacements: a currently underestimated problem. J Bone Joint Surg. 1998;80:568–72.
16. Mackowiak PA, Jones SR, Smith JW. Diagnostic value of sinus-tract cultures in chronic osteomyelitis. JAMA. 1978;239:2772–5.

Chapter 5
Classification of Prosthetic Joint Infections

Rihard Trebše and Anže Mihelič

Abstract This chapter presents the development of classification systems for PJI and the rationale behind them. Their features are discussed and compared for the reader to understand the strengths and the weaknesses. The most important and widely used is presented and discussed in some detail.

Keywords Classification • Infections • Symptoms • Presentation

5.1 Introduction

Clinical presentation of prosthetic joint infections (PJI) is highly varied. The disease may present as a fulminating sepsis immediately after the implantation or anytime later during the implant life, or it may be clinically completely silent. Frequently PJI is an accidental finding during the evaluation or revision of a presumably aseptically failed artificial joint. Because of diverse clinical presentations and courses and different approaches to diagnosis and treatment, PJI need to be classified into groups. Despite the presence of various clinical variables that could have been used for classification, it seems that time between primary implantation and the development of symptoms is the most clinically useful determinant for grouping since it guides the treatment mode selection. Mode of infection development is the second most important element for classification systems (Table 5.1).

R. Trebše, M.D., Ph.D. (✉) • A. Mihelič, M.D.
Department for Bone Infections and Adult Reconstructions,
Orthopaedic Hospital Valdoltra,
Jadranska cesta 31, Ankaran SI-6286, Slovenia
e-mail: rihard.trebse@ob-valdoltra.si; anze.mihelic@ob-valdoltra.si

R. Trebše (ed.), *Infected Total Joint Arthroplasty*,
DOI 10.1007/978-1-4471-2482-5_5, © Springer-Verlag London 2012

Table 5.1 Classification of prosthetic joints infections

Classification	Features
Depending on the source of infection	
Perioperative	Inoculation of the organism during surgery or immediately after it
Hematogenous	Inoculation from remote source via blood or lymph vessels
From nearby focus (contiguous)	Direct inoculation from nearby focus (e.g., stab wound, adjacent osteomyelitic focus, skin and soft tissue infections, psoas abscess)
Depending on the time of development of symptoms	
Early infections (<1 month)	Obtained during surgery or in the first after days, usually highly virulent organisms (e.g., *Staphylococcus aureus* or Gram-negative germs)
Delayed and/or silent infections (1–24 months)	Mostly perioperative, low virulent organisms (e.g., KNS or *Propionibacterium acnes*)
Late infections (>24 months)	Mostly hematogenic or lymphogenic from remote sources, including silent perioperative

5.2 Classification Systems

First classification of PJI was published by Coventry [1]. It was based on analysis of THA infections. He divided infections into acute postoperative, resulting from contamination during surgery; delayed, developed at least 8 weeks after surgery, usually silent and clinically poorly expressed; and late-hematogenic, which can develop at any time after the surgery and are generally acute in nature. The classification system was later supplemented by Fitzgerald [2]. It is currently the most frequently used system [9]. This classification is based on symptom duration which means that precisely specified onset of symptoms is necessary. This is sometimes difficult to determine. The system is thus less suitable for silent or "low-grade" infection, where symptoms are not significant in the beginning and the onset time is difficult to define. Silent infections are inoculated during surgery and can cause only pain and early loosening or not even this. Frequently there are no laboratory signs of inflammation.

The classification ignores infections attained in other ways like those acquired through stab wounds or by propagation from a nearby septic focus, such as infection of the hip through psoas abscess originating from the spine, or those caused by skin necrosis or wound breakdown over an implant.

Presently the modification of the classification by Toms [7] seems to be more appropriate. Early, acute infections are defined as infections that develop within the first 6 weeks after implantation. Delayed infection includes silent, chronic, and clinically ill expressed, regardless of the time of onset. Late infections begin with sudden onset in patients who had previously not had any problems with the artificial joint. Tsukajama et al. suggested additional fourth type, unexpectedly positive intraoperative microbiological samples, if, during the presumed aseptic revision of artificial hip, at least five samples were taken and at least two of them were positive with the same germ [8].

To improve the accuracy of the diagnosis of PJI and for determination of its severity, Zimmerli has developed a scoring system that included also radiologic, laboratory, and other parameters. It was intended to upgrade the classification systems and become a basis for the analysis of treatment successes. The scoring system has not become widely accepted in clinical practice and research work. The reason lays probably in its low specificity [9].

5.3 The Classification According to Fitzgerald

Considering the time of development and clinical presentation, we classify infections of artificial joints after Fitzgerald's classification into three groups:

5.3.1 Early Infections

Early infections develop in the first month after surgery and are usually manifested by severe pain in the affected joint, elevated body temperature, and effusion. Wound healing may be impaired early after the development of infection, with redness, swelling, and warmness in implant surroundings. During infection clinically important cellulitis or tissue necrosis with purulent discharging fistula can develop in the proximity of the implant. With time the fistula epithelizes and chronifies. Mobility and function of the joint are greatly impaired, and the condition may also limit patient ambulation ability if lower limb joint is involved. After the discharging fistula has formed, systemic symptoms usually subside. Only in rare occasions septicemia develops in the presence of an open fistula. Untreated infection with fistula can persist for years, and occasionally it may even heal spontaneously [4]. PJI leads to gradual loosening of the artificial joint with pain. Loosening is not evident in all patients. Tsukajama reported loosening in 59 % out of 106 infected hips [8]. Rarely, systemic signs of sepsis emerge before the local signs and symptoms develop, especially in immunocompromised patients and virulent microbes of exogenous origin.

5.3.2 Delayed Infections

Delayed infections can develop at any time, by definition between 1 and 24 months after surgery. Such a patient is usually never completely free of pain since the early postoperative period. With time pain may (but not necessarily) escalate, and it is often dependent on the level of joint exertion. In some cases the infection develops later, at any time after implantation, and is manifested by gradual pain development and limited mobility. There may be also a gradual development of a discharging sinus and/or implant loosening. *Low-grade infections* may present with pain only without other symptoms and/or early loosening, or there is only loosening. They are clinically and by laboratory examination very difficult to distinguish from aseptic implant loosening [6]. Poorly virulent microbes such as coagulase-negative *staphylococci* and anaerobes like *P. acnes* are the usual causative agents. Delayed infections can potentially be clinically silent with no laboratory manifestation. They may not cause even an early loosening and can be an occasional finding at revision decades after primary implantation [8].

5.3.3 Late Infections

Late infections usually develop two or more years after implantation of the artificial joint or at any time and are mostly of hematogenous origin. The most common source of bacteremia are the microbes from the skin, respiratory, urinary tract, and periodontal tissue. *Sreptococci, S. aureus*, and Gram-negative germs are the most frequent causative agents. Clinical presentation is usually fulminant, resembling early postoperative infections.

In a recent retrospective study, Giulieri et al. reported 29 % early, 41 % delayed, and 30 % late infections in a series of 63 infected artificial joints presenting within 16 years of study period [3]. Murdoch demonstrated that *S. aureus* bacteremia caused implant infection in 15 out of 44 patients with artificial joint and that it can occur at any time during the lifetime [5]. According to some calculations the incidence of such an infection is supposed to be around 0.2 % per artificial joint per year.

References

1. Coventry MB. Treatment of infections occurring in total hip surgery. Orthop Clin North Am. 1975;6:991–1003.
2. Fitzgerald Jr RH, Nolan DR, Ilstrup DM, Van Scoy RE, Washington JA, Coventry MB. Deep wound sepsis following total hip arthroplasty. J Bone Joint Surg Am. 1977;59:847–55.
3. Giulieri SG, Graber P, Ochsner P, Zimmerli W. Management of infection associated with total hip arthroplasty according to a treatment algorithm. Infection. 2004;32:222–8.
4. Hunter G, Dandy D. The natural history of the patient with an infected total hip replacement. J Bone Joint Surg Br. 1977;59:293–7.
5. Murdoch DR, Roberts SA, Fowler Jr VG. Infection of orthopedic protheses after *Saphylococcus aureus* bacteremia. Clin Infect Dis. 2001;32:647–9.
6. Steckelberg JM, Osmon DR. Prosthetic joint infection. In: Bisno AL, Waldvogel FA, editors. Infections associated with indwelling medical devices. 3rd ed. Washington, DC: American Society for Microbiology; 2000.
7. Toms AD, Davidsom D, Masri BA, Duncan CP. The management of periprosthetic infection in total joint arthroplasty. J Bone Joint Surg Br. 2006;88:149–55.
8. Tsukajama DT, Estrada R, Gustilo RB. Infections after total hip arthroplasty: a study of the treatment of one hundred and six infections. J Bone Joint Surg Am. 1996;78:512–23.
9. Zimmerli W, Ochsner PE. Management of infection associated with prosthetic joints. Infection. 2003;31:99–108.

Chapter 6
The Epidemiology of Total Joint Arthroplasty Infections

David J. Jaekel, Kevin L. Ong, Edmund C. Lau, and Steven M. Kurtz

Abstract Prosthetic joint infection (PJI) is a rare occurrence following joint arthroplasty, which has a significant impact on the patient population. This chapter critically reviews the literature to form a consensus on the epidemiology of PJI within total joint arthroplasty. PJI occurs in 0.7–1.1 % of total knee (TKA) and hip arthroplasty (THA) cases in the USA and internationally but is projected to grow to 6.5–6.8 % by 2030. The infection rate for TKA is higher than for THA and is performed almost twice as much. Infection is diagnosed within the first year for 60 % of primary surgeries, and the vast majority of cases occur within 2 years. Among reasons for revision, infection is projected to become the most frequent and is currently around 25 % of revisions for TKA and 15 % for THA. Infection is also more prevalent after previous revision for infection and can occur in 10–33 % of those cases. The largest risk factors for concern were found to be gender, BMI > 50, extended length proce-

D.J. Jaekel, M.S., Ph.D. (✉)
School of Biomedical Engineering, Science and Health Systems, Drexel University,
3401 Market Street, Suite 300, Philadelphia, PA 19104, USA
e-mail: djj25@drexel.edu

K.L. Ong, Ph.D., P.E.
Department of Biomedical Engineering, Exponent, Inc.,
3401 Market Street, Suite 300, Philadelphia, PA 19104, USA
e-mail: kong@exponent.com

E.C. Lau, M.S.
Department of Epidemiology and Computation Biology, Exponent, Inc.,
149 Commonwealth Drive, Menlo Park, CA 94025, USA
e-mail: elau@exponent.com

S.M. Kurtz, Ph.D.
School of Biomedical Engineering, Science and Health Systems, Drexel University,
3401 Market Street, Suite 300, Philadelphia, PA 19104, USA and

Department of Biomedical Engineering, Exponent, Inc.,
3401 Market Street, Suite 300, Philadelphia, PA 19104, USA
e-mail: skurtz@exponent.com

R. Trebše (ed.), *Infected Total Joint Arthroplasty*,
DOI 10.1007/978-1-4471-2482-5_6, © Springer-Verlag London 2012

35

dures, lack of antibiotic bone cement, and comorbidities. Other arthroplasty procedures such as total disk replacement and total shoulder arthroplasty have similar
infection rates to TKA that range from 1.3 to 3.8 %. In contrast though, total elbow
arthroplasty can have infection rates as high as 12 %, which may be a result of the
subcutaneous nature of the elbow joint and its surrounding thin soft tissue envelope.

Keywords Projections • Incidence • Hip • Knee • Elbow • Shoulder

6.1   Introduction

Total joint arthroplasty (total knee [TKA], total hip arthroplasty [THA], etc.) is
one of the most cost-efficient and effective clinical procedures in terms of reducing pain and enhancing mobility and function of patients with advanced arthritis.
Implant designs and surgical techniques are continuously being advanced to
extend implant life while reducing negative outcome to the patient [1–4]. Despite
these improvements, the burden of revision for TKA and THA (defined as the
percentage of revisions as function of the total number of primary and revision
arthroplasties performed) has not lowered with time and even increased with some
procedures [5–8]. A number of factors are related to the increase in revision,
which include increasing volume of primary procedures, better implant longevity,
and increasing number of procedures in younger and more active patient populations [9, 10]. Additionally, recent studies by Kurtz et al. project the number of
primary and revision THA to double and TKA to grow substantially by a factor of
5 by 2030 [7, 11].

As discussed previously throughout this book, revision of an implanted total
joint replacement for infection is a rare but devastating complication that is associated with longer hospital stay, increased hospital cost, and higher morbidity. Due to
how the infection manifests, it is difficult to cure and is nonresponsive to systemic
antibiotics. While short-term infection risks were originally reported as low as 0.2
and 0.4 % for THA and TKA, respectively [12, 13], thousands of patients are still
presented with a painful complication and are an economic burden for hospitals
because of inadequate reimbursement [14, 15]. To further understand the complete
impact infection revisions have on society, it is crucial to define its incidence and
risk. Information on infection incidence in regard to total joint arthroplasty has
been analyzed from various sources ranging from single-center studies to large-
scale multi-institution studies and national registries.

Other chapters in this book have and will discuss the development and progression of total joint infection across implanted devices, but the purpose of this chapter is to catalogue the incidence of infection in total joint arthroplasty within
populations across the globe and define what risk factors have the highest influence
on infection revision in the future. Databases and international registries are the
largest sources for documenting clinical utilization and procedures performed, and
thus are first summarized and compared for infection rates. We also review the
influence of various risk factors, antibiotic cement use, and device type on infection

development. Finally, infection rates after revision surgeries are summarized to compare with their primary counterparts.

6.2 Registries

International registries represent a vast and consistent source of data regarding the utilization of total joint replacement in Australia and Europe. A registry is more than a data repository for basic clinical, patient, and implant data regarding the implantation and revision of total joint replacements. Where registries have been established, the information is a tool providing continuous feedback to clinicians to drive the constant enhancement of surgical procedures. Sweden first established orthopedic implant registries in the 1970s, which later spread across Europe and to Australia. Early establishment allows the Swedish registry to currently be able to chronicle the growth of knee arthroplasty from the start of the procedure within their hospital system.

National registries are significant in providing perspective on the current use and outcome of total joint replacement across the globe; however, registries are not the only tool to measure the utilization of arthroplasty procedures. For example, neither the United States nor Germany currently has in place a national registry for joint replacements. In the following section, administrative databases for countries without a full registry are described. These databases provide necessary information concerning the current use of total joint arthroplasty that is otherwise unavailable in these countries.

6.3 Public Data Sources

Administrative claims databases are an important source of data for total joint replacements, even in countries with an established registry. An administrative claims database can collect a sampling of electronic hospital discharge records, or as with the Medicare database, the complete insurance claim history for individual patients. Specific hip and knee replacement procedures are classified in these databases by hospitals in accordance with the codes from the 9th Revision of the International Classification of Diseases, Clinical Modification. Claims filed by surgeons and clinics often use Current Procedural Terminology (CPT) codes. In the United States, three public sources of administration claims data are available and are summarized in the following sections.

6.3.1 National Hospital Discharge Survey

The National Hospital Discharge Survey (NHDS)[16] is a survey conducted annually by the National Center for Health Statistics (NCHS). This survey program was started in 1965 and has continuously recorded a statistically representative sample of hospitalization from nonfederal and nonmilitary short-stay community hospitals across the United States. It is currently the oldest and most well-established inpatient discharge database available in the USA. NHDS has grown in the past decade to include from 430 to 490 hospitals and collect ~300,000 discharge records sampled per year. The NHDS database includes patient demographics (e.g., age, gender), disease diagnosis, performed procedure, resource utilization, and institutional characteristics.

6.3.2 Nationwide Inpatient Sample

Established in 1988 by the Healthcare Cost and Utilization Project (HCUP) of the Agency of Healthcare Quality and Research (AHRQ), the Nationwide Inpatient Sample (NIS) has a far larger sample size in terms of both discharge records and number of hospitals in comparison to the NHDS [17]. Specifically, the NIS includes twice the number of hospitals and collects 25 times more records with an average of five to eight million records per year. The NIS annually samples 20 % of US inpatient hospital stays. NIS is able to capture patient, payer, and hospitalization factors, including charges, cost, and reimbursement information during hospitalization, which facilitates the evaluation of economic impact of specific diagnoses and procedures.

6.3.3 Medicare

Made available by the Center for Medicare and Medicaid Services (CMS), the 5 % Medicare Limited Data Set (LDS) consists of seven components: hospital inpatient, hospital outpatient, home health agency, skilled nursing facility, hospice care, physician carrier (Part B), and durable medical equipment. LDS also tracks the date of death or the rare withdrawal of a patient from the program with a denominator file. Medicare beneficiaries in the LDS are identified with an encrypted identification number that is link through all aspects of the database as well as time. For this reason, utilization of healthcare resources by a patient can be traced through different systems such as inpatient, outpatient, or home hospice care. Medicare data is also available in the 100 % format, i.e., for all Medicare beneficiaries. Of the seven file components, the inpatient, outpatient, home health agency, skilled nursing facility, and hospice care data are available in the 100 % format, but not the physician carrier and durable medical equipment data.

6.4 Infection Incidence

6.4.1 Infection Incidence in Primary Joint Arthroplasty

Historically, the number of total knee arthroplasty procedures has been greater than the number of total hip arthroplasties performed, and thus, when Kurtz et al. analyzed

NIS data from 1990 to 2004 in the USA, it was expected that the number of infections would follow similar trends. By 2004, which is the last year incorporated in this study, ~5,838 knee arthroplasties were revised for infection, while only an estimated 3,352 hip arthroplasties were revised for infection (Tables 6.1 and 6.2) [18].

Kurtz et al. also calculated the revision burden for infections as a proportion of the total number of primary and revision arthroplasties performed, and in 2004, the infection burden for THA and TKA were 1.23 and 1.21 %, respectively. In addition, NIS data revealed that the infection burden for both hip and knee arthroplasties almost doubled from 1990 to 2004. The trend of increasing infection burden with time was statically significant ($p < 0.0001$) and grew annually at a rate of nearly 5 % (Fig. 6.1) [18]. The average infection burden across the sampled years was similar at 0.88 % for THA and 0.92 % for TKA; however, the burden was significantly lower for THA [18]. Further analysis of the NIS data yielded model projections of this trend continuing in the near future and infection burden reaching 6.5 % for THA and 6.8 % for TKA by 2030 (Fig. 6.2) [19]. The NIS data also showed a steep decline in length of hospital stay for patients, which could influence the chance of discovering an early infection within the initial hospital stay and delay the infection to a revision procedure [18].

Single institution studies in the USA indicated similar incidence of infection in their patient groups. Pulido et al. monitored 9,245 patients and measured an overall incidence of 0.7% with joint specific incidence of 1.1% for TKA and 0.3% for THA (Tables 6.3 and 6.4) [20]. Malinzak et al. reported infection rates of 0.52 and 0.47 % for TKA and THA, respectively, after monitoring 8,494 cases from 1991 to 2004 [21]. When specifically looking at the Medicare LDS and thus limiting the population to ages over 65, infection occurred in 2.01 % of TKA [22] and 2.22 % for THA [23]. This could indicate higher risk for infection with increasing age, which will be discussed further in the next section.

Internationally, hospitals and clinics were also subjected to a incidence of infection at nearly 1 % (Tables 6.3 and 6.4) [24–27]. In the case of total knee arthroplasty, infection occurred in 0.8–0.9 % of cases in Finland when observed from single institution studies or analysis of the Finnish Arthroplasty Register from 1997 to 2006 [25, 26]. Similarly, a single institution study in Japan from 1995 to 2006 had infection occur in 0.8 % of TKA procedures [27]. For THA, an analysis of the Norwegian Arthroplasty Register data from 2005 to 2006 revealed an infection incidence of 0.7 % [24]. Studies in the United States and abroad suggest that infection rates for the general population are similar and are estimated to range from ~0.7 to 1.1 %. Overall, infections are still rare occurrences but have a significant impact on morbidity and resource utilization. As number of revisions meet or exceed projected increases, infection will have an increasing impact on the population of arthroplasty patients [18].

6.4.2   Time to Revision

Infection can develop at various times after primary joint replacement surgery and can range from 2 weeks postoperatively to over 3 years [20, 23, 24, 27, 28].

Table 6.1 Infection burden and resource utilization from patients with both primary and revision hip replacement surgeries

| Year | No infection | | | With infection | | | Percent surgery with infection | Lower 95 % surgery with infection | Upper 95 % surgery with infection |
	Noninfected procedures	Average total charge	Average stay (days)	Infected procedures	Average total charge	Average stay (days)			
1990	163,818	$39,057	10.6	1,104	$67,415	22.2	0.66 %	0.51 %	0.80 %
1991	165,908	$39,531	9.8	922	$82,258	21.1	0.54 %	0.43 %	0.65 %
1992	178,757	$39,598	9.0	1,192	$72,182	17.7	0.66 %	0.56 %	0.77 %
1993	167,648	$36,559	8.1	1,154	$79,147	20.2	0.67 %	0.54 %	0.81 %
1994	177,128	$35,294	7.0	1,207	$65,147	14.9	0.66 %	0.51 %	0.82 %
1995	175,767	$32,556	6.3	1,092	$54,720	13.4	0.61 %	0.50 %	0.73 %
1996	182,786	$31,343	5.5	1,350	$55,249	12.1	0.71 %	0.60 %	0.83 %
1997	188,358	$31,748	5.1	1,534	$54,224	10.7	0.79 %	0.68 %	0.90 %
1998	187,984	$30,456	4.8	1,797	$48,793	10.0	0.92 %	0.75 %	1.10 %
1999	189,888	$30,782	4.8	1,844	$51,014	10.2	0.94 %	0.79 %	1.10 %
2000	199,937	$32,589	4.7	1,989	$59,955	10.8	0.96 %	0.82 %	1.11 %
2001	224,631	$34,046	4.7	2,398	$60,596	10.6	1.04 %	0.91 %	1.18 %
2002	238,958	$35,696	4.5	2,879	$64,839	10.8	1.17 %	1.01 %	1.32 %
2003	235,684	$39,261	4.4	2,878	$73,658	11.2	1.17 %	1.03 %	1.32 %
2004	262,089	$39,654	4.3	3,352	$70,378	9.7	1.23 %	1.07 %	1.40 %

Based on data from Kurtz et al. [18]

Table 6.2 Infection burden and resource utilization from patients with both primary and revision knee replacement surgeries

Year	No infection			With infection			Percent surgery with infection	Lower 95 % surgery with infection	Upper 95 % surgery with infection
	Noninfected procedures	Average total charge	Average stay (days)	Infected procedures	Average total charge	Average stay (days)			
1990	175,789	$35,578	9.7	1,090	$59,491	18.3	0.63 %	0.52 %	0.74 %
1991	200,698	$35,910	9.0	1,197	$54,295	15.7	0.61 %	0.49 %	0.74 %
1992	237,165	$35,340	8.2	1,629	$58,560	14.9	0.71 %	0.59 %	0.84 %
1993	232,067	$33,394	7.4	1,470	$53,109	15.7	0.65 %	0.53 %	0.76 %
1994	256,174	$32,808	6.4	1,577	$43,594	10.5	0.63 %	0.54 %	0.73 %
1995	263,169	$30,095	5.6	1,793	$43,868	10.3	0.69 %	0.58 %	0.81 %
1996	293,850	$29,316	5.0	2,105	$38,420	8.5	0.74 %	0.63 %	0.85 %
1997	313,111	$29,565	4.6	2,479	$43,568	8.3	0.82 %	0.71 %	0.92 %
1998	292,706	$28,560	4.4	2,771	$40,331	8.0	0.98 %	0.85 %	1.11 %
1999	307,938	$28,890	4.3	2,984	$43,279	7.4	1.00 %	0.87 %	1.12 %
2000	324,100	$29,446	4.3	3,051	$45,231	7.7	0.97 %	0.86 %	1.08 %
2001	359,755	$30,750	4.3	3,644	$53,109	9.1	1.04 %	0.93 %	1.15 %
2002	402,247	$32,245	4.1	4,273	$51,459	8.3	1.09 %	0.96 %	1.22 %
2003	429,459	$34,507	4.0	5,324	$57,202	8.1	1.26 %	1.11 %	1.40 %
2004	490,180	$35,769	3.9	5,838	$56,275	7.6	1.21 %	1.07 %	1.36 %

Based on data from Kurtz et al. [18]

Nonetheless, it is crucial to understand in which periods most infections occur to accurately enhance future preventative measures. In a study of 9,245 patients in the USA, Pulido et al. reported that 27 % of infected total joint arthroplasties occurred within the first 30 days, while 65 % of infection diagnoses were revised within the first year. The average time to diagnosis was ~1.2 years [20]. In the retrospective analysis by Malinzak, 83.7 % of infections were diagnosed within

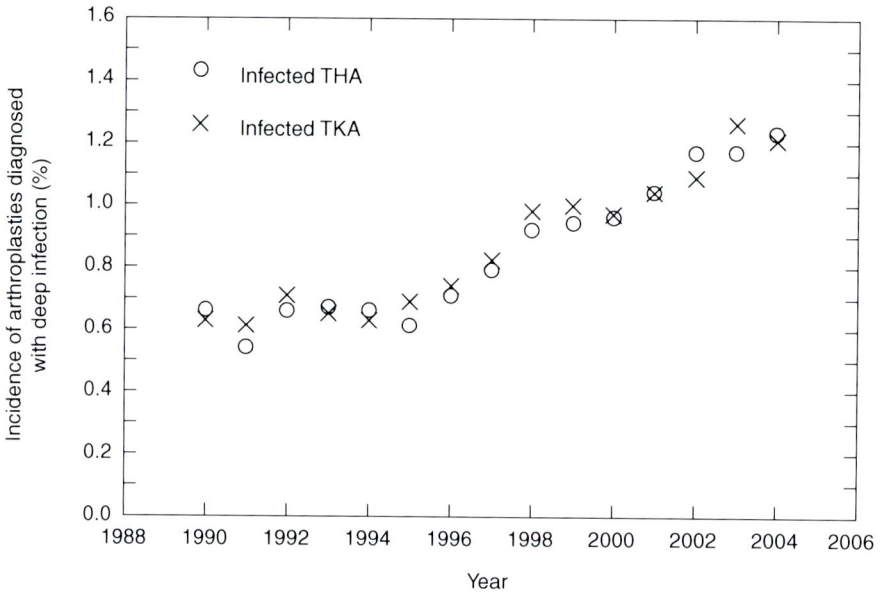

Fig. 6.1 The incidence of diagnosis of periprosthetic infection for total knee and total hip arthroplasties within the United States from 1994–2004. Based on figure from Kurtz et al. [18]

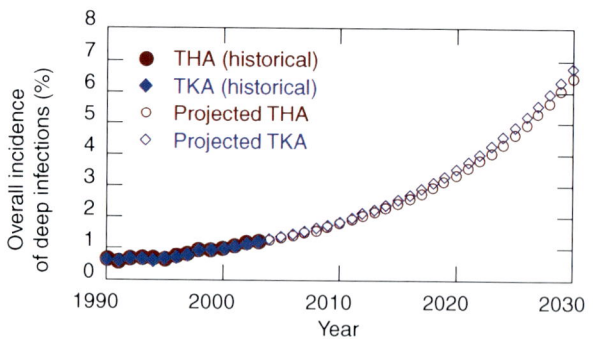

Fig. 6.2 The projected overall incidence of infection among all arthroplasties, including both primary and revision, up to the years 2030. Based on figure from Kurtz et al. [19]

Table 6.3 Infection rates for total hip arthroplasty

Country	Infection rate (%)	Time period analyzed	Literature source	Data source
USA	0.88	1990–2004	Kurtz et al. [18]	NIS
USA	1.23	2004	Kurtz et al. [18]	NIS
USA	0.3	2001–2006	Pulido et al. [20]	Single institution
USA	0.47	1991–2004	Malinzak et al. [21]	Single institution
USA	2.22	1997–2006	Ong et al. [23]	Medicare 5 %
Norway	0.7	2005–2006	Dale at al. [24]	Norwegian registry

Table 6.4 Infection rates for total knee arthroplasty

Country	Infection rate (%)	Time period analyzed	Literature source	Data source
USA	0.92	1990–2004	Kurtz et al. [18]	NIS
USA	1.21	2004	Kurtz et al. [18]	NIS
USA	1.1	2001–2006	Pulido et al. [20]	Single institution
USA	0.52	1991–2004	Malinzak et al. [21]	Single institution
USA	2.01	1997–2006	Kurtz et al. 2010 [22]	Medicare 5 %
Finland	0.8	2002–2006	Jamsen et al. [26]	Single institution
Finland	0.9	1997–2006	Jamsen et al. [25]	Finnish Arthroplasty Register
Japan	0.8	1995–2006	Susuki et al. [27]	Single institution

2 years with an average time to infection of 9.6 months [21]. For patients over 65 years of age, the 5 % Medicare sampling showed 73–77 % of all THA and TKA were diagnosed with infection within 2 years of primary surgery [22, 23]. Specifically for TKA, the incidence of infection was 1.55 % within 2 years but dropped to 0.46 % between 2 and 10 years post-surgery [22]. In congruence with the US data on TKA, the Finnish Arthroplasty Register had 68 % of patients from 1997 to 2004 diagnosed with periprosthetic joint infections within the first year [25, 26]. Though not reporting analysis of diagnosis in terms of years, Suzuki et al. found that infection developed within 3 months in 65 % of primary TKA cases at their institution in Japan [27]. In Norway, the Norwegian Arthroplasty Register noted a median time to revision for infection with primary THA of 47 days (range 4–1,782 days) [24]. The incidence of revision for infection also increased rapidly in the first year after surgery in the population observed by the Australian Joint Replacement Registry, yet declined beyond 1 year [29]. Even though the sources of the data range in region and scope, the consensus shows that greater than 60 % of infections are detected within 1 year of surgery and an overwhelming majority is diagnosed within 2 years.

6.4.3   Infection Incidence Within Revision Surgery

Again, these rates may seem low, but when comparing infection to other reasons for implant failure, infection is projected to be one of the dominant reasons for revision in both total knee and total hip arthroplasties. Based on NIS data from 1990 to 2003, Kurtz et al. modeled the growth of infection as a cause for revision surgery. The number of infections after THA was predicted to increase from 3,400 in 2005 to an estimated 46,000 in 2030. Since, historically, knee arthroplasty is performed in larger numbers, infections after TKA were predicted to increase from 6,400 in 2005 to 175,500 in 2030. In addition to number of revisions, the model projected the fraction of revisions performed for infection of THA to increase from 8.4% in 2005 to 47.5% in 2030. Likewise, the model projected the fraction of revisions performed for infection of TKA to increase from 16.8% in 2005 to 65.5% in 2030 (Fig. 6.3) [19]. The model suggest that, if the present trend is maintained, by 2016, 50% of the hospital expenditure on revisions would be spent on revising infected cases, and by 2025 for THA [19].

A later analysis of NIS data from 2005 to 2006 revealed that infection was the third most frequent reason for revision for THA with 14.8 % of revisions and the most frequent for TKA with 25.2 % [30, 31] (Table 6.5). Infection was the most common indication for arthrotomy and removal of prosthesis for THA (74.3 %) and TKA (79.1 %). For both arthroplasty types, the incidence within revision was larger than originally projected in the model by Kurtz et al. and may indicate faster growth rate than expected [19, 30, 31]. The Australian National Joint Replacement Registry 2010 annual report indicated infection as the third most prevalent revision reason for THA at 15.4 % and the second most for TKA at 17.1 % [29]. Similarly, 15–20 % of THA revisions in Norway from 2007 to 2010 were due to infection [32], and 17 % of THA in Sweden in 2008 were due to infection [33]. An estimated 20 % of TKA revisions were caused by infection in the Swedish population in 2001 [34]. Although, compared to other revision reasons in Sweden, incidence of infection decreased from 25.9 % during the first 2 years postoperatively to 2.9 % after 10 years.

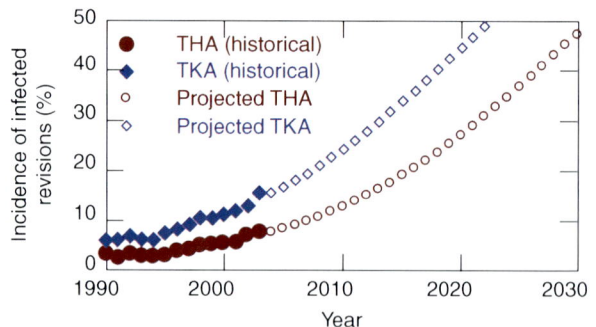

Fig. 6.3 Projections of the incidence of infection within revision arthroplasty procedure up to 2030. Based on figure from Kurtz et al. [19]

Table 6.5 Incidence of infection in reasons for revision

Country	Hip/knee	% of revisions	Time period	Source	Data type
USA	Hip	8.4	1990–2004	Kurtz et al. 2007 [19]	NIS
USA	Hip	14.8	2005–2006	Bozic et al. [31]	NIS
Australia	Hip	8.2	2010	National Arthroplasty Registry [29]	Registry
Norway	Hip	15–20	2009	National Arthroplasty Registry [32]	Registry
Sweden	Hip	10.8	2008	National Arthroplasty Registry [34]	Registry
USA	Knee	16.7	1990–2004	Kurtz et al. 2007 [19]	NIS
USA	Knee	25.2	2005–2006	Bozic et al. [30]	NIS
Australia	Knee	15.4	2010	National Arthroplasty Registry[29]	Registry
Sweden	Knee	~20	2011	National Arthroplasty Register [34]	Registry

The same trends are also observed in revised ultra-high-molecular-weight poly-ethylene (UHMWPE) hip cup liners. In a study of 212 revised acetabular liners, the most frequent reason for revision was loosening (35 %), instability (28 %), and infection (21 %) [28]. In almost all cases and sources of data represented, infection is preceded by aseptic loosening as a more frequent cause of revision. The only exception is the Bozic et al. study in which infection was the most common reason for TKA revision (25.2 %) and was followed by loosening (16.1 %). Recently, researchers proposed that in some cases of aseptic loosening and poor fixation, subclinical infections are the real cause [35–37]. Loosening has been suspected as septic loosening when bacteria were recovered from aseptically loose implants by more vigorous methods for detecting surface bacteria like polymerase chain reaction assays and implant sonication [35–37]. With more accurate techniques for diagnosis of infected arthroplasty components, infection may become the primary cause of revision surgery. However, even without these methods, within two decades, periprosthetic infection has the potential to become the most prevalent implant failure mode for total joint replacement procedures in the United States and abroad.

6.4.4   *Infection After Revision Surgery*

Infection of a primary arthroplasty device is already a taxing ordeal because of pain, increased hospital stay, and the two-stage exchange process. In addition to these consequences, infection is also associated with higher reinfection rates [25, 38–40]. Revised TKA, regardless of revision reasons, is linked to lower infection-free survival rates than primary procedures and have an infection rate of ~8.25 % (based on the Finnish Arthroplasty Register) [25]. Knee arthroplasty devices specifically revised for infection, however, have infection rates ranging from 10 to 33 % [38–40].

Many studies on reinfection suffer from small cohort sizes, which may explain the variability in infection rate. The largest study thus far was conducted at the Mayo Clinic and focused on 368 patients from 1998 to 2006 who had TKA revised previously for infection [40]. 15.8 % of the patients developed reinfection, and 86 % of cases were categorized as late chronic infections. The median time to reinfection was 3.6 years (range: 0.01–7.82 years), and the only significant risk factor associated was chronic lymphedema [40]. The findings fall in the ranges previously reported for reinfection and highlight the long-term effects of developing total joint infection.

6.5 Risk Factors

Various patient risk factors have been associated with periprosthetic joint infection ranging from gender to allogenic blood transfusion (Table 6.6) [13, 14, 20–27, 41, 42]. Previously in this chapter, TKA was noted to have a slight but significantly higher infection rates than THA [18, 20, 21], yet a more commonly found risk factor was gender. In eight studies reviewing risk factors for infection and in multiple international registries, males were at higher risk than their female counterparts [13, 22–27, 33, 34, 43]. The Australian Hip and Knee Registry 2010 report found that at 9 years, the cumulative incidence of infection was 1.3 % for males and only 0.6 % for females [29]. In a retrospective review of 2022 primary TKA, Suzuki et al. suggested the difference in infection rates could be due to difference in the pH level of the skin, sebum induction, and skin thickness between genders [27]. Dale et al. proposed the disparities could be cause by differences in referral thresholds or bacterial flora between sexes [24].

Elevated body mass index (BMI) was also commonly listed as a risk factor for PJI [20, 21, 23, 27, 41, 42]. In the retrospective analysis of 6108 THA and TKA patients by Malinzak et al., BMI greater than 50 was associated with an infection rate of 7.0 %, BMI greater than 40 but less than 50 was 1.1 %, and less than 40 was 0.47 %. If isolating TKA patients, BMI over 40 was 3.3 times more likely to become an infection when compared to BMI less than 40. The exact cause of this increased odds ratio for knee surgery is currently unknown but is significantly linked with BMI and obesity [21].

Longer duration procedures have also increased the risk of PJI in arthroplasty patients and could possibly be due to increased wound exposure to bacteria (*Staphylococci*, *Escherichia. coli*, etc.) and other virulent organisms that are causative agents for PJI [20, 22, 23, 44]. Patients, who were receiving public assistance, were also at higher risk of infection [18, 22, 23, 45]. Ong et al. suggested that the patient's socioeconomic status could indicate nutritional level, obesity, and existence of comorbidities that would predispose patients for risk of PJI [23]. Similarly, revision infection rates of primary TKA were increased at large nonteaching urban hospitals as opposed to rural and teaching institutions [18, 30]. However, it is more likely attributed to treatment patterns for revision surgery instead of directly to the institution. Urban nonteaching hospitals are often referral centers for revision (including infection) where primary surgery was performed elsewhere [18].

Table 6.6 Risk factors that are commonly associated with periprosthetic joint infection summarized from the literature

Male gender
BMI/obesity
Longer duration procedures
Receiving public assistance
Diabetes
Larger urban nonteaching hospitals
Lack of antibiotic bone cement
ASA risk score >2
Preexisting comorbidities
Postoperative complications
Rheumatoid arthritis
Revision TKA
Increased blood loss
Age
Emergency vs. planned surgery
Previous open reduction/internal fixation
Preop nutritional status
Urinary tract infection
Allogenic blood transfusion

The use of bone cement can likewise impact the chance of infection in both hip and knee arthroplasty [24–26, 46]. For TKA, the exclusion of antibiotic bone cement is one of the strongest determinates for revision of either primary or revision procedures [25]. Analysis of the Finnish Arthroplasty Registry observed fewer infections when antibiotics were delivered from bone cement and IV in combination, although, lack of bone cement alone showed a much more dramatic effect [25]. Multiple reviews of clinical results for THA have also shown up to a 50 % higher chance on infection when antibiotic bone cement was excluded [24, 46]. Antibiotic cement has even been shown to reduce infection rate in elbow arthroplasty from 11 to 5 % in certain cases [47]. Bone cement allows for the direct delivery of antibiotics to the surface of implants and local tissue, while antibiotics administered intravenously may not be adequate enough to reduce infection.

Diabetes has been listed as a risk factor in multiple studies; however, a review of 751,340 primary and revision hip and knee arthroplasties by Bolognesi et al. discovered no increase in occurrence of infections in diabetic patients [21, 23, 48, 49]. Diabetes has been highly correlated with high BMI, and glucose levels can be elevated after surgery or trauma, which may influence diabetes as a risk factor [21]. Patient management of the disease may also explain the discrepancy between diabetes as a risk factor. Marchant et al. retrospectively compared patients from 1998 to 2005 in the NIS with controlled and uncontrolled diabetes mellitus and found a much higher chance of developing a wound infection when the diabetes was inadequately controlled (odds ratio: 2.28) [49]. Management of diabetes was not factored in to risk analysis in other studies in the literature.

The American Society of Anesthesiologists physical status classification system (ASA) assesses the physical fitness of a patient prior to surgery. In the literature, ASA scores greater than 2 have been linked as a risk factor for infection [20, 24, 26]. ASA being a risk factor signifies that the incidence of infection increases with even minor comorbidities. Preexisting comorbidities previously have been connected to poor functional outcomes and more complications postoperatively [22, 23]. Ong et al. and Kurtz et al. also identified comorbidities as one of the primary risk factors for increased incidence of PJI as measured by the modified Charlson index [22, 23]. Interestingly, postoperative complications, which were linked to comorbidities of a patient prior to surgery, were also a risk factor for PJI in studies by Bozic and Ries and Jamsen et al. [14, 25].

The Norwegian and the Finnish Arthroplasty Registers both listed a diagnosis of rheumatoid arthritis (RA), as compared to osteoarthritis (OA), as a significant risk factor for infection [25, 26, 32]. One study of 2,647 patients reported an incidence of infection of 2.45 % for RA and 0.82 % for OA from 2002 to 2006 [26]. Other noted risk factors for PJI mentioned in the literature were increased blood loss [14], increased age [24], emergency vs. planned surgery [24], revision TKA [25], race [13], previous open reduction or fixation surgery [27], nutritional status [50], urinary tract infection [20], and allogenic blood transfusion (Table 6.6) [20].

Many studies of risk factors in the literature utilized the Charlson comorbidity index to identify the presence of patient comorbidities, but Bozic et al. proposed that the Charlson index does not help define the impact of specific diseases on patient outcomes, especially in elderly populations [51]. The limitation with using this index is patients with different combinations of preexisting conditions may still have similar Charlson scores. To alleviate this limitation in elderly populations, Bozic et al. used the 5 % national sample of the Medicare database to detect associations between infection and specific preexisting medical comorbid conditions for TKA patients. A Cox regression was used to evaluate the link between infection and 29 separate comorbidities. After adjusting for the effects from all 29 comorbidities, 13 conditions showed a significant effect on risk of infection following TKA. In order of significance, the conditions with the highest risk of PJI were congestive heart failure, chronic pulmonary disease, preoperative anemia, diabetes, depression, renal disease, pulmonary circulation disorders, obesity, rheumatologic disease, psychoses, metastatic tumor, peripheral vascular disease, and valvular disease (Table 6.7). The 5 % Medicare sample, compared to other databases, allowed for the identification of specific disorders as risk factors for infection. The focus of this research was to provide a basis for superior clinical decision-making between surgeons and patient populations over 65 years in age [51].

Since bearing surfaces for hip replacements are made from multiple material types, Bozic et al. was also able to compare infection rates between material couplings used for bearing surfaces [41]. Bearing surfaces for replacement hips are typically either metal on polyethylene (M-PE), metal on metal (M-M), or ceramic on ceramic (C-C), and these three bearing types were compared using the 2005–2007 100 % Medicare inpatient claims. After adjusting for patient and hospital factors, M-M bearings were at a higher risk for infection when compared with C-C

Table 6.7 Risk factors in elderly Medicare patients with TKA compiled from Bozic et al. [51]

Risk factor for PJI	Adjusted hazard ratio
Congestive heart failure	1.28
Chronic pulmonary disease	1.22
Preoperative anemia	1.26
Diabetes	1.19
Depression	1.28
Renal disease	1.38
Pulmonary circulation disorders	1.42
Obesity	1.22
Rheumatologic disease	1.18
Psychosis	1.26
Metastatic tumor	1.59
Peripheral vascular disease	1.13
Valvular disease	1.15

bearings (0.59 % vs. 0.32 %, respectively). The infection risks between M-M and M-PE bearings and between C-C and M-PE bearings were not found to be significantly different. Although the findings between bearing cohorts were significant, the clinical impact remains uncertain [41].

6.6 Additional Total Joint Replacements: Spine, Shoulder, and Elbow

By far, hip and knee arthroplasties are the most common form of total joint replacements and thus have the largest amount of data collected on the incidence of infection. Nonetheless, studies have emerged cataloging the development of infection following total disk replacements (TDR), total shoulder arthroplasty (TSA), and total elbow arthroplasty (TEA). Late infection on TDR is a rare occurrence even when compared to THA and TKA [52, 53]. In a review of 7170 TDR procedures using the NIS from 2005 to 2006, only 1.3 % of revision cases (2/165 revisions) were device-related infections. Incidence of infection was significantly lower than reported for THA (9.6 % of revisions) and TKA (17.4 % of revision) in the same period of data. Admittedly, the demographics and overall health status of the patient groups vary considerably between arthroplasty procedures. Nonetheless, the NIS data still suggests that the infection burden for disk replacement surgery is lower than other arthroplasty procedures.

Though there is a lack of large multicenter or national database studies, a systematic review of 84 articles in English, French, German, and Spanish recapitulated the results of clinical complications for TSA [54]. The analysis uncovered that infection occurred in 30 cases in 14 studies for an incidence of infection of ~3.8 %. Infection was the second most common complication and was only preceded by instability at

4.7 % of cases [54]. Even though the review was a summation of results from multiple sources, infection rates for shoulder replacements were comparable to other forms of arthroplasty.

Infection rates reported after primary elbow replacement range from as low as 1 to as high as12.5% and are generally regarded as higher than other major joint arthroplasty procedures [47, 55, 56]. Infection rates are considerably increased as the result of the subcutaneous nature of the elbow joint residing within a thin soft tissue envelope [55, 56]. In addition, large portions of patients undergoing TEA are immunocompromised as well as having poor soft tissue quality as a side effect of medication used in treatment for rheumatoid arthritis, traumatic arthritis, or from previous surgeries [56]. Known risk factors for PJI include previous elbow operations, a history of infections, rheumatoid arthritis (Class IV), psychiatric disorders, and wound drainage postoperatively. To a lesser degree, patients with psoriatic arthritis, immunocompromised conditions, and diabetes are at a high risk [55]. Infection rates as high as 31 % have been recorded for patient groups diagnosed previously with multiple comorbid risk factors such as rheumatoid arthritis and prior surgical intervention [55, 57].

6.7   Economic Impact of Infections

In addition to being difficult to treat and growing in incidence among revision reasons, data has shown there is also a greater economic burden for infected revisions than other common revision reasons. In a retrospective study of arthroplasty patients from March 2001 to December 2002, Bozic and Ries found that, compared to primary arthroplasty or revision for aseptic loosening, infected hip arthroplasty was associated with significantly higher number of days in the hospital, total hospital costs, and total outpatient charges [14]. Specifically, the direct medical costs for revision of THA because of infection were 2.8 times higher than revision for aseptic loosening and 4.8 times higher than primary THA [14]. Similar results were reported in France, where Klouche et al. reported that revision of septic THA was 2.6 times more costly than aseptic revisions and 3.6 times more than primary THA [58]. Kurtz et al. analyzed the NIS from 1990 to 2004, and for both TKA and THA, the ratio of hospital charges for infected arthroplasty was 1.52 and 1.76 times higher than uninfected arthroplasty, respectively, and was associated with 1.87 and 2.21 times longer length of stay, respectively [18].

The economic burden of infection arthroplasties is also felt directly by hospitals. A study by Hebert et al. uncovered that infected TKA utilized two times more hospital resources than their revision counterparts, while inadequate reimbursements resulted in a net loss to the hospital of $30,000 per Medicare patient and $15,000 per standard patient [59]. Furthermore, the costs discussed are direct medical costs, and only one piece of the economic impact of infected THA. In most cases, infection was linked to longer hospital stay and increased outpatient visits, which would require a longer-term leave of absence from work and impact daily activities and quality of life of the patients [18]. Increased costs only further eluci-date the severity and wide-reaching impact of infection as compared to other arthro-plasty complications.

6.8 Summary

In summary, a thorough review of the literature discovered infection currently afflicts ~1 % of joint arthroplasty patients worldwide and is expected to grow as patient populations increase in size and expand into younger cohorts. Infection is poised to be the most frequent reason for revision and is associated with higher hospital costs and longer inpatient stay. As this number of arthroplasty patients begins to multiple in the coming years, the financial impact of infected revisions will be felt through the health community because of inadequate reimbursement procedures. New devices and technology will hopefully help to curb the increasing trends of infection, and thus it is critical to identify the primary factors that influence infection to design techniques and methods to specifically address these problems. The most commonly reported risk factors were found to be gender, BMI > 50, extended length procedures, lack of antibiotic bone cement, and comorbidities. With the information available, physicians can begin to target effective strategies to reduce infection in higher risk groups and with preexisting patient conditions.

References

1. Berger RA, Rosenberg AG, Barden RM, Sheinkop MB, Jacobs JJ, Galante JO. Long-term fol-lowup of the Miller-Galante total knee replacement. Clin Orthop Relat Res. 2001;388:58–67.
2. Indelli PF, Aglietti P, Buzzi R, Baldini A. The Insall-Burstein II prosthesis: a 5- to 9-year fol-low-up study in osteoarthritic knees. J Arthroplasty. 2002;17:544–9.
3. Quintana JM, Arostegui I, Escobar A, Azkarate J, Goenaga JI, Lafuente I. Prevalence of knee and hip osteoarthritis and the appropriateness of joint replacement in an older population. Arch Intern Med. 2008;168:1576–84.
4. Rorabeck CH, Murray P. Cost effectiveness of revision total knee replacement. Instr Course Lect. 1997;46:237–40.
5. Berry DJ, Harmsen WS, Cabanela ME, Morrey BF. Twenty-five-year survivorship of two thou-sand consecutive primary Charnley total hip replacements: factors affecting survivorship of acetabular and femoral components. J Bone Joint Surg Am. 2002;84:171–7.
6. Bourne RB, Maloney WJ, Wright JG. An AOA critical issue. The outcome of the outcomes movement. J Bone Joint Surg Am. 2004;86-A:633–40.
7. Kurtz SM, Ong K, Lau E, Mowat F, Halpern M. Projections of primary and revision hip and knee arthroplasty in the United States from 2005 to 2030. J Bone Joint Surg Am. 2007; 89(4):780–5.
8. Soderman P, Malchau H, Herberts P. Outcome after total hip arthroplasty: part I. General health evaluation in relation to definition of failure in the Swedish National Total Hip Arthroplasty register. Acta Orthop Scand. 2000;71:354–9.
9. Maloney WJ. National joint replacement registries: has the time come? J Bone Joint Surg Am. 2001;83-A:1582–5.

10. Saleh KJ, Santos ER, Ghomrawi HM, Parvizi J, Mulhall KJ. Socioeconomic issues and demographics of total knee arthroplasty revision. Clin Orthop Relat Res. 2006;446:15–21.
11. Kurtz SM, Ong KL, Lau E, Manley MT. Current and projected utilization of total joint replacement. In: Ducheyne P, Healy K, Hutmacher DW, Grainger DW, Kirkpatrick CJ, editors. Comprehensive biomaterials. Oxford: Elsevier Science; 2011.
12. Katz JN, Barrett J, Mahomed NN, Baron JA, Wright RJ, Losina E. Association between hospital and surgeon procedure volume and the outcomes of total knee replacement. J Bone Joint Surg Am. 2004;86-A:1909–16.
13. Mahomed NN, Barrett J, Katz JN, Baron JA, Wright J, Losina E. Epidemiology of total knee replacement in the United States Medicare population. J Bone Joint Surg Am. 2005;87: 1222–8.
14. Bozic KJ, Ries MD. The impact of infection after total hip arthroplasty on hospital and surgeon resource utilization. J Bone Joint Surg Am. 2005;87:1746–51.
15. Sculco TP. The economic impact of infected joint arthroplasty. Orthopedics. 1995;18:871–3.
16. National Hospital Discharge Survey. National Center for Health Statistics. http://www.cdc. gov/nchs/nhds/about_nhds.htm (2009).
17. The Nationwide Inpatient Sample (NIS). Healthcare Cost and Utilization Project (HCUP): Agency for Healthcare Research and Quality. http://www.hcup-us.ahrq.gov/nisoverview.jsp (2008).
18. Kurtz SM, Lau E, Schmier J, Ong KL, Zhao K, Parvizi J. Infection burden for hip and knee arthroplasty in the United States. J Arthroplasty. 2008;23:984–91.
19. Kurtz SM, Ong KL, Schmier J, Mowat F, Saleh K, Dybvik E, Karrholm J, Garellick G, Havelin LI, Furnes O, Malchau H, Lau E. Future clinical and economic impact of revision total hip and knee arthroplasty. J Bone Joint Surg Am. 2007;89 Suppl 3:144–51.
20. Pulido L, Ghanem E, Joshi A, Purtill JJ, Parvizi J. Periprosthetic joint infection: the incidence, timing, and predisposing factors. Clin Orthop Relat Res. 2008;466:1710–5.
21. Malinzak RA, Ritter MA, Berend ME, Meding JB, Olberding EM, Davis KE. Morbidly obese, diabetic, younger, and unilateral joint arthroplasty patients have elevated total joint arthroplasty infection rates. J Arthroplasty. 2009;24:84–8.
22. Kurtz SM, Ong KL, Lau E, Bozic KJ, Berry D, Parvizi J. Prosthetic joint infection risk after TKA in the Medicare population. Clin Orthop Relat Res. 2010;468:52–6.
23. Ong KL, Kurtz SM, Lau E, Bozic KJ, Berry DJ, Parvizi J. Prosthetic joint infection risk after total hip arthroplasty in the Medicare population. J Arthroplasty. 2009;24:105–9.
24. Dale H, Skramm I, Lower HL, Eriksen HM, Espehaug B, Furnes O, Skjeldestad FE, Havelin LI, Engesaeter LB. Infection after primary hip arthroplasty. Acta Orthop. 2011;82:646–54.
25. Jamsen E, Huhtala H, Puolakka T, Moilanen T. Risk factors for infection after knee arthroplasty. A register-based analysis of 43,149 cases. J Bone Joint Surg Am. 2009;91:38–47.
26. Jamsen E, Varonen M, Huhtala H, Lehto MU, Lumio J, Konttinen YT, Moilanen T. Incidence of prosthetic joint infections after primary knee arthroplasty. J Arthroplasty. 2010;25:87–92.
27. Suzuki G, Saito S, Ishii T, Motojima S, Tokuhashi Y, Ryu J. Previous fracture surgery is a major risk factor of infection after total knee arthroplasty. Knee Surg Sports Traumatol Arthrosc. 2011;19:2040–4.
28. Kurtz SM, Medel FJ, MacDonald DW, Parvizi J, Kraay MJ, Rimnac CM. Reasons for revision of first-generation highly cross-linked polyethylenes. J Arthroplasty. 2010;25:67–74.
29. Graves S, Davidson D, de Steiger R, Tomkins A. Annual report 2010. Australian National Joint Replacement Registry. Adelaide: Australian Orthopaedic Association; 2010.
30. Bozic KJ, Kurtz SM, Lau E, Ong K, Chiu V, Vail TP, Rubash HE, Berry DJ. The epidemiology of revision total knee arthroplasty in the United States. Clin Orthop Relat Res. 2010;468:45–51.
31. Bozic KJ, Kurtz SM, Lau E, Ong K, Vail TP, Berry DJ. The epidemiology of revision total hip arthroplasty in the United States. J Bone Joint Surg Am. 2009;91:128–33.
32. Annual report 2010. The Norwegian Arthroplasty Register. Bergen: Centre of Excellence of Joint Replacements; 2010.

33. Garellick G, Karrholm J, Rogmark C, Herberts P. Annual report 2008. Swedish Hip Arthroplasty Register. Göteborg: Department of Ortopaedics, Sahlgrenska University Hospital; 2009
34. Lidgien L, Sundberg M, Dahl AW, Robertsson O. Annual report 2010. The Swedish Knee Arthroplasty Register. Lund: Department of Orthopedics, Lund University Hospital; 2010.
35. Dempsey KE, Riggio MP, Lennon A, Hannah VE, Ramage G, Allan D, Bagg J. Identification of bacteria on the surface of clinically infected and non-infected prosthetic hip joints removed during revision arthroplasties by 16S rRNA gene sequencing and by microbiological culture. Arthritis Res Ther. 2007;9:R46.
36. Ince A, Rupp J, Frommelt L, Katzer A, Gille J, Lohr JF. Is "aseptic" loosening of the prosthetic cup after total hip replacement due to nonculturable bacterial pathogens in patients with low-grade infection? Clin Infect Dis. 2004;39:1599–603.
37. Kobayashi N, Procop GW, Krebs V, Kobayashi H, Bauer TW. Molecular identification of bacteria from aseptically loose implants. Clin Orthop Relat Res. 2008;466:1716–25.
38. Azzam K, McHale K, Austin M, Purtill JJ, Parvizi J. Outcome of a second two-stage reimplantation for periprosthetic knee infection. Clin Orthop Relat Res. 2009;467:1706–14.
39. Hanssen AD, Osmon DR. Evaluation of a staging system for infected hip arthroplasty. Clin Orthop Relat Res. 2002;403:16–22.
40. Kubista B, Hartzler RU, Wood CM, Osmon DR, Hanssen AD, Lewallen DG. Reinfection after two-stage revision for periprosthetic infection of total knee arthroplasty. Int Orthop. 2011;36(1):65–71.
41. Bozic KJ, Ong K, Lau E, Kurtz SM, Vail TP, Rubash HE, Berry DJ. Risk of complication and revision total hip arthroplasty among Medicare patients with different bearing surfaces. Clin Orthop Relat Res. 2010;468:2357–62.
42. Swierstra BA, Vervest AM, Walenkamp GH, Schreurs BW, Spierings PT, Heyligers IC, van Susante JL, Ettema HB, Jansen MJ, Hennis PJ, de Vries J, Muller-Ploeger SB, Pols MA. Dutch guideline on total hip prosthesis. Acta Orthop. 2011;82:567–76.
43. Parvizi J, Johnson BG, Rowland C, Ereth MH, Lewallen DG. Thirty-day mortality after elective total hip arthroplasty. J Bone Joint Surg Am. 2001;83-A:1524–8.
44. Smabrekke A, Espehaug B, Havelin LI, Furnes O. Operating time and survival of primary total hip replacements: an analysis of 31,745 primary cemented and uncemented total hip replacements from local hospitals reported to the Norwegian Arthroplasty Register 1987–2001. Acta Orthop Scand. 2004;75:524–32.
45. Webb BG, Lichtman DM, Wagner RA. Risk factors in total joint arthroplasty: comparison of infection rates in patients with different socioeconomic backgrounds. Orthopedics. 2008;31: 445.
46. Parvizi J, Saleh KJ, Ragland PS, Pour AE, Mont MA. Efficacy of antibiotic-impregnated cement in total hip replacement. Acta Orthop. 2008;79:335–41.
47. Kim JM, Mudgal CS, Konopka JF, Jupiter JB. Complications of total elbow arthroplasty. J Am Acad Orthop Surg. 2011;19:328–39.
48. Bolognesi MP, Marchant Jr MH, Viens NA, Cook C, Pietrobon R, Vail TP. The impact of diabetes on perioperative patient outcomes after total hip and total knee arthroplasty in the United States. J Arthroplasty. 2008;23:92–8.
49. Marchant Jr MH, Viens NA, Cook C, Vail TP, Bolognesi MP. The impact of glycemic control and diabetes mellitus on perioperative outcomes after total joint arthroplasty. J Bone Joint Surg Am. 2009;91:1621–9.
50. Font-Vizcarra L, Lozano L, Rios J, Forga MT, Soriano A. Preoperative nutritional status and post-operative infection in total knee replacements: a prospective study of 213 patients. Int J Artif Organs. 2011;34:876–81.
51. Bozic KJ, Lau E, Kurtz S, Ong K, Berry DJ. Patient-related risk factors for postoperative mortality and periprosthetic joint infection in Medicare patients undergoing TKA. Clin Orthop Relat Res. 2012;470:130–7.
52. Gerometta A, Rodriguez Olaverri JC, Bittan F. Infection and revision strategies in total disc arthroplasty. Int Orthop. 2011;36(2):471–4.

53. Kurtz SM, Lau E, Ianuzzi A, Schmier J, Todd L, Isaza J, et al. National revision burden for lumbar total disc replacement in the United States: epidemiologic and economic perspectives. Spine 2010;35:690–6.

54. Zumstein MA, Pinedo M, Old J, Boileau P. Problems, complications, reoperations, and revisions in reverse total shoulder arthroplasty: a systematic review. J Shoulder Elbow Surg/Am Shoulder Elbow Surg. 2011;20:146–57.

55. Beadel G, King G. Revision elbow arthroplasty. In: Williams GR, Yamaguchi K, Ramsey ML, Galatz LM, editors. Shoulder and elbow arthroplasty. Philadelphia: Lippincott Williams and Wilkins; 2005. p. 428.

56. Voloshin I, Schippert DW, Kakar S, Kaye EK, Morrey BF. Complications of total elbow replacement: a systematic review. J Shoulder Elbow Surg/Am Shoulder Elbow Surg. 2011;20: 158–68.

57. Morrey BF, Bryan RS. Infection after total elbow arthroplasty. J Bone Joint Surg Am. 1983;65:330–8.

58. Klouche S, Sariali E, Mamoudy P. Total hip arthroplasty revision due to infection: a cost analysis approach. Orthop Traumatol Surg Res. 2010;96:124–32.

59. Hebert CK, Williams RE, Levy RS, Barrack RL. Cost of treating an infected total knee replacement. Clin Orthop Relat Res. 1996;331:140–145.

Chapter 7
Septic Complications in Arthroplasty

Gerold Labek

Abstract In the present chapter incidence of revision in primary and revision total hip and knee arthroplasty is presented mainly based on registry data. The information is then discussed separately for primary and revision arthroplasty focusing on the septic reasons for revision. Influence of registries on improvement of joint arthroplasty outcomes is discussed as well.

Keywords Complications • Hip • Knee • Infection

7.1 Introduction and Risk Factors for Infection

Septic complications are very burdensome to the patient, and the therapy involves high costs for the health care system.

On-topic statements from large datasets can only be made on the basis of average values, whereas a wide range of variation has to be taken into account in the assessment of individual situations.

The risk of infection depends on several risk factors. Apart from a reduced immune response due to steroid therapy, HIV, advanced age, alcoholism, renal or hepatic impairment, diabetes mellitus, or rheumatoid arthritis, obesity and prior knee surgery are also risk factors for increased rates of complications [1–8]. Increased rates of infection must of course also be expected in patients after a septic incident or osteomyelitis.

G. Labek, M.D.
Department of Orthopaedic Surgery, Innsbruck Medical University,
Anichstr. 35, Innsbruck 6020, Austria
e-mail: gerold.labek@i-med.ac.at

R. Trebše (ed.), *Infected Total Joint Arthroplasty*,
DOI 10.1007/978-1-4471-2482-5_7, © Springer-Verlag London 2012

7.2 Epidemiology

7.2.1 Primary Arthroplasty

Clinical studies report revision rates of between 0.39 and 0.7 % due to septic complications after total arthroplasty interventions [3, 9–11].

Direct comparison of data from clinical studies and register data is not possible in all respects. The most essential difference is the definition of the case of failure. In registers the removal or exchange of at least one part of the implant is a prerequisite so that – in contrast to some clinical studies – debridement and soft tissue surgery are not included.

Nevertheless the average rates are higher in registers. Tables 7.1 and 7.2 show the average value from high-quality registers worldwide, adjusted for number of cases and follow-up period of the respective datasets.

Following aseptic loosening, the most frequent reason for revision, septic loosening is the second most common cause after total knee replacement. This compli-

Table 7.1 Risks and reasons for revision after primary total hip arthroplasty

Reason for revision	Reason for revision in (%) of all revisions	Frequency after primary surgery in (%)	Absolute frequency risk after primary surgery 1/x patients
Aseptic loosening	55.24	7.94	13
Dislocation	11.79	1.69	59
Septic loosening	7.45	1.07	93
Periprosthetic fracture	6.07	0.87	115
Wear	4.18	0.78	128
Pain for no other reason	3.74	0.52	193
Implant fracture	2.48	0.31	323

Source: All most recent National Arthroplasty Register reports worldwide in 2009 that publish the actual reason of revision (Sweden, Norway, Canada, Finland, Australia)

Table 7.2 Risks and reasons of revision after primary total knee arthroplasty

Reason for revision	Reason for revision in (%) of all revisions	Frequency after primary surgery in (%)	Absolute frequency risk after primary surgery 1/x patients
Aseptic loosening	29.83	2.44	41
Septic loosening	14.93	1.63	61
Pain for no other reason	9.49	0.89	112
Wear	8.15	0.65	153
Instability	6.23	0.50	200
Implant fracture	4.73	0.43	234
Periprosthetic fracture	3.07	0.24	417

Source: All most recent National Arthroplasty Register reports worldwide in 2009 that publish the actual reason of revision (Sweden, Norway, Canada, Finland, Australia)

cation occurs in 1.63 % of patients after primary implantation in the course of their lives. That means that 1 out of 61 patients is affected.

The incidence after total hip replacement is slightly lower at 1.07 %, which corresponds to 1 out of 93 patients. After aseptic loosening and dislocation, septic complications rank third among the most common causes of revision surgery of the hip.

Chronologically, the occurrence of complications is not at all a linear process. There is an accumulation of infections and dislocations in the first few years after primary surgery. About 20 % of all revisions within the first 3 years have to be performed due to septic complications, which are therefore approximately as frequent as dislocations after hip arthroplasty.

In Sweden, which has one of the best quality monitoring systems in the world, the timeline shows a significant reduction in complication rate initially after launch of the register (see Table 7.3). However, after a low in revision frequency of about 0.5 % for those patients who had undergone primary surgery in 1987, a slight increase in complication rates was subsequently observed.

Owing to stringent quality improvement measures, a marked decrease in complication rate was achieved from 4 % around 1980 down to approximately 0.5 % nowadays. However, it seems that in the last few years, further improvement has hardly been feasible (see Figure 7.1).

Unicompartmental knee replacements on average exhibit considerably lower rates of septic complications than total knee or hip replacement (see Figure 7.2).

Differences between the sexes have been observed particularly for knee arthroplasty. Males are more frequently affected than females; in the case of total knee arthroplasty, the differences are statistically significant (see Figure 7.3).

7.2.2   Septic Complications at Revision Surgery

The recording of septic complications after revision surgery involves methodological challenges. To ensure correct statistical evaluation, the patients' previous medical history must be captured. Since the end point for analyses is a re-revision, large and well-controlled patient collectives are a basic requirement. In practice, this can only be achieved by means of high-quality national or regional arthroplasty registers. The initial situation of individual patients may vary considerably, which again can only be taken into consideration through the large number of patients covered in registers.

The probably best paper in this context was published by the Norwegian Arthroplasty Register [12]. Even though the issue of septic complications is not the main focus of this publication and septic complications were excluded from further evaluation, a few essential data can be derived from the facts given. 5,137 out of 78,534 patients after primary total hip arthroplasty had to undergo revision surgery. 375 of them had to be excluded from further analysis due to septic complications. This corresponds to an incidence of 7.3 %.

After revision of 599 patients, 76 new infections (= 12.7 %) occurred. Out of the 98 patients who even had to undergo a third reoperation, another 12 had to be revised once again for newly developed infections (= 12.2 %).

Table 7.3 Incidence of revision surgery after primary surgery in Sweden

Number of revisions per reason and time to revision only the first revision, primary THRs 1979–2008

Reason for revision	0–3 years		4–6 years		7–10 years		>10 years		Total	Share
Aseptic loosening	2,810	43.2%	3,593	81.7%	5,174	86.1%	6,268	86.0%	17,845	73.7%
Dislocation	1,312	20.2%	231	5.3%	207	3.4%	259	3.6%	2,009	8.3%
Deep infection	1,335	20.5%	215	4.9%	153	2.5%	100	1.4%	1,803	7.5%
Fracture	415	6.4%	240	5.5%	343	5.7%	517	7.1%	1,515	6.3%
Technical error	464	7.1%	26	0.6%	17	0.3%	12	0.2%	519	2.1%
Implant fracture	56	0.9%	74	1.7%	108	1.8%	117	1.6%	355	1.5%
Pain only	67	1.0%	11	0.3%	4	0.1%	7	0.1%	89	0.4%
Miscellaneous	41	0.6%	9	0.2%	5	0.1%	9	0.1%	64	0.3%
Total	6,500	100%	4,399	100%	6,011	100%	7,289	100%	24,199	100%

Source: Swedish National Hip Arthroplasty Register, Annual Report 2008

Fig. 7.1 Risk for revision after THA due to deep infection over time in Sweden (*Source*: Swedish National Hip Arthroplasty Register, Annual Report 2008)

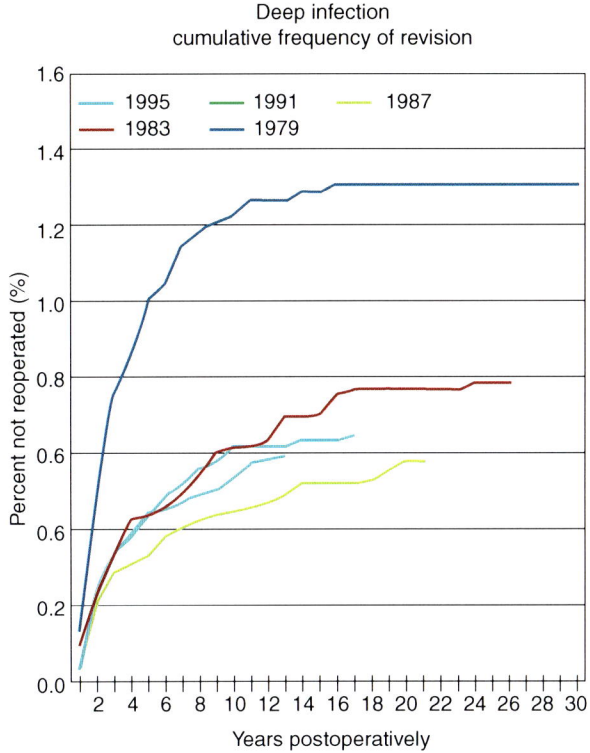

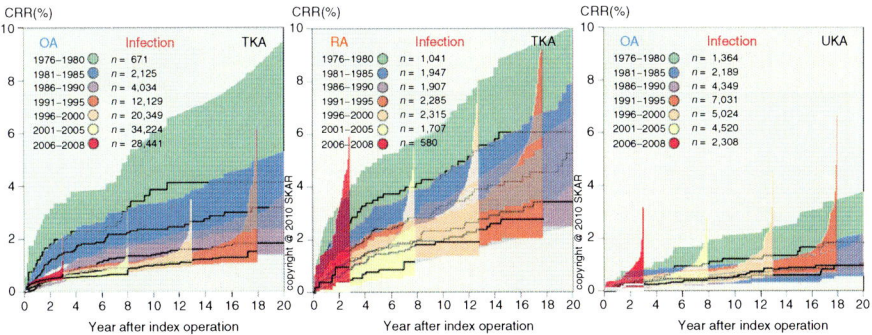

Fig. 7.2 Risk for revision after knee arthroplasty due to deep infection over time in Sweden. Comparing the *CRR*, using only revision for infection as end point, we find an improvement with time for both *TKA* and *UKA*. However, the CRR for infection in 2006–2008 seems to have increased somewhat as compared to 2001–2005 (*Source*: Swedish Knee Arthroplasty Register, Annual Report 2010)

If we add these values and assume a complication rate of 1 % after primary surgery, we would have to suppose that septic complications occurred in one third of patients after the third revision.

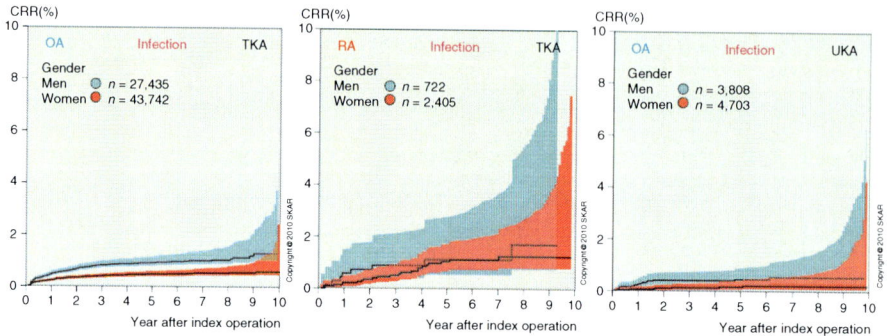

Fig. 7.3 Gender distribution of septic complications after knee arthroplasty in Sweden. Using as the end point revision for infection, the *CRR* (1999–2008) shows in *TKA* for *OA* that men are more affected than women (*RR* 2.0). The same tendency is true for *RA*, although not significant. *UKA* with its smaller implant size does better than the larger *TKA*, but even in *UKA* men have 2.9 times the risk of women of becoming revised for infection. In *TKA*, patients with *RA* are more affected than those with *OA* (*RR* 1.7) (*Source*: Swedish Knee Arthroplasty Register, Annual Report 2010)

An older publication by the Norwegian Register suggests that there are an unknown number of chronic septic loosenings which are documented as aseptic revisions. Otherwise, it would hardly be explicable why different antibiotic regimes are associated with a different risk of revision for aseptic loosening as the end point [13].

Evaluation of these data should also consider the diagnostic options available in 1997. It should, however, be critically analyzed whether all low-grade septic complications can be safely diagnosed nowadays.

Regarding the success rates of the different treatment methods, only rough estimations can be made based on the data available.

7.2.3   *Treatment of Infections*

A recently published meta-analysis provides a good overview of the literature dealing with this topic [14].

Basically, there are several treatment options which are primarily used according to the symptoms.

Debridement with simultaneous implant retention is most commonly used in the case of short-term symptoms; published eradication rates range from 26 to 71 %.

One-stage revisions are mainly performed using antibiotic-loaded bone cement, with good published success rates of more than 90 %. However, this procedure puts high demands on surgeons and microbiologists during the entire therapy.

Two-stage revisions represent the gold standard among treatment options. The published success rates are similar to those of single-stage revisions, whereas the inclusion criteria for patients usually vary. The treatment regimens in the time interval until reimplantation differ as well. However, in most cases high-dose, antibiogram-adapted antibiotic regimens are recommended for 6 weeks. The majority of studies recommend reimplantation after 6–12 weeks, depending on the extent of pathogen eradication.

Spacers of antibiotic-loaded cement or articulating spacers are a sensible option to achieve high local antibiotic levels, maintain the patient's mobility as far as possible, and reduce soft tissue contraction. Nevertheless, impaired mobility is still a frequent, long-term, and restricting outcome of two-stage revision, particularly in the case of knee arthroplasty.

Excision arthroplasty or enucleation may be used as a salvage procedure in case of severely damaged bone substance and multiple therapy failure, but only few comparative studies are available on the outcome. Ganse et al., however, report on largely identical clinical outcome of about 60 points in the HHS for each group at 52 months for two-stage revisions and excision arthroplasty of the hip [15].

As a general rule, methodological weaknesses should be considered in quite a number of clinical studies dealing with this topic. The numbers of cases are mostly relatively small; statistical power is often low. The parameters collected sometimes show considerable deviations and interobserver variability.

An established standard can therefore not be derived from the data currently available, not even for clearly defined patient groups.

7.3 Conclusions

Comprehensive analysis of the data available reveals considerable differences in outcome after primary arthroplasty in various countries. Owing to stringent quality control and regular feedback to the treating physicians, Sweden managed to halve the revision rate within a decade. This is true for both the overall revision rate and septic complications. Recently founded registers, where these mechanisms have not fully developed yet, show higher absolute values. Relative risk data analyses reveal that in nearly all countries approximately 10 % of all revisions are due to septic complications.

However, even under favorable circumstances about one revision after primary implantation must be expected in consequence of septic complications per 200 primary interventions. Biofilm-forming bacteria represent a particular challenge [16].

In the past few years, an increasing occurrence of multiresistant pathogens and small colony variants have been observed that will probably be a continuing challenge in diagnosis and therapy also in the future and can only partly be compensated by improved laboratory techniques.

Apart from advances in the diagnosis and therapy of infections, ancient surgical principles should not be forgotten either. The operation time, the number of persons present in the operating theater, the observance of hygienic guidelines, or the soft tissue trauma following the intervention – all these factors have an influence on the complication rate as well. Standardized procedures, as well as the good collaboration of all persons involved, can make a substantial contribution to improving the results. The surgeon's awareness and willingness to act as a model are essential in this process.

However, the most important impact factor for septic complications is the number of revision surgeries required – regardless of their causes.

References

1. Wilson MG, et al. Infection as a complication of total knee-replacement arthroplasty. Risk factors and treatment in sixty-seven cases. J Bone Joint Surg Am. 1990;72(6):878–83.
2. Berbari EF, et al. Risk factors for prosthetic joint infection: case control study. Clin Infect Dis. 1998;27(5):1247–54.
3. Peersman G, et al. Infection in total knee replacement: a retrospective review of 6489 total knee replacements. Clin Orthop Relat Res. 2001;392:15–23.
4. Chiu FY, et al. Cefuroxime-impregnated cement at primary total knee arthroplasty in diabetes mellitus. A prospective, randomized study. J Bone Joint Surg Br. 2001;83(5):691–5.
5. Meding JB, et al. Total knee replacement in patients with diabetes mellitus. Clin Orthop Relat Res. 2003;416:208–16.
6. Winiarsky R, et al. Total knee arthroplasty in morbidly obese patients. J Bone Joint Surg Am. 1998;80(12):1770–4.
7. Amin AK, et al. Does obesity influence the clinical outcome at 5 years following total knee replacement for osteoarthritis? J Bone Joint Surg Br. 2006;88(3):335–40.
8. Krushell RJ, et al. Primary total knee arthroplasty in morbidly obese patients: a 5 to 14 year follow-up study. J Arthroplasty. 2007;22(6 Supp 2):77–80.
9. Blom AW, et al. Infection after total knee arthroplasty. J Bone Joint Surg Br. 2004;86(5):688–91.
10. Hanssen AD, Rand JA. Evaluation and treatment of infection at site of total hip and knee arthroplasty. Instr Course Lect. 1999;48:111–22.
11. Pulido L, et al. Periprosthetic joint infection: the incidence, timing and predisposing factors. Clin Orthop Relat Res. 2008;446(7):1710–5.
12. Lie SA, et al. Failure rates for 4762 revision total hip arthroplasties in the Norwegian Arthroplasty Register. J Bone Joint Surg Br. 2004;86(4):504–9.
13. Espehaug B, et al. Antibiotic prophylaxis in total hip arthroplasty. Review of 10,905 primary cemented total hip replacements reported to the Norwegian Arthroplasty Register, 1987–1995. J Bone Joint Surg Br. 1997;79(4):590–5.
14. Senthi S, et al. Infection in total hip replacement: meta-analysis. Int Orthop (SICOT). 2011;35:253–60.
15. Ganse B, et al. Two-stage hip revision arthroplasty: the role of the excision arthroplasty. Eur J Orthop Surg Traumatol. 2008;18(3):223–8.
16. Stewart PS, Costerton JW. Antibiotic resistance of bacteria in biofilms. Lancet. 2001;358(9276):135–8.

Chapter 8
Perioperative Antibiotic Prophylaxis in Total Joint Arthroplasty

Nataša Faganeli

Abstract In this chapter an overview is given about the rationale of perioperative antibiotic prophylaxis in total joint arthroplasty. Currently there are only level 1a recommendations for primary joint replacements, while the recommendations for revision joint replacements are still missing because of complexity and heterogeneity of this cases and lack of randomized controlled trials as well. Current literature and available data are reviewed, and recommendations are summarized.

Keywords Antibiotic • Prophylaxis • Timing • Prosthetic joints

8.1 Background

Surgical site infection (SSI) is a healthcare-associated infection in which a wound infection occurs after a surgical procedure. The infection may range from superficial to deep and organ-space infection [1]. According to the National Healthcare Safety Network report between the years 2006 and 2008, the SSI rate in hip replacements varied from 0.67–2.4 % to 0.58–1.6 % in knee replacements in the United States [2]. European Centre for Disease Prevention and Control reports a cumulative incidence of surgical site infections in hip prosthesis of 1.2 % in Europe for the year 2007 [3]. Rates of SSI for ankle replacement have been reported as high as 15 %, 1.2 % for elbow replacement, and 0.7 % for shoulder replacement [4–6].

SSI after orthopedic surgical procedures is one of the most costly complications due to hospital readmissions, extended hospital length of stay, need of additional surgical procedures, convalescent or nursing home care between procedures and outcomes that are worse than those in uninfected cases [5, 7]. Whitehouse and colleagues estimate that orthopedic SSIs prolong total hospital stay by a median of 2 weeks per patient, double rehospitalization rates, and increase healthcare costs by more than 300 %. Patients with orthopedic SSIs have substantially greater physical limitations and significant decrease in their quality of life [8].

N. Faganeli, Pharm.D.
Department of Pharmacy, Orthopedic Hospital Valdoltra,
Jadranska cesta 31, Ankaran SI-6280, Slovenia
e-mail: natasa.faganeli@ob-valdoltra.si

R. Trebše (ed.), *Infected Total Joint Arthroplasty*,
DOI 10.1007/978-1-4471-2482-5_8, © Springer-Verlag London 2012

Supported by strong evidence the perioperative antibiotic prophylaxis is highly recommended for primary total joint arthroplasty [1, 9–14] to limit the incidence of serious infectious consequences. The majority of the available data supporting antibiotic prophylaxis is derived from studies that included patients undergoing total hip or total knee arthroplasty. There is a lack of data regarding the efficacy of the antibiotic prophylaxis for elbow, shoulder, and ankle arthroplasty. By analogy we assume that the same antibiotic prophylaxis can be applied [5].

It must be emphasized that perioperative antibiotic prophylaxis is not intended to sterilize tissues, but to reduce the microbial burden of intraoperative contamination to a level that cannot overwhelm host defenses [14]. From this point of view, it is clear that surgical antibiotic prophylaxis consists of a brief course of antibiotics that begins before the start of a surgical procedure and is discontinued very shortly postoperatively, if continued at all, after the procedure.

The efficacy of perioperative antibiotic prophylaxis is achieved only with appropriate administration of prophylactic antibiotic and includes the correct antibiotic selection, timing, dosing, and discontinuation. Nevertheless other factors, such as surgeon's experience and technique, instrument sterilization issues, preoperative preparation, and underlying medical conditions of the patient, may have a strong impact on SSI rates [15].

Practice Points

- Perioperative antibiotic prophylaxis is a standard for all patients undergoing primary total joint replacement.
- The efficacy of perioperative antibiotic prophylaxis is achieved only with appropriate antibiotic selection, timing, dosing, and discontinuation.
- Surgical antibiotic prophylaxis is an adjunct, not a substitute, for good surgical technique.
- Routine prophylactic antibiotic should not be used for antibiotic treatment.

Patients with joint replacements who are having invasive procedures are at increased risk of hematogenous seeding of their prosthesis. The most critical period is during the first 2 years after surgery. According to the American Academy of Orthopedic Surgeons (AAOS), all patients with joint replacement should receive antibiotic prophylaxis before high-risk dental procedures in 2 years after the replacement, and high-risk patient should receive antibiotic prophylaxis before high-risk dental procedures for the lifelong period. AAOS also generally recommends antibiotic prophylaxis before gastrointestinal or genitourinary tract procedures [16, 17].

8.2 Common Surgical Pathogens

SSIs following total joint arthroplasty are primarily caused by skin flora or exogenous airborne microorganisms. The most common pathogens are *Staphylococcus aureus*, *Staphylococcus epidermidis*, and other types of coagulase-negative staphylococci, while *Enterococcus*, *Streptococcus*, and Gram-negative organisms such as *Pseudomonas* species and *Klebsiella* species are less common [18]. A contributing factor for SSIs in joint arthroplasty surgery is the ability of *Staphylococcus* species to create the bacterial biofilm on the surface of the orthopedic implant. The biofilm shields bacteria from antibiotic action and increases their antibiotic resistance capabilities.

The agents chosen for antibiotic prophylaxis should have excellent activity against the most common surgical pathogens. The selection is influenced by the development of resistance and patient colonization. The prevalence of methicillin-resistant *S. aureus* (MRSA) and especially methicillin-resistant coagulase-negative staphylococci (CoNS) is increasing steadily. Preoperative mupirocin decolonization as an adjunction to perioperative antibiotic prophylaxis showed significant decreases in SSIs after joint replacements [5].

8.3 The Choice of the Antibiotic

There is no data supporting superiority of one class of antibiotics over another for antibiotic prophylaxis in total joint replacements [9]. The selection of prophylactic antibiotic should be based on its spectrum of action, pharmacokinetics and safety profile, local resistance patterns, availability, and nevertheless cost.

Cefazolin, the first-generation cephalosporin, is the most commonly studied and used for perioperative antibiotic prophylaxis in primary total joint replacement. Recently cefuroxime, the second-generation cephalosporin, has been recommended for total hip arthroplasty [19]. In generally cefazolin is preferred because of its greater intrinsic activity against staphylococci; narrower side-effect profile and antimicrobial spectrum; excellent distribution profiles in the bone, muscle, and synovia; and much lower cost.

In case of a serious allergy or adverse reaction to β-lactams, clindamycin is currently the preferred alternative [18, 20], although there are few data supporting its use for routine prophylaxis [13]. However, clindamycin provides less reliable coverage against CoNS. In case of high institutional incidence of infections due to methicillin-resistant CoNS, vancomycin should be used for antibiotic prophylaxis in patient with confirmed β-lactam allergy [5, 19].

History consistent with "true allergy" (i.e., urticaria, hypotension, bronchospasm, angioedema) or of a serious drug reaction (i.e., drug fever, toxic epidermolysis) to β-lactams is the key information to obtain because they represent the absolute contraindication to administration of cephalosporins. However, if patient reports a drug fever or rush, in the absence of anaphylaxis, with penicillins, then cephalosporins can be given safely [21]. Use of intraoperative "test dosing" is not supported by the literature and will not prevent potential anaphylaxis. It should be emphasized that anaphylaxis is not dose dependent; the test dose can result in anaphylaxis up to 1 h after the application [22].

Practice Points

- You need to distinguish between nonimmune-mediated drug reactions and immune-mediated reactions.
- If patient reports a drug fever or rush, in the absence of anaphylaxis, with penicillins, then cephalosporins can be given safely.

- If a history of a severe penicillin allergy (i.e., hypotension, difficulty breathing) exists, the alternative antibiotic such as clindamycin should be used.
- It is unfair to label a patient as "penicillin allergic" when the history is equivocal.

In patients with previous history of MRSA infection, at institutions with high rate of MRSA (>10 %) and methicillin-resistant *Staphylococcus epidermidis* (MRSE) (>20 %) orthopedic SSIs, and in patients colonized with MRSA, vancomycin should be used as prophylactic antibiotic [5]. Vancomycin has adequate activity against the most common high-resistant pathogens involved in orthopedic SSIs and reaches high concentrations in the bone, synovia, and muscle within minutes after administration [23]. On the other hand, vancomycin does not cover Gram-negative pathogens and anaerobes. The use of vancomycin along with cefazolin or gentamicin is in practice in some institutions, but is not supported by relevant data [12].

Patients at high risk for carriage of MRSA should be screened before elective joint arthroplasty, while universal screening is controversial. Preoperative decolonization with intranasal mupirocin may be used as adjunctive measure in patients undergoing elective joint arthroplasty who are known to be carriers or infected with MRSA [5, 20, 24].

Practice Points

- The selection of the prophylactic antibiotic should be based on antimicrobial data, local resistance patterns, and patient allergies and consistent with current recommendation.
- Vancomycin should be reserved for treatment of known infections, not for routine prophylaxis.
- Vancomycin for antibiotic prophylaxis should only be used for patients with known colonization with MRSA or in facilities with recent MRSA outbreaks.
- In case of confirmed β-lactam allergy type I, vancomycin should be used for antibiotic prophylaxis only in high institutional incidence of infections due to CoNS.

The intravenous administration of prophylactic antibiotic is unambiguous while it assures rapid, reliable, and predictable serum and tissue concentration.

8.4 Timing of Initial Dose

There is ample data in literature to support the recommended timing of the first parenteral dose of antibiotic within 60 min prior to surgical incision [25]. It is imperative to administer the antibiotic in this time range to achieve adequate serum and tissue concentration at the incision site at the time of incision and throughout of the procedure. The adequate concentration means concentration above minimal inhibitory concentration (MIC) of the likely pathogens for the procedure.

Pharmacokinetic properties of antibiotic must be taken in consideration to complete infusion within the target time.

Standard practice in the clinical settings is the application of parenteral cefazolin at the induction of anesthesia as intermittent infusion over 20–30 min. The principle is valid for application of parenteral beta-lactam and clindamycin. Vancomycin solution must be administered at a rate of 10 mg/min or less to avoid infusion-related events (i.e., "red man" syndrome). For prophylaxis vancomycin should be started 1–2 h before initiation of operation (usually already on the ward) as intermittent infusion over 60 min. It is imperative to completely infuse antibiotic solution before surgical incision.

When a proximal tourniquet is used, the antibiotic infusion has to be completely infused before inflation of the tourniquet. Some authors suggest waiting 10 min before tourniquet inflation [18].

8.5 Dosing

It is generally accepted that the dosage of an antibiotic required for prophylaxis is the same as that for the therapy of infection. Based on available date there is no conclusive recommendation for weight-based antimicrobial dosing for antimicrobial prophylaxis [5].

The recommended dose for cefazolin is 1 g i.v. for patients who weigh < 80 kg and 2 g i.v. for patients who weigh > 80 kg. In case of sever renal impairment (creatinine clearance < 35 mL/min), the dosage must be half of the usual dose [26].

The recommended dose for clindamycin is 600 mg i.v. No dosage adjustment is required in renal impairment [27].

The recommended dose for vancomycin is 1 g i.v. (10–15 mg/kg body weight). In renal impairment, start with usual dose; re-dosing interval, if needed, must be adjusted [28].

8.6 Intraoperative Repeat Dose

Intraoperative re-dosing is based on serum and tissue concentration-time profile of prophylactic antibiotic [5, 26–28]. The concentration of prophylactic antibiotic must be above MIC on the incision site throughout of the procedure for continued effect. Additional intraoperative doses of antibiotic are recommended if the operation exceeds two half-lives of the antibiotics administered preoperatively: cefazolin every 3–5 h, clindamycin every 3–6 h, and vancomycin every 6–12 h. Re-dosing may not be warranted in patients with prolonged half-life because of renal impairment.

Intraoperative re-dosing is also warranted if prolonged or excessive bleeding occurs (>1500 mL) [5].

8.7   Duration

The duration of antibiotic prophylaxis in total joint arthroplasty is still controversial. Evidence is mounting that continuation of antibiotic prophylaxis beyond 24 h after surgery is not likely to be beneficial. However, since there is insufficient evidence to support single-dose regimens, the current recommendation is that the duration of prophylaxis should not exceed 24 h [5, 10]. According to their pharmacokinetic profiles, a 24-h regimen in patients with normal renal function for cefazolin is 1–2 g i.v. every 6–8 h, for clindamycin 600 mg i.v. every 8 h, and for vancomycin 1 g (10–15 mg/kg body weight) i.v. repeated once after 12 h.

There is no evidence to support the benefit of prolong antibiotic prophylaxis until all drains are removed [19].

8.8   Antibiotic-Loaded Bone Cement

While antibiotic-loaded bone cement (ALBC) has not been shown to be superior to intravenous antibiotics, there is evidence that their combination is more effective than i.v. prophylactic antibiotic alone in reducing the risk of SSI [29]. Premixed commercial ALBCs are standardized in accordance to specific scientific and technical requirements and have superior mechanical and elution properties relative to hand-mixed ALBC. Therefore, only industrial preparations are appropriate for this purpose. The aminoglycosides (gentamicin and tobramycin) and lincosamides (clindamycin and erythromycin) are the only antibiotics available in commercial ALBC. They have appropriate physical and elution profiles, with broad antimicrobial coverage and a low incidence of allergy. There is no evidence to support superiority of one antibiotic in bone cement over another. The U.S. Food and Drug Administration (FDA) has approved premixed antibiotic bone cements only for use in second-stage revision of total joint arthroplasty, but not as prophylaxis in routine primary joint arthroplasties. There are different opinions about the routine use of ALBC in primary joint arthroplasty [5, 13, 30]. However, due to lack of controlled trials, the clinical efficacy of ALBC in primary implantation remains uncertain. Nevertheless ALBCs in conjunction with i.v. antibiotic prophylaxis are widely used worldwide for the prevention of infection in primary joint arthroplasty [20, 31–33].

8.9   Antibiotic Prophylaxis in Revision Joint Arthroplasty

There is no evidence to guide antibiotic prophylaxis in the revision joint arthroplasty. It has become common practice to withhold administration of prophylactic antibiotics before obtaining intraoperative cultures during revision joint arthroplasty in patients with a presumed PJI if the pathogen has not been identified by preoperative aspiration [34]. There is a concern that the use of perioperative antibiotic prophylaxis will result in false-negative intraoperative culture results, leading in suboptimal diagnosis and treatment of infection for these patients. Delaying antibiotics after the optimal period may on the other hand predispose not-infected patients for an infection or already infected cases for an additional infection [25]. Recent data showed that the administration of perioperative antibiotics in cases with known infection did not interfere with the isolation of the infected organism. The authors suggest the perioperative antibiotic prophylaxis should not be withheld in cases with known infection or those without clinical evidence of infection. Withholding antibiotic prophylaxis may be of benefits in those with clinical suspicion of infection in which preoperative aspiration has been negative. Still the practice of withholding prophylactic antibiotics remains theoretical and warrants further study [35–37].

Another issue is the choice of prophylactic antibiotic in revision joint arthroplasty. There is a concern about efficacy of cephalosporins (i.e., cefazolin), usually used for antibiotic prophylaxis in primary joint arthroplasty, because of changed resistance pattern. Some authors suggest adding vancomycin i.v. or gentamicin i.v. to routine prophylactic antibiotic protocol [38]. However, it should be kept in mind that the role of perioperative antibiotic prophylaxis is to prevent the intraoperative contamination to progress in SSI and not for treatment of current infection. The choice of prophylactic antibiotic in revision joint arthroplasty should be based on the same principles as in primary procedures, i.e., on antimicrobial data, local resistance patterns, and patient allergies.

Combining intravenous antibiotic prophylaxis with antibiotic-impregnated bone cement seems advisable in revision joint arthroplasty [39].

The recommendations for perioperative antibiotic prophylaxis are summarized in Table 8.1.

8.10 Conclusions

Supported by strong evidence the perioperative antibiotic prophylaxis is highly recommended for primary total joint arthroplasty. The majority of available supporting data include total hip or total knee arthroplasty. There is a lack of data about the efficacy data for elbow, shoulder, and ankle arthroplasty; however, the same antibiotic prophylaxis can be applied.

The efficacy of perioperative antibiotic prophylaxis is achieved only with appropriate administration of prophylactic antibiotic and includes appropriate antibiotic selection, timing, dosing, and discontinuation. The anesthesiologist should be responsible for administering the antibiotics to optimize appropriate timing.

Choice of prophylactic antibiotic should be consistent with current recommendations; however, it should consider the institutional range of antimicrobial susceptibility patterns. Sound clinical judgment must be exercised to recognize the unusual cases in which alternative approach is necessary.

Table 8.1 Recommendations for perioperative antibiotic prophylaxis in TJA

Choice	Cefazolin	If patient reports a drug fever or rush, in the absence of anaphylaxis, with penicillins, then cephalosporins can be given safely
	Clindamycin	In case of β-lactam allergy type I and low institutional incidence of methicillin-resistant CoNS
	Vancomycin	In case of β-lactam allergy type I and high institutional incidence of methicillin-resistant CoNS
		Known colonization with MRSA or in facilities with recent MRSA outbreaks
Timing	Cefazolin, clindamycin	At the induction of anesthesia as intermittent infusion over 20–30 min (completely infused before inflation of the tourniquet)
	Vancomycin	1–2 h before initiation of operation (usually already on the ward) as intermittent infusion over 60 min (completely infused before inflation of the tourniquet)
Dosing	Cefazolin 1 g i.v. weight < 80 kg	Half of the usual dose in creatinine clearance <35 mL/min
	Cefazolin 2 g i.v. weight > 80 kg	
	Clindamycin 600 mg i.v.	No dosage adjustment needed in renal impairment
	Vancomycin 1 g i.v.	In renal impairment, start with usual dose; re-dosing interval, if needed, must be adjusted
Intraoperative re-dosing	Cefazolin after 3–5 h	Re-dosing needed in case of:
	Clindamycin after 3–6 h	Prolonged surgery
	Vancomycin after 6–12 h	Blood loss > 1500 mL
Duration	Cefazolin 1–2 g i.v./6–8 h	Duration should not exceed 24 h!
	Clindamycin 600 mg i.v./8 h	
	Vancomycin 1 g (10–15 mg/kg) i.v. repeated once after 12 h	

Nevertheless surgical antibiotic prophylaxis is an adjunct, not a substitute, for good surgical technique.

There are different opinions about the routine use of ALBCs in primary joint arthroplasty. However, ALBC in conjunction with i.v. antibiotic prophylaxis are widely used worldwide for the prevention of infection in primary joint arthroplasty.

Currently due to the heterogeneity and complexity of most revision cases as well as a lack of randomized controlled trials, there are no clear recommendations for antibiotic prophylaxis for hip revision arthroplasty. The choice of prophylactic antibiotic in revision joint arthroplasty should be based on the same principles as in primary procedures, i.e., on antimicrobial data, local resistance patterns, and patient allergies. Based on recent date perioperative antibiotic prophylaxis in revision joint arthroplasty should not be withheld in cases with known infection or those without clinical evidence of infection.

Combining intravenous antibiotic prophylaxis with antibiotic-impregnated cement seems advisable in revision joint arthroplasty.

The cephalosporins (cefazolin) are currently preferred antibiotics with proven efficacy and safety profile for antibiotic prophylaxis in total joint arthroplasty.

In case of proven type I allergy to β-lactams, clindamycin should be used. Vancomycin should be limited for cases of MRSA colonization or previous history of MRSA or MRSE infection and outbreaks of MRSA or MRSE surgical site infections. Vancomycin would be an acceptable alternative in case of proven type I allergy to β-lactams only in high institutional incidence of infections due to methicillin-resistant CoNS.

Take Home Messages
- Perioperative antibiotic prophylaxis is standard for primary joint arthroplasty.
- Perioperative antibiotic prophylaxis should be in accordance not only with current recommendations, but also with periodica.
- The anesthesiologist should be responsible for administering the antibiotics to optimize appropriate timing and dosing.
- Perioperative antibiotic prophylaxis should not exceed the 24-h postoperative period.
- There is no evidence to support the benefit of prolong antibiotic prophylaxis until all drains are removed.
- Antibiotic loaded bone cement in conjunction with i.v. antibiotic prophylaxis seems advisable for the prevention of infection in primary joint arthroplasty.
- Because of standardized elution and mechanical properties only commercial antibiotic loaded bone cement should be used.
- There are no clear recommendations for antibiotic prophylaxis for hip revision arthroplasty. The choice of prophylactic antibiotic in revision joint arthroplasty should be based on the same principles as in primary procedures and not misused as antimicrobial therapy.
- Prophylactic preoperative antibiotics should not be withheld in patients at lower probability for periprosthetic joint infection and those with an established diagnosis of periprosthetic joint infection who are undergoing reoperation.

References

1. National Collaborating Centre for Women's and Children's Health. Surgical site infection: prevention and treatment of surgical site infection. London (UK): National Institute for Health and Clinical Excellence (NICE); October 2008. p. 142.

2. Edwards JR, Peterson KD, Mu Y, et al. National Healthcare Safety Network (NHSN) report: data summary for 2006 through 2008, issued December 2009. Am J Infect Control. 2009;37:783–805.

3. European Centre for Disease Prevention and Control. Annual epidemiological report on communicable diseases in Europe. Stockholm: European Centre for Disease Prevention and Control; 2009.

4. Gougoulias N, Khanna A, Maffulli N. How successful are current ankle replacements? A systematic review of the literature. Clin Orthop Relat Res. 2010;468:199–208.

5. American Society of Health-System Pharmacists. Draft therapeutic guidelines on antimicrobial prophylaxis in surgery. 2011. http://www.ashp.org/DocLibrary/Policy/PracticeResources/Orthopedics-ForPublicComment.aspx. Accessed 10 June 2011.

6. Bohsali KI, Wirth MA, Rockwood Jr CA. Complications of total shoulder arthroplasty. J Bone Joint Surg Am. 2006;88-A(10):2279–92.

7. Bosco 3rd JA, Slover JD, Haas JP. Perioperative strategies for decreasing infection: a comprehensive evidence-based approach. J Bone Joint Surg Am. 2010;92:232–9.

8. Whitehouse JD, Friedman ND, Kirkland KB, Richardson WJ, Sexton DJ. The impact of surgical site infections following orthopedic surgery at a community hospital and a university hospital: adverse quality of life, excess length of stay, and extra cost. Infect Control Hosp Epidemiol. 2002;23:183–9.

9. AlBuhairan B, Hind D, Hutchinson A. Antibiotic prophylaxis for wound infections in total joint arthroplasty. J Bone Joint Surg Br. 2008;90-B:915–9.

10. American Academy of Orthopaedic Surgeons. Information statement: recommendations for the use of intravenous antibiotic prophylaxis in primary total joint arthroplasty. http://www.aaos.org/about/papers/advistmt/1027.asp. Accessed 12 Dec 2010.

11. Association for Professionals in Infection Control and Epidemiology. APIC elimination guide: guide to the elimination of orthopedic surgical site infections. 2010. http://www.apic.org/downloads/ortho_guide.pdf. Accessed 29 Aug 2011.

12. Meehan J, Jamali AA, Nguyen H. Prophylactic antibiotics in hip and knee arthroplasty. J Bone Joint Surg Am. 2009;91:2480–90.

13. Bratzler DW, Houck PM, for the surgical Infection Prevention Guidelines Writers Workgroup. Antimicrobial prophylaxis for surgery: an Advisory Statement from the National Surgical Infection Prevention Project. Clin Infect Dis. 2004;38:1706–15.

14. Mangram AJ, Horan TC, Pearson ML, Silver LC, Jarvis WR, the Hospital Infection Control Practices Advisory Committee. Guideline for the prevention of surgical site infection, 1999. Infect Control Hosp Epidemiol. 1999;20:247–80.

15. Hansen AD, Osmon DR, Nelson CL. Prevention of deep prosthetic joint infection. J Bone Joint Surg Am. 1996;78-A(3):458–71.

16. Bosco 3rd JA, Slover JD, Haas JP. Perioperative strategies for decreasing infection: a comprehensive evidence-based approach. An Instructional Course Lecture, American Academy of Orthopaedic Surgeons. J Bone Joint Surg Am. 2010;92(1):232–9.

17. American Academy of Orthopedic Surgeons. Information statement: antibiotic prophylaxis for bacteremia in patients with joint replacements. February 2009. Available at: http://www.aaos.org/about/papers/advistmt/1033.asp. Accessed 12 Mar 2011.

18. Gradl G, Horn C, Postl LK, Miethke T, Gollwitzer H. Antibiotic prophylaxis in primary and revision hip arthroplasty: what is the evidence? Orthopade. 2011;40(6):520–7.

19. Bratzler DW, Hunt DR. The surgical infection prevention and surgical care improvement projects: national initiatives to improve outcomes for patients having surgery. Clin Infect Dis. 2006;43(3):322.

20. Matar WY, Jafari SM, Restrepo C, Austin M, Purtill JJ, Parvizi J. Preventing infection in total joint arthroplasty. J Bone Joint Surg Am. 2010;92 Suppl 2:36–46.

21. DePestel DD, Benninger MS, Danziger L, LaPlante KL, May C, Luskin A, Pichichero M, Hadley JA. Cephalosporin use in treatment of patients with penicillin allergies. J Am Pharm Assoc (2003). 2008;48(4):530–40. Review. Erratum in: J Am Pharm Assoc (2003). 2008;48(5):572.

22. James M, Martinez EA. Antibiotics and perioperative infections. Best Pract Res Clin Anaesthesiol. 2008;22(3):571–84.

23. Eshkenazi AU, Garti A, Tamir L, Hendel D. Serum and synovial vancomycin concentrations following prophylactic administration in knee arthroplasty. Am J Knee Surg. 2001;14(4):221–3.
24. Harbarth S, Fankhauser C, Schrenzel J, Christenson J, Gervaz P, Bandiera-Clerc C, Renzi G, Vernaz N, Sax H, Pittet D. Universal screening for methicillin-resistant Staphylococcus aureus at hospital admission and nosocomial infection in surgical patients. JAMA. 2008;299(10):1149–57.
25. Classen DC, Evans RS, Pestotnik SL, Horn SD, Menlove RL, Burke JP. The timing of prophylactic administration of antibiotics and the risk of surgical-wound infection. N Engl J Med. 1992;326(5):281.
26. Cefazolin. In: Lexi-Drugs Online [Internet Database]. Hudson: Lexi-Comp, Inc.
27. Clindamycin. In: Lexi-Drugs Online [Internet Database]. Hudson: Lexi-Comp, Inc.
28. Vancomycin. In: Lexi-Drugs Online [Internet Database]. Hudson: Lexi-Comp, Inc.
29. Engesaeter LB, Lie SA, Espehaug B, Furnes O, Vollset SE, Havelin LI. Antibiotic prophylaxis in total hip arthroplasty: effects of antibiotic prophylaxis systemically and in bone cement on the revision rate of 22,170 primary hip replacements followed 0–14 years in the Norwegian Arthroplasty Register. Acta Orthop Scand. 2003;74(6):644–51.
30. Jiranek W. Antibiotic-loaded cement in total hip replacement: current indications, efficacy, and complications. Orthopedics. 2005;28 Suppl 8:s873–7.
31. American Academy of Orthopedic Surgeons. Information statement: antibiotic laden cement: current state of the art. May 2007. Available at: http://www.aaos.org/news/bulletin/may07/clinical7.asp. Accessed 29 Aug 2011.
32. de Beer J, Petruccelli D, Rotstein C, Weening B, Royston K, Winemaker M. Antibiotic prophylaxis for total joint replacement surgery: results of a survey of Canadian orthopedic surgeons. Can J Surg. 2009;52(6):E229–34.
33. NHS QIS. Antibiotic prophylaxis in surgery. A national clinical guideline. July 2008. Scottish Intercollegiate Guidelines Network. Edinburgh: SIGN; July 2008. www.sign.ac.uk
34. Achermann Y, Vogt M, Leunig M, Wüst J, Trampuz A. Improved diagnosis of periprosthetic joint infection by multiplex PCR of sonication fluid from removed implants. J Clin Microbiol. 2010;48(4):1208–14.
35. Ghanem E, Parvizi J, Clohisy J, Burnett S, Sharkey PF, Barrack R. Perioperative antibiotics should not be withheld in proven cases of periprosthetic infection. Clin Orthop Relat Res. 2007;461:44–7.
36. Burnett RS, Aggarwal A, Givens SA, McClure JT, Morgan PM, Barrack RL. Prophylactic antibiotics do not affect cultures in the treatment of an infected TKA. A prospective trial. Clin Orthop Relat Res. 2010;468:127–34.
37. American Academy of Orthopaedic Surgeons. Board of Directors. The diagnosis of periprosthetic joint infections of the hip and knee. Guideline and evidence report. June 2010.
38. Sharma D, Douglas J, Coulter C, Weinrauch P, Crawford R. Microbiology of infected arthroplasty: implications for empiric peri-operative antibiotics. J Orthop Surg (Hong Kong). 2008;16(3):339–42.
39. Jämsen E, Huhtala H, Puolakka T, Moilanen T. Risk factors for infection after knee arthroplasty. A register-based analysis of 43,149 cases. J Bone Joint Surg Am. 2009;91(1):38–47.

Chapter 9
Risk Factors for Prosthetic Joint Infections

René Mihalič and Matevž Topolovec

Abstract Prosthetic joint infection (PJI) is one of the most devastating complications in the field of orthopedic surgery. Risk factors for PJI can be divided in two groups: patient-related risk factors and procedure-related risk factors. This chapter presents and discusses the most important risk factors in both groups. Recommendations about the measures to reduce the risk for PJI to the lowest possible level are presented and argued.

Keywords Patient • Immunosuppression • Risk factors • Diabetes • Body mass index

9.1 Introduction

It is important to identify and investigate risk factors for surgical site infections (SSI) because infections have adverse affects on health and functional status of the patients and use up valuable health care resources. Investigators have identified and examined risk factors for SSI using univariate and multivariate analyses. Consequently multiple risk factors for orthopedic SSI have been identified.

Risk factors for total joint infection can be divided in two groups. In the first group, there are risk factors that are in direct conjunction with patient condition – patient-related factors (Table 9.1). In the second group, there are factors that are related to the operative procedure, divided in preoperative and intraoperative – procedure-related factors (Table 9.1).

In every surgical wound there is a conflict between bacteria that invade the surgical wound and patient's defense mechanisms that rely on his/her immune system.

R. Mihalič, M.D. (✉) • M. Topolovec, M.D.
Bone Infection and Adult Reconstruction Surgery, Orthopaedic Hospital Valdoltra,
Jadranska cesta 31, Ankaran 6280, Slovenia
e-mail: rene.mihalic@ob-valdoltra.si; matevz.topolovec@ob-valdoltra.si

R. Trebše (ed.), *Infected Total Joint Arthroplasty*,
DOI 10.1007/978-1-4471-2482-5_9, © Springer-Verlag London 2012

Patient-related factors	Procedure-related factors
Age	Preoperative shaving
Obesity	Preoperative skin antisepsis
Diabetes mellitus and hyperglycemia	Hand scrubbing and washing
Smoking	Surgical drapes
Malnutrition	Surgical gloves
Compromised immune system	Surgical face masks
Rheumatic or autoimmune diseases	Surgical foot wear and theater floors
Nonsteroidal anti-inflammatory drugs (NSAIDs)	Surgical gowns
Corticosteroids	
Disease-modifying antirheumatic drugs (DMARDs)	
Biologic agents	
Coexisting infection in a remote body site	Operating-room environment
	Movement of medical personnel in operating room
	Surgical instruments
	Surgical technique
	Duration of operation
	Antibiotic prophylaxis

Table 9.1 Patient-related and procedure-related factors that may increase the risk for SSI

Altemeier and Culbertson [1] have pointed out that wound infection is the result of the equation:

$$Risk of SSI = \frac{Dose of bacterial contamination \times virulence}{Resistance of patient}$$

For most SSIs, the source of pathogens is the endogenous flora of the patient's skin, mucous membranes, or hollow viscera [1]. Exogenous sources of SSI pathogens include surgical personnel (especially members of the surgical team) [2, 3], operating-room environment (including air), and all tools, instruments, and materials brought to the sterile field during an operation [4]. On the other hand, endogenous sources include diseases and physical conditions that can adversely influence the immune system of the patient and in this respect increase the risk for SSI.

Many of these risk factors in both groups can be eliminated or modified to reduce the risk for SSI. It is important that not only orthopedic surgeons but also other members of medical teams are instructed about the measures to reduce the risk factors for SSI as much as possible.

9.2 Patient-Related Factors

Patient characteristics may affect the incidence of SSI. We can identify patients at increased risk for developing SSI during the operation by identifying the following patient-related factors.

9.2.1 Age

Many studies reported increased risk of SSI with increasing age [5–7]. Immune system dysfunction and accumulation of comorbid conditions with increasing age may be the reason for the finding. Other studies concluded that age alone was not an independent risk factor for SSI [8, 9]. A study performed by Kaye et al. [10] revealed that risk of infection is linearly increasing until age of 65 years. After this age, risk of infection is decreasing by 1.2 % for each additional year. The explanation for this phenomenon could be that frail old patients are less frequently treated by surgical interventions than their healthy peers. This may have resulted in the selection of a relatively healthy group among older patients at decreased risk of SSI, compared with the group of younger patients where healthy and sicker peers are operated on. These findings can lead us to a conclusion that biological age, determined by comorbidities and immune competence, is more important than chronological age when considering the risk for infection.

9.2.2 Obesity

Several studies have shown that obesity, defined as body mass index (BMI) of ≥ 30 kg/m^2, represents a risk factor for infection in joint replacement surgery [11–15]. A study performed by Namba et al. demonstrated that the risk of an infection was 6.7 times higher in obese patients who underwent total knee replacement and 4.7 times higher in those selected for total hip replacement [16]. Waisbren et al. showed in their study that body fat share (BFS) is more sensitive and the precise measure for determining SSI risk than BMI because it reflects more accurately body composition [17]. In their study they defined obesity if BFS in men was higher than 25 % and in women, higher than 31 %. Obesity defined by those BFS criteria was associated with a fivefold increased SSI risk. There are several hypotheses that explain how obesity is related to increased rate of SSI. Increased frequency of hematoma formation and subsequent prolonged drainage due to greater extent of surgical dissection [15], low tissue levels of prophylactic antibiotics due to improper dose adjustment to weight [18], fat tissue hypoperfusion with decreased tissue oxygenation and reduced oxygen tension with consequent decreased oxidative killing potential of neutrophils against pathogens [19] are among the most important. Killing potential of neutrophils against pathogens in combination with antibiotic prophylaxis is especially important for reducing risk for SSI at the time of bacterial contamination following skin incision.

It is possible to reduce the SSI risk for patients in this group by controlling weight, applying an appropriate dose of perioperative prophylactic antibiotics, and controlling serum glucose level in those with diabetes.

9.2.3 Diabetes Mellitus and Hyperglycemia

Diabetes has been associated with an increased risk of SSI in all orthopedic fields [20–22]. The reason for higher SSI risk may lay, in part, in the impact of the disease on patient's physiology, but it is more likely that particularly the effects of perioperative hyperglycemia are even more detrimental [21, 23, 24]. The study performed by Jämsen et al. revealed that patients with glucose levels higher than 7 mmol/L had a fourfold higher risk for total knee replacement infection when compared to patients with glucose levels below 6.1 mmol/L [21]. Further research is needed to evaluate the optimal perioperative glucose levels. We think that patients with uncontrolled diabetes mellitus are not appropriate candidates for elective orthopedic surgery before their blood glucose level is under control.

9.2.4 Smoking

Tobacco use is a very important risk factor for serious postsurgical complications, especially for complications related to wound healing [25]. Tobacco use delays primary wound healing and may increase the risk of SSI [26]. Tobacco products cause microvascular vasoconstriction and together with carbon monoxide found in cigarette smoke, which generates nonfunctional carboxyhemoglobin by binding to hemoglobin, contribute to tissue hypoxia [27]. According to the recommendations of US Center for Disease Control and Prevention (CDC), patients undergoing elective surgery should abstain from using tobacco products for at least 30 days before surgery [4, 28]. Our recommendation stands that cessation should be lifelong or at least until the operative wound is healed.

9.2.5 Malnutrition

Poor nutritional status is a well-known risk factor for deep infection after a variety of orthopedic surgical procedures [27, 29]. Optimizing nutrition is important to ensure proper immune function and postoperative wound healing [18]. Patients at risk for malnutrition are those who have gastrointestinal diseases, renal failure, and cancer; who are abusing alcohol; and especially group of patients with advanced age. Some useful and readily available parameters which define malnutrition are a BMI lower than 18.4 kg/m^2, a total lymphocyte count of <1,800/μL, a total serum albumin level of <35 g/L, or a total serum transferrin level of <180 g/L [30]. Green et al. revealed in their study that patients who matched the criteria for malnutrition have been associated with an increased rate of wound complications [29]. German hospitals' malnutrition study revealed that every fourth hospitalized patient in their country is malnourished [31]. This important finding revealed that malnutrition is an underestimated issue even in developed countries. When there is objective evidence of malnutrition in patient undergoing elective orthopedic procedure, preoperative and postoperative nutritional support should be provided. The aim is to improve the total lymphocyte count and to increase the albumin and transferrin levels which positively influence wound healing potential and consequently reduce the risk of infection. In perioperative period patients should obtain sufficient protein intake and daily vitamin and mineral supplementation [18, 32, 33].

9.2.6 *Human Immunodeficiency Virus (HIV)*

Basic science studies have shown that impaired immune defenses make patients susceptible to common surgical pathogens and opportunistic microorganisms [34]. However, most of the clinical studies did not demonstrate a greater incidence of early postoperative complications in asymptomatic HIV-positive patients in comparison to HIV-negative patients [35]. HIV-positive patients may be at increased risk for late hematogenous infection as host immune defense diminishes with the progression of the disease [35]. Therefore, regular medical attention; prophylactic antibiotic therapy prior to dental, orthopedic, or other invasive procedures; and early recognition and treatment of possible infections are essential. Studies from non-orthopedic surgical fields have suggested that specific risk factors exist and include an absolute lymphocyte CD4 count of <200 cells/μL and viral load of >10,000 copies/mL [18].

HIV-positive patients who are candidates for elective orthopedic procedures should be carefully assessed, focusing particularly on their immune status, including CD4 lymphocyte count, history of opportunistic infection, serum albumin level, nutritional state, and general health [35]. The risk is reduced if patient has no history of opportunistic infection, CD4 lymphocyte count of >200 cells/μL, polymorphonuclear leukocyte count of >1,000 cells/μL, serum albumin concentration of >25 g/L, and no signs of cutaneous anergy [35].

9.2.7 *Rheumatic Disease*

Patients with rheumatoid arthritis (RA) who are scheduled for total joint arthroplasty have a two- to threefold greater risk of acquiring a postoperative infection than patients with primary osteoarthritis [18, 36–38]. Those patients are frequently treated with complex drug regimes that include NSAIDs, corticosteroids, methotrexate, DMARDs, and biologic agents. All of those drugs have direct or indirect influence on wound healing and potential risk of infection. Because of complexity of the disease and complexity of drug treatment regimens, there are yet no evidence-based recommendations about perioperative drug administration protocols. According to the available data, we suggest the following:

- *NSAIDs* decrease inflammation and pain through two known mechanisms. By inhibiting cyclooxygenase (COX)-1 and (COX)-2, NSAIDs inhibit the transformation of arachidonic acid to prostaglandins, prostacyclin, and thromboxanes [37]. With this mechanism they are inhibiting platelet function and increasing risk of intraoperative and postoperative bleeding, which may lead to increased risk of a postoperative infection. The second known mechanism of action is the inhibition of white cell activation which may lead to decreased cell immunity. Use of these medications should be discontinued according to their half-lives before elective orthopedic surgery. It is recommended that they should be discontinued three to five half-lives before surgery [39].

- *Corticosteroids* are very frequently used medications in treatment of RA. Perioperative management of corticosteroids is a very important issue in reduction of infection risk. It involves setting a balance between the minimal amount of corticosteroids necessary to reduce joint inflammation and unnecessarily high levels that might lead to perioperative complications. Excessive use can produce immunosuppression, increased protein catabolism, and stifled inflammatory response, all of which can lead to poor wound healing and increased risk of infection. Conversely, inadequate levels can lead to disease flares and adrenal insufficiency [37, 40]. We recommend all patients on chronic corticosteroid therapy to receive their regular dose of corticosteroids perioperatively. The use of stress-dose corticosteroids remains controversial [41]. To our knowledge, there are no evidence-based guidelines about the use of stress-dose corticosteroids. Our recommendation stands that stress-dose corticosteroids should not be prescribed routinely, but individually, according to the length of steroid treatment time, cumulative steroid dose, and anticipated stress level of surgery.

- *DMARDs* are defined as medications that retard or halt the progression of rheumatic disease [42]. This group of medications consists of methotrexate, leflunomide, sulfasalazine, hydroxychloroquine, intramuscular gold, and penicillamine. *Methotrexate* administration is a mainstay of therapy in RA because of its long-term efficacy, tolerability, low cost, and response rate exceeding 60 % [43]. It is most often selected DMARD for initial therapy in RA [44]. Methotrexate is a folate analogue with anti-inflammatory properties resulting from a decrease in cytokine production, including interleukin IL-1, IL-8, and tumor necrosis factor (TNF) [37]. When the medication is discontinued, the patient runs the risk of flares within 4 weeks. In general, use of methotrexate should not be discontinued perioperatively. Only in patients with renal insufficiency, uncontrolled diabetes mellitus, and liver or lung disease methotrexate should be discontinued perioperatively for 1 week [37]. In patients with RA and no other associated chronic disease mentioned above, treatment with methotrexate is not associated with greater risk of infection [45, 46]. *Leflunomide* is an inhibitor of pyrimidine synthesis and targets rapidly dividing cells, such as lymphocytes. Its half-life is approximately 2 weeks. Large placebo-controlled studies comparing leflunomide and methotrexate suggest that both drugs have similar efficacy [47]. There is little evidence in the literature about leflunomide influence on potential infection risk. One study revealed that leflunomide increases the risk of early wound healing complications [48], but another study revealed that there is no association with higher infection risk [49]. Because of its mechanism of action and its half-life, we recommend that leflunomide should be discontinued 2 weeks prior elective orthopedic surgery. There is no evidence-based data available when to restart leflunomide therapy after surgery. We recommend to reintroduce it as late as possible after surgery, but not before patient is stable and operative wound is healed. Further well-designed trials are needed to get more precise data about infection risk and perioperative therapy regimes. *Other DMARDs* are usually used as potential adjuncts to first-line RA medications. They have usually low potency and low toxicity and have not been associated with increased infection risk [50]. In general, those drugs should not be discontinued perioperatively.

- *Biologic agents* are a group of medications acting as tumor necrosis factor alpha (TNF-α) or interleukin-1 (IL-1) antagonists. They are decreasing host's inflammatory response and are suppressing host's defense against infection. There are many conflicting data about perioperative use of biologic agents in elective orthopedic surgery. Many studies revealed no differences in wound healing and postoperative infection rates comparing patients who continued biologic agents' therapy and patients who discontinued therapy [51–53]. On the other hand, there are many studies which revealed the opposite [54–56] including data about late prosthetic joint infections occurring immediately after administration of biologic agents [57, 58]. This may reveal a serious risk of immune suppression caused by these drugs. The majority of articles highlighted the need for large, good quality trials to be conducted. Current evidence base is poor and insufficient to enable definitive guidelines regarding the use of biologic agents perioperatively with regard to postoperative infection and wound healing problems. We recommend that biologic agents should be withdrawn for about four half-lives preoperatively [59], but the optimal time period for withholding therapy is still undetermined [60]. According to available data and immunosuppressive nature of these drugs, we recommend that the therapy should not be started before the patient is stable, out of anergic phase, and the wound is healed.

9.2.8 Coexisting Infection in a Remote Body Site

Coexisting infection in a remote body site is thought to be a risk factor for prosthetic joint infection. An elevated leukocyte count with left shifted differential and elevated C-reactive protein (CRP) level should raise the suspicion of an underlying infection in patients with no known inflammatory disease. Particularly important are inflammations and bacterial foci in oral cavity. All of them can progress into potential sources of infection in early postoperative period and for many years following implantation, as well [61–63]. Other potential sources of PJI are urinary, respiratory and gastrointestinal tract infections, chronic osteomyelitis, bacterial skin infections, and venous ulcers. We recommend postponing the elective orthopedic surgery until the remote body site infection is healed, if at all possible. Additional recommendation is to adopt a proper antibiotic prophylaxis prior to planned invasive procedures in patients with orthopedic implants.

9.3   Procedure-Related Factors

In 1867 Lister [64] published the first reports of antisepsis in surgery, demonstrating the immediate clinical benefit from reduction of airborne organisms. In the 1960s Charnley [65] introduced the concept of ultraclean air systems. In order to prevent or to minimize perioperative infection, we must consider the available evidence regarding the use of preoperative antibiotics, preoperative skin preparation of the patient and the surgeon, operating-room issues, theater discipline and protocols, wound closure, operative drainage, and use of dressings.

9.3.1   Preoperative Shaving

Preoperative shaving of the surgical site is a common practice. However, we must be aware of micro-abrasions of the skin caused by shaving which may support the multiplication of bacteria, particularly if undertaken several hours before surgery. A meta-analysis by the Cochrane group [66] showed that the relative risk of a surgical site infection following hair removal with a razor was significantly higher than that following hair removal with clippers (relative risk, 2.02; 95 % confidence interval, 1.21–3.36) [66]. Furthermore, the analysis showed no difference in the rate of postoperative infections between procedures preceded by hair removal and those performed without hair removal. Shaving immediately before the operation compared to shaving within 24 and >24 h preoperatively was associated with decreased SSI rates [67]. Whenever hair is removed, clippers, rather than a razor, should be used at the time of surgery [68].

9.3.2   Preoperative Skin Antisepsis

Skin antiseptics are used to reduce the number of microorganisms on the skin around the incision in order to reduce the probability of SSI. Several antiseptic agents are available for preoperative preparation of the skin. Most commonly used agents are iodophors, alcohol-containing products, and chlorhexidine gluconate solution. A meta-analysis from Cochrane group [69] showed no difference in efficacy among skin antiseptics used in clean surgery. Also Adams et al. [70] demonstrated that all compared antiseptics achieved a log10 reduction factor of 5. Important is also the effect on wound healing process. Cooper et al. [71] found that povidone-iodine is extremely toxic to fibroblasts and keratinocytes. According to the recommendation of Fletcher et al. [72], chlorhexidine surgical scrub provides a prolonged reduction in skin contamination with less toxicity and skin irritation compared with povidone-iodine. The same was also concluded in a recent meta-analysis from Noorani [73].

9.3.3   Hand Scrubbing and Washing

Surgical hand scrubbing and washing is also a usual step in the preparation for surgery. Washing with soaps has become obsolete because much higher reduction of bacterial counts is obtained with antiseptics, like alcohol solutions. The optimal antiseptic agent for surgical hand scrubbing and washing has not been established. Parienti et al. [74] found no difference in infection rates when comparing aqueous alcohol hand rubs with that of traditional povidone-iodine or chlorhexidine gluconate scrubbing with a scrub brush. Not only the antimicrobial activity but also its acceptability by operating-room personnel after repeated use is important. Widmer et al. [75] favor the use of alcohol-based hand rubs for surgical hand preparation. Moreover, operating staff tolerated alcohol solutions better than other antiseptics. Although the proper duration for surgical hand rub is also not known, traditional practices recommend different time protocols [75]. Time recommended by the manufacturer, usually 2–6 min, is the time recommended to consider [27, 75, 76].

9.3.4   Surgical Drapes

Sterile surgical drapes are used to create a barrier between the surgical field and potential sources of bacteria. French et al. [77] compared the adhesive plastic surgical drapes and cloth surgical drapes. They found that plastic adhesive drape prevents penetration and lateral migration of the skin bacteria and reduces wound contamination. In use are also impregnated plastic drapes (e.g., iodophor-impregnated plastic drapes) to be attached on expected incision site. However, according to the literature the use of iodophor-impregnated surgical drapes decreases skin contamination but does not appear to reduce infection rates [78, 79].

9.3.5   Surgical Gloves

Initially, gloves were used to protect surgeons, only then they recognized that gloves can also protect the patient [80]. Because of the high incidence of perforation common

Fig. 9.1 Surgical face mask

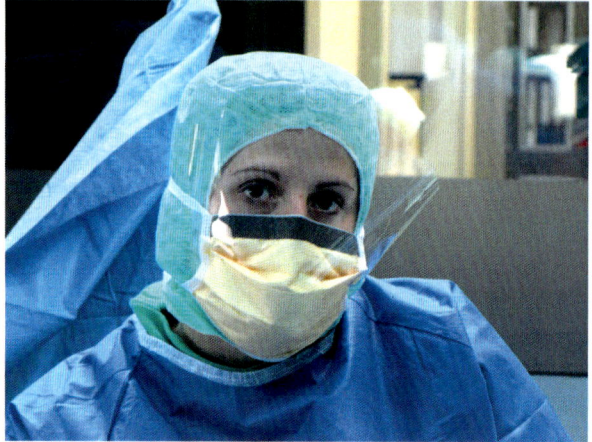

to orthopedic surgery, surgeons wear two pairs of gloves [81, 82]. Also changing gloves at regular intervals can reduce the incidence of glove perforation and contamination [83]. Moreover, for draping, only a separate pair of outer gloves should be used [81].

9.3.6   Surgical Face Masks

Usage of surgical face mask in the modern operating suite became a standard practice (Fig. 9.1). It protects both the patient from bacteria expelled from the respiratory tract of the wearer and the wearer's nose and mouth from exposure to the patient's fluids. However, some studies questioned the efficacy of surgical masks in reducing SSI risk [84, 85]. But reports, like the report of Gaillard et al. [86], reinforce the role of surgical masks in SSI prevention. Nevertheless, wearing a mask can be beneficial due to a greater awareness of HIV and other blood-borne viruses.

9.3.7   Surgical Foot Wear and Theater Floors

Theater shoes and floors represent potential sources for postoperative infections. Up to 15 % of bacteria found in the air are re-dispersed floor bacteria [87]. However, Knochen et al. [88] believed that frequent disinfection and cleaning of floors is not necessary if a laminar airflow ventilation system is installed. Surgical shoes have been the subject of investigation, too. The use of dedicated theater shoes by surgical staff is recommended [89]. Changing shoes and other clothes should be done as far from the operating theater as possible [90].

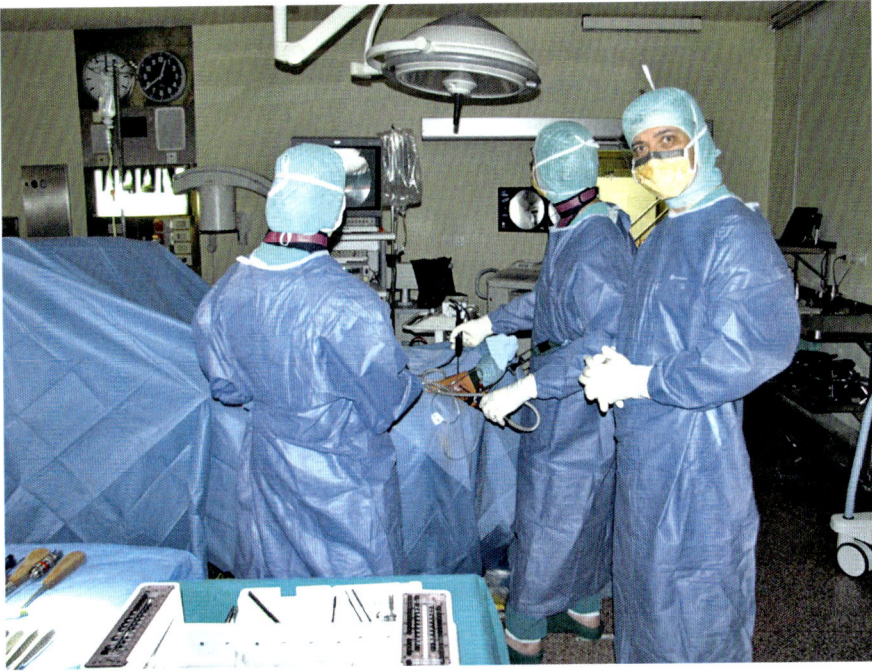

Fig. 9.2 Operating-room environment. Surgical team performing arthroscopic-assisted ankle fusion (photo courtesy of Rihard Trebše)

9.3.8 Surgical Gowns

Gowns are worn by all scrubbed surgical team members and are used to prevent direct contact transfer of potentially infective agents between surgical team and the patient. Surgical gowns are fabricated from either reusable or single-use materials. A cost/benefit analysis from Baykasoğlu [91] shows that single-use gown and drape sets provide the highest benefit rates. Regardless of the material used, they should be impermeable to liquids and viruses [4, 92]. However, surgeon should avoid repetitive touching of the surgical gown with their gloves [92, 93].

9.3.9 Operating-Room Environment

Although many preoperative and intraoperative measures have been shown to reduce SSI rates, many consider the operating-room environment to be the most important one (Fig. 9.2). Laminar airflow and use of UV radiation have been suggested as measures that reduce not only bacterial counts but also rates of SSI. Laminar airflow results in a significant reduction in rates of bacterial wound contamination [94]. However, a significant decrease in infection rate has not been shown. Surprisingly, Brandt et al. [95] showed that operating room with laminar airflow did no benefit on reducing SSI and was even associated with a significantly higher risk for severe SSI after hip arthroplasty. However, the position of the surgical team and the wound with respect to the laminar airflow unit seems to be important, too [96]. The laminar flow unit can be placed horizontally or vertically.

Clean air in the operating room can also result from the use of ultraviolet (UV) light. UV light kills bacteria on the surfaces of the operating theater and in the air rather than simply decreasing bacteria counts [97]. Berg et al. [98] showed that UV light was more effective than the ultraclean air enclosure. As concluded by Ritter et al. [99], when safety precautions are considered, UV lighting appears to be an effective way to lower the risk of infection in the operating room during joint replacement surgery.

9.3.10 Movement of Medical Personnel in Operating Room

Medical personnel including surgeons, anesthesiologists, nurses, and also the technicians, students, and porters represent a major source of bacterial contamination [100, 101]. Ritter et al. [102] also found that microbiological counts increased significantly when the doors of operating room were left open. Moreover, Babkin et al. [103] recognized significant traffic through the OR door as risk factors for SSI. Consequently the number and activity of medical personnel in the operating theater should be kept to a minimum level.

9.3.11 Surgical Instruments

Instrument contamination can also represent a potential route for infection (Fig. 9.3). Chosky et al. [104] showed a 28-fold decrease in contamination of surgical instruments by preparing the instruments in the ultraclean air theater rather than in a conventional plenum-ventilated preparation room. A positive correlation between the time instruments were left open and their contamination was also proven. [105]. Furthermore, covering the instruments reduced contamination rates [104, 105].

However, special attention must be given to splash basins, suckers, irrigation solutions, and light handles [92, 106, 107] because they are frequently contaminated objects in the operative field.

9.3.12 Surgical Technique

Good surgical technique is believed to reduce the risk of SSI. To explain this concept, there are many issues that need further consideration. One is irrigation of the

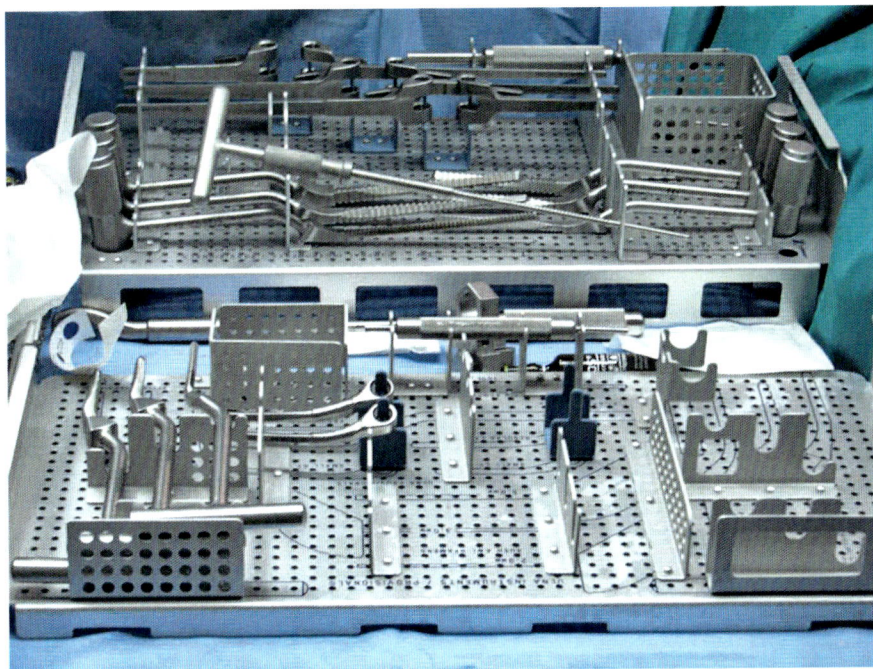

Fig. 9.3 Surgical instruments for total elbow arthroplasty (photo courtesy of Rihard Trebše)

wound. The main debate is whether to use a high-pressure pulsatile lavage or a low-pressure and bulb syringe lavage. Several studies have shown that high-pressure pulsatile lavage is more effective than low-pressure pulsatile lavage or bulb syringe lavage [108, 109]. However, there is a general concern that high- or low-pressure pulsatile lavage may result in deep bacterial seeding in bone that can cause greater musculoskeletal damage [110–112]. As concluded by Fletcher [72], low-pressure irrigation should be used if contamination is minimal. Many solutions containing bacitracin, neomycin, and soap were tested in comparison with normal saline solution. The data is confusing. Anglen et al. [113] showed significant advantage of soap solution over antibiotic irrigant or saline alone in removing *Staphylococcus epidermidis* from metallic surfaces. In contrast, a study by Owens et al. [114] showed that the highest rebound in bacteria counts (120 %) was measured in the soap group and the lowest for normal saline solution (68 %). Another remarkable issue is the long-lasting debate regarding drainage of the wound. A meta-analysis from Parker et al. [115] indicated that closed suction drainage increases the transfusion requirements and represent no major benefits. However, Kim et al. [116] support the view that a wound drain reduces drainage, ecchymosis formation, and erythema. They agree that either use or nonuse of suction drainage does not affect the incidence of wound complication or infection after total hip arthroplasty. Drinkwater and Neil [117] concluded that if the drain is used, the optimal time in place should not exceed 24 h.

Other operative steps like maintaining effective hemostasis, proper dead space closure, application of topical antiseptics and antimicrobials to surgical incisions prior to their closure, usage of different surgical techniques, etc., may have an effect on developing SSI, but the discussion about these questions is beyond the scope of this chapter.

9.3.13 Duration of Operation

Many studies that involved large numbers of cases have shown that duration of operation is an independent risk factor for periprosthetic joint infection [118–120].

9.3.13.1 Postoperative Issues

The risk for developing a SSI does not stop when the operation is over and the wound is closed. Proper wound care and dressing technique are necessary to reduce the risk for an infection. The dressing should be permeable, waterproof, transparent, absorbent, and flexible [121]. The use of antibacterial dressing can limit bacterial growth and may reduce the risk of an infection as well [122]. When the dressings are changed, the wound should be cleaned with saline solution or tap water rather than with antiseptics [71, 123]. Overall, it is important to keep the wound clean and dry.

9.4 Conclusion

There are few issues that can so severely compromise a patient outcome as PJI. PJI can lead to severe morbidity and even death of a patient. Despite all the measures taken, the risk of infection remains ever present.

Infection occurs when the number and virulence of a pathogen overcome the physiologic capability of the host to respond. To decrease the risk of PJI, we must be aware of potential extrinsic and intrinsic risk factors (procedure- and patient-related factors). Our task is to reduce those risk factors as much as possible to insure the optimal conditions for the conduction of operative therapy and postoperative management.

References

1. Altemeier WA, Culbertson WR. Surgical infection. In: Moyer C et al., editors. Surgery; principles and practice. 3rd ed. Philadelphia: JB Lippincott Co.; 1965.
2. Albrich WC, Harbarth S. Health-care workers: source, vector, or victim of MRSA? Lancet Infect Dis. 2008;8:289–301.
3. Hughes SP, Anderson FM. Infection in the operating room. J Bone Joint Surg Br. 1999;81: 754–5.

4. Mangram AJ, Horan TC, Pearson ML, Silver LC, Jarvis WR. Guideline for prevention of surgical site infection, 1999. Hospital Infection Control Practices Advisory Committee. Infect Control Hosp Epidemiol. 1999;20:250–78.

5. De Boer AS, Mintjes-de Groot AJ, Severijnen AJ, van den Berg JM, van Pelt W. Risk assessment for surgical-site infections in orthopedic patients. Infect Control Hosp Epidemiol. 1999; 20:402–7.

6. Delgado-Rodriguez M, Gomez-Ortega A, Sillero-Arenas M, Llorca J. Epidemiology of surgical-site infections diagnosed after hospital discharge: a prospective cohort study. Infect Control Hosp Epidemiol. 2001;22:24–30.

7. Scott JD, Forrest A, Feuerstein S, Fitzpatrick P, Schentag JJ. Factors associated with postoperative infection. Infect Control Hosp Epidemiol. 2001;22:347–51.

8. Olsen MA, Lock-Buckley P, Hopkins D, Polish LB, Sundt TM, Fraser VJ. The risk factors for deep and superficial chest surgical-site infections after coronary artery bypass graft surgery are different. J Thorac Cardiovasc Surg. 2002;124:135–45.

9. Malone DL, Genuit T, Tracy JK, Gannon C, Napolitano LM. Surgical site infections: reanalysis of risk factors. J Surg Res. 2002;103:89–95.

10. Kaye KS, Schmit K, Pieper C, Sloane R, Caughlan KF, Sexton DJ, Schmader KE. The effect of increasing age on the risk of surgical site infection. J Infect Dis. 2005;191: 1056–62.

11. Dowsey MM, Choong PF. Obesity is a major risk factor for prosthetic infection after primary hip arthroplasty. Clin Orthop Relat Res. 2008;466:153–8.

12. Luebbeke A, Moons KGM, Garavaglia G, et al. Outcomes of obese and nonobese patients undergoing revision total hip arthroplasty. Arthritis Rheum. 2008;59:738–45.

13. Dowsey MM, Choong PF. Obese diabetic patients are at substantial risk for deep infection after primary TKA. Clin Orthop Relat Res. 2009;467:1577–81.

14. Samson AJ, Mercer GE, Campbell DG. Total knee replacement in the morbidly obese: a literature review. ANZ J Surg. 2010;80:595–9.

15. Patel VP, Walsh M, Sehgal B, Preston C, DeWal H, Di Cesare PE. Factors associated with prolonged wound drainage after primary total hip and knee arthroplasty. J Bone Joint Surg Am. 2007;89:33–8.

16. Namba RS, Paxton L, Fithian DC, Stone ML. Obesity and perioperative morbidity in total hip and total knee arthroplasty patients. J Arthroplasty. 2005;20 Suppl 3:46–50.

17. Waisbren E, Rosen H, Bader AM, Lipsitz SR, Rogers Jr SO, Eriksson E. Percent body fat and prediction of surgical site infection. J Am Coll Surg. 2010;210:381–9.

18. Moucha CS, Clyburn T, Evans RP, Prokuski L. Modifiable risk factors for surgical site infection. J Bone Joint Surg Am. 2011;93:398–404.

19. Kabon B, Nagele A, Reddy D, Eagon C, Fleshman JW, Sessler DI, Kurz A. Obesity decreases perioperative tissue oxygenation. Anesthesiology. 2004;100:274–80.

20. Olsen MA, Nepple JJ, Riew KD, Lenke LG, Bridwell KH, Mayfield J, Fraser VJ. Risk factors for surgical site infection following orthopaedic spinal operations. J Bone Joint Surg Am. 2008;90:62–9.

21. Jämsen E, Nevalainen P, Kalliovalkama J, Moilanen T. Preoperative hyperglycemia predicts infected total knee replacement. Eur J Intern Med. 2010;21:196–201.

22. Edmonston DL, Foulkes GD. Infection rate and risk factor analysis in an orthopaedic ambulatory surgical center. J Surg Orthop Adv. 2010;19:174–6.

23. Mraovic B, Suh D, Jacovides C, Parvizi J. Perioperative hyperglycemia and postoperative infection after lower limb arthroplasty. J Diabetes Sci Technol. 2011;5:412–8.

24. Marchant Jr MH, Viens NA, Cook C, Vail TP, Bolognesi MP. The impact of glycemic control and diabetes mellitus on perioperative outcomes after total joint arthroplasty. J Bone Joint Surg Am. 2009;91:1621–9.

25. Møller AM, Villebro N, Pedersen T, Tønnesen H. Effect of preoperative smoking intervention on postoperative complications: a randomised clinical trial. Lancet. 2002;359:114–7.

26. Nagachinta T, Stephens M, Reitz B, Polk BF. Risk factors for surgical wound infection following cardiac surgery. J Infect Dis. 1987;156:967–73.

27. American Academy of Orthopaedic Surgeons Patient Safety Committee, Evans RP. Surgical site infection prevention and control: an emerging paradigm. J Bone Joint Surg Am. 2009;91 Suppl 6:2–9.
28. Cierny G, Rao N. Procedure-related reduction of the risk of infection. In: Cierny G, McLaren AC, Wongworawat MD, editors. Orthopaedic knowledge update: musculoskeletal infection. Rosemont: American Academy of Orthopaedic Surgeons; 2009.
29. Greene KA, Wilde AH, Stulberg BN. Preoperative nutritional status of total joint patients. Relationship to postoperative wound complications. J Arthroplasty. 1991;6:321–5.
30. Dobbins RL, Wilson JD. Nutritional requirements and assessment. In: Fauci AS, Braunwald E, Isselbacher KJ, Wilson JD, Martin JB, Kasper DL, Hauser SL, Longo DL, editors. Harrison's principles of internal medicine. 14th ed. New York: McGraw-Hill; 1998.
31. Pirlich M, Schütz T, Norman K, Gastell S, Lübke HJ, Bischoff SC, Bolder U, Frieling T, Güldenzoph H, Hahn K, Jauch KW, Schindler K, Stein J, Volkert D, Weimann A, Werner H, Wolf C, Zürcher G, Bauer P, Lochs H. The German hospital malnutrition study. Clin Nutr. 2006;25:563–72.
32. Fairfield KM, Fletcher RH. Vitamins for chronic disease prevention in adults: scientific review. JAMA. 2002;287:3116–26.
33. Fletcher RH, Fairfield KM. Vitamins for chronic disease prevention in adults: clinical application. JAMA. 2002;287:3127–9.
34. Gurkan I, Wenz JF. Perioperative infection control: an update for patient safety in orthopedic surgery. Orthopedics. 2006;29:329–39.
35. Luck Jr JV, Logan LR, Benson DR, Glasser DB. Human immunodeficiency virus infection: complications and outcome of orthopaedic surgery. J Am Acad Orthop Surg. 1996;4:297–304.
36. Luessenhop CP, Higgins LD, Brause BD, Ranawat CS. Multiple prosthetic infections after total joint arthroplasty. Risk factor analysis. J Arthroplasty. 1996;11:862–8.
37. Howe CR, Gardner GC, Kadel NJ. Perioperative medication management for the patient with rheumatoid arthritis. J Am Acad Orthop Surg. 2006;14:544–51.
38. Jämsen E, Huhtala H, Puolakka T, Moilanen T. Risk factors for infection after knee arthroplasty. A register-based analysis of 43,149 cases. J Bone Joint Surg Am. 2009;91:38–47.
39. Robinson CM, Christie J, Malcolm-Smith N. Nonsteroidal antiinflammatory drugs, perioperative blood loss, and transfusion requirements in elective hip arthroplasty. J Arthroplasty. 1993;8:607–10.
40. Oelkers W. Adrenal insufficiency. N Engl J Med. 1996;335:1206–12.
41. Lamberts SW, Bruining HA, de Jong FH. Corticosteroid therapy in severe illness. N Engl J Med. 1997;337:1285–92.
42. O'Dell JR. Therapeutic strategies for rheumatoid arthritis. N Engl J Med. 2004;350:2591–602.
43. Bathon JM, Martin RW, Fleischmann RM, Tesser JR, Schiff MH, Keystone EC, Genovese MC, Wasko MC, Moreland LW, Weaver AL, Markenson J, Finck BK. A comparison of etanercept and methotrexate in patients with early rheumatoid arthritis. N Engl J Med. 2000;343:1586–93.
44. Mikuls TR, O'Dell J. The changing face of rheumatoid arthritis therapy: results of serial surveys. Arthritis Rheum. 2000;43:464–5.
45. Grennan DM, Gray J, Loudon J, Fear S. Methotrexate and early postoperative complications in patients with rheumatoid arthritis undergoing elective orthopaedic surgery. Ann Rheum Dis. 2001;60:214–7.
46. Loza E, Martinez-Lopez JA, Carmona L. A systematic review on the optimum management of the use of methotrexate in rheumatoid arthritis patients in the perioperative period to minimize perioperative morbidity and maintain disease control. Clin Exp Rheumatol. 2009;27:856–62.
47. Olsen NJ, Stein CM. New drugs for rheumatoid arthritis. N Engl J Med. 2004;350:2167–79.
48. Fuerst M, Möhl H, Baumgärtel K, Rüther W. Leflunomide increases the risk of early healing complications in patients with rheumatoid arthritis undergoing elective orthopedic surgery. Rheumatol Int. 2006;26:1138–42.

49. Tanaka N, Sakahashi H, Sato E, Hirose K, Ishima T, Ishii S. Examination of the risk of continuous leflunomide treatment on the incidence of infectious complications after joint arthroplasty in patients with rheumatoid arthritis. J Clin Rheumatol. 2003;9:115–8.
50. Pieringer H, Stuby U, Biesenbach G. Patients with rheumatoid arthritis undergoing surgery: how should we deal with antirheumatic treatment? Semin Arthritis Rheum. 2007;36:278–86.
51. Hirano Y, Kojima T, Kanayama Y, Shioura T, Hayashi M, Kida D, Kaneko A, Eto Y, Ishiguro N. Influences of anti-tumour necrosis factor agents on postoperative recovery in patients with rheumatoid arthritis. Clin Rheumatol. 2010;29:495–500.
52. den Broeder AA, Creemers MC, Fransen J, de Jong E, de Rooij DJ, Wymenga A, de Waal-Malefijt M, van den Hoogen FH. Risk factors for surgical site infections and other complications in elective surgery in patients with rheumatoid arthritis with special attention for anti-tumor necrosis factor: a large retrospective study. J Rheumatol. 2007;34:689–95.
53. Talwalkar SC, Grennan DM, Gray J, Johnson P, Hayton MJ. Tumour necrosis factor alpha antagonists and early postoperative complications in patients with inflammatory joint disease undergoing elective orthopaedic surgery. Ann Rheum Dis. 2005;64:650–1.
54. Kawakami K, Ikari K, Kawamura K, Tsukahara S, Iwamoto T, Yano K, Sakuma Y, Tokita A, Momohara S. Complications and features after joint surgery in rheumatoid arthritis patients treated with tumour necrosis factor-alpha blockers: perioperative interruption of tumour necrosis factor-alpha blockers decreases complications? Rheumatology (Oxford). 2010;49:341–7.
55. Ruyssen-Witrand A, Gossec L, Salliot C, Luc M, Duclos M, Guignard S, Dougados M. Complication rates of 127 surgical procedures performed in rheumatic patients receiving tumor necrosis factor alpha blockers. Clin Exp Rheumatol. 2007;25:430–6.
56. Giles JT, Bartlett SJ, Gelber AC, Nanda S, Fontaine K, Ruffing V, Bathon JM. Tumor necrosis factor inhibitor therapy and risk of serious postoperative orthopedic infection in rheumatoid arthritis. Arthritis Rheum. 2006;55:333–7.
57. Yurube T, Takahi K, Owaki H, Fuji T, Kurosaka M, Doita M. Late infection of total knee arthroplasty inflamed by anti-TNFalpha, Infliximab therapy in rheumatoid arthritis. Rheumatol Int. 2010;30:405–8.
58. Mori S, Tomita Y, Horikawa T, Cho I, Sugimoto M. Delayed spinal infection after laminectomy in a patient with rheumatoid arthritis interruptedly exposed to anti-tumor necrosis factor alpha agents. Clin Rheumatol. 2008;27:937–9.
59. Ward M, Liang MH, Burns T, Singh G. RA treatment study group: improvement in RA management. Joint Bone Spine. 2009;76:435–7.
60. Crawford M, Curtis JR. Tumor necrosis factor inhibitors and infection complications. Curr Rheumatol Rep. 2008;10:383–9.
61. Kaar TK, Bogoch ER, Devlin HR. Acute metastatic infection of a revision total hip arthroplasty with oral bacteria after noninvasive dental treatment. J Arthroplasty. 2000;15:675–8.
62. LaPorte DM, Waldman BJ, Mont MA, Hungerford DS. Infections associated with dental procedures in total hip arthroplasty. J Bone Joint Surg Br. 1999;81:56–9.
63. Waldman BJ, Mont MA, Hungerford DS. Total knee arthroplasty infections associated with dental procedures. Clin Orthop Relat Res. 1997;343:164–72.
64. Lidwell OM. Joseph Lister and infection from the air. Epidemiol Infect. 1987;99:568–78.
65. Charnley J. A clean-air operating enclosure. Br J Surg. 1964;51:202–5.
66. Tanner J, Woodings D, Moncaster K. Preoperative hair removal to reduce surgical site infection (review). Cochrane Database Syst Rev. 2006;3:CD004122.
67. Seropian R, Reynolds BM. Wound infections after preoperative depilatory versus razor preparation. Am J Surg. 1971;121:251–4.
68. Pfiedler Enterprises. Preoperative hair removal: impact on surgical site infections. A nursing continuing education self-study activity. http://www.pfiedler.com/1091/index.html (2008). Accessed 23 Sept 2011.
69. Edwards PS, Lipp A, Holmes A. Preoperative skin antiseptics for preventing surgical wound infections after clean surgery (review). Cochrane Database Syst Rev. 2004;3:CD003949.
70. Adams D, Quayum M, Worthington T, Lambert P, Elliott T. Evaluation of a 2% chlorhexidine gluconate in 70% isopropyl alcohol skin disinfectant. J Hosp Infect. 2005;61:287–90.

71. Cooper ML, Laxer JA, Hansbrough JF. The cytotoxic effects of commonly used topical antimicrobial agents on human fibroblasts and keratinocytes. J Trauma. 1991;31:775–82.

72. Fletcher N, Sofianos D, Berkes MB, Obremskey WT. Prevention of perioperative infection. J Bone Joint Surg Am. 2007;89:1605–18.

73. Noorani A, Rabey N, Walsh SR, Davies RJ. Systematic review and meta-analysis of preoperative antisepsis with chlorhexidine versus povidone-iodine in clean-contaminated surgery. Br J Surg. 2010;97:1614–20.

74. Parienti JJ, Thibon P, Heller R, Le Roux Y, von Theobald P, Bensadoun H, Bouvet A, Lemarchand F, Le Coutour X. Antisepsie Chirurgicale des mains Study Group. Hand-rubbing with an aqueous alcoholic solution vs traditional surgical hand-scrubbing and 30-day surgical site infection rates: a randomized equivalence study. JAMA. 2002;288:722–7.

75. Widmer AF, Rotter M, Voss A, Nthumba P, Allegranzi B, Boyce J, Pittet D. Surgical hand preparation: state-of-the-art. J Hosp Infect. 2010;74:112–22.

76. O'Shaughnessy M, O'Malley VP, Corbett G, Given HF. Optimum duration of surgical scrub-time. Br J Surg. 1991;78:685–6.

77. French ML, Eitzen HE, Ritter MA. The plastic surgical adhesive drape: an evaluation of its efficacy as a microbial barrier. Ann Surg. 1976;184:46–50.

78. Geelhoed GW, Sharpe K, Simon GL. A comparative study of surgical skin preparation methods. Surg Gynecol Obstet. 1983;157:265–8.

79. Ritter MA, Campbell ED. Retrospective evaluation of an iodophor-incorporated antimicrobial plastic adhesive wound drape. Clin Orthop Relat Res. 1988;228:307–8.

80. Klenerman L. The evolution of orthopaedic surgery. London: The Royal Society of Medicine Press; 1998.

81. McCue SF, Berg EW, Saunders EA. Efficacy of double-gloving as a barrier to microbial contamination during total joint arthroplasty. J Bone Joint Surg Am. 1981;63:811–3.

82. Sanders R, Fortin P, Ross E, Helfet D. Outer gloves in orthopaedic procedures. Cloth compared with latex. J Bone Joint Surg Am. 1990;72:914–7.

83. Al-Maiyah M, Bajwa A, Mackenney P, Port A, Gregg PJ, Hill D, Finn P. Glove perforation and contamination in primary total hip arthroplasty. J Bone Joint Surg Br. 2005;87:556–9.

84. Tunevall TG. Postoperative wound infections and surgical face masks: a controlled study. World J Surg. 1991;15:383–7.

85. Orr NW. Is a mask necessary in the operating theatre? Ann R Coll Surg Engl. 1981;63:390–2.

86. Gaillard T, Gaillard C, Martinaud C, Védy S, Pons S, Brisou P. Epidemic surgical site infections attributable to incorrect use of face masks. J Hosp Infect. 2009;71:192–3.

87. Hambraeus A, Bengtsson S, Laurell G. Bacterial contamination in a modern operating suite. 3. Importance of floor contamination as a source of airborne bacteria. J Hyg. 1978;80:169–74.

88. Knochen H, Hübner NO, Below H, Assadian O, Külpmann R, Kohlmann T, Hildebrand K, Clemens S, Bartels C, Kramer A. Influence of floor disinfection on microbial and particulate burden measured under low turbulence air flow in ophthalmological operation theatres. Klin Monbl Augenheilkd. 2010;227:871–8.

89. Amirfeyz R, Tasker A, Ali S, Bowker K, Blom A. Theatre shoes – a link in the common pathway of postoperative wound infection? Ann R Coll Surg Engl. 2007;89:605–8.

90. Nagai I, Kadota M, Takechi M, Kumamoto R, Ueoka M, Matsuoka K, Jitsukawa S. Studies on the mode of bacterial contamination of an operating theatre corridor floor. J Hosp Infect. 1984;5:50–5.

91. Baykasoğlu A, Dereli T, Yilankirkan N. Application of cost/benefit analysis for surgical gown and drape selection: a case study. Am J Infect Control. 2009;37:215–26.

92. Davis N, Curry A, Gambhir AK, Panigrahi H, Walker CR, Wilkins EG, Worsley MA, Kay PR. Intraoperative bacterial contamination in operations for joint replacement. J Bone Joint Surg Br. 1999;81:886–9.

93. Howard JL, Hanssen AD. Principles of a clean operating room environment. J Arthroplasty. 2007;22:6–11.

94. Knobben BA, van Horn JR, van der Mei HC, Busscher HJ. Evaluation of measures to decrease intra-operative bacterial contamination in orthopaedic implant surgery. J Hosp Infect. 2006;62:174–80.

95. Brandt C, Hott U, Sohr D, Daschner F, Gastmeier P, Rüden H. Operating room ventilation with laminar airflow shows no protective effect on the surgical site infection rate in orthopedic and abdominal surgery. Ann Surg. 2008;248:695–700.

96. Salvati EA, Robinson RP, Zeno SM, Koslin BL, Brause BD, Wilson Jr PD. Infection rates after 3175 total hip and total knee replacements performed with and without a horizontal unidirectional filtered air-flow system. J Bone Joint Surg Am. 1982;64:525–35.

97. Taylor GJ, Bannister GC, Leeming JP. Wound disinfection with ultraviolet radiation. J Hosp Infect. 1995;30:85–93.

98. Berg M, Bergman BR, Hoborn J. Ultraviolet radiation compared to an ultra-clean air enclosure. Comparison of air bacteria counts in operating rooms. J Bone Joint Surg Br. 1991;73:811–5.

99. Ritter MA, Olberding EM, Malinzak RA. Ultraviolet lighting during orthopaedic surgery and the rate of infection. J Bone Joint Surg Am. 2007;89:1935–40.

100. Ritter MA, Eitzen H, French ML, Hart JB. The operating room environment as affected by people and the surgical face mask. Clin Orthop Relat Res. 1975;111:147–50.

101. Bethune DW, Blowers R, Parker M, Pask EA. Dispersal of *Staphylococcus aureus* by patient and surgical staff. Lancet. 1965;1(7383):480–3.

102. Ritter MA. Operating room environment. Clin Orthop Relat Res. 1999;369:103–9.

103. Babkin Y, Raveh D, Lifschitz M, Itzchaki M, Wiener-Well Y, Kopuit P, Jerassy Z, Yinnon AM. Incidence and risk factors for surgical infection after total knee replacement. Scand J Infect Dis. 2007;39:890–5.

104. Chosky SA, Modha D, Taylor GJ. Optimisation of ultraclean air. The role of instrument preparation. J Bone Joint Surg Br. 1996;78:835–7.

105. Dalstrom DJ, Venkatarayappa I, Manternach AL, Palcic MS, Heyse BA, Prayson MJ. Time-dependent contamination of opened sterile operating-room trays. J Bone Joint Surg Am. 2008;90:1022–5.

106. Robinson AH, Drew S, Anderson J, Bentley G, Ridgway GL. Suction tip contamination in the ultraclean-air operating theatre. Ann R Coll Surg Engl. 1993;75:254–6.

107. Anto B, McCabe J, Kelly S, Morris S, Rynn L, Corbett-Feeney G. Splash basin bacterial contamination during elective arthroplasty. J Infect. 2006;52:231–2.

108. Svoboda SJ, Bice TG, Gooden HA, Brooks DE, Thomas DB, Wenke JC. Comparison of bulb syringe and pulsed lavage irrigation with use of a bioluminescent musculoskeletal wound model. J Bone Joint Surg Am. 2006;88:2167–74.

109. Brown LL, Shelton HT, Bornside GH, Cohn Jr I. Evaluation of wound irrigation by pulsatile jet and conventional methods. Ann Surg. 1978;187:170–3.

110. Kalteis T, Lehn N, Schröder HJ, Schubert T, Zysk S, Handel M, Grifka J. Contaminant seeding in bone by different irrigation methods: an experimental study. J Orthop Trauma. 2005;19:591–6.

111. Bhandari M, Schemitsch EH. High-pressure irrigation increases adipocyte-like cells at the expense of osteoblasts in vitro. J Bone Joint Surg Br. 2002;84:1054–61.

112. Wheeler CB, Rodeheaver GT, Thacker JG, Edgerton MT, Edilich RF. Side-effects of high pressure irrigation. Surg Gynecol Obstet. 1976;143:775–8.

113. Anglen J, Apostoles PS, Christensen G, Gainor B, Lane J. Removal of surface bacteria by irrigation. J Orthop Res. 1996;14:251–4.

114. Owens BD, White DW, Wenke JC. Comparison of irrigation solutions and devices in a contaminated musculoskeletal wound survival model. J Bone Joint Surg Am. 2009;91:92–8.

115. Parker MJ, Roberts CP, Hay D. Closed suction drainage for hip and knee arthroplasty. A meta-analysis. J Bone Joint Surg Am. 2004;86-A:1146–52.

116. Kim YH, Cho SH, Kim RS. Drainage versus nondrainage in simultaneous bilateral total hip arthroplasties. J Arthroplasty. 1998;13:156–61.

117. Drinkwater CJ, Neil MJ. Optimal timing of wound drain removal following total joint arthroplasty. J Arthroplasty. 1995;10:185–9.

118. Ong KL, Kurtz SM, Lau E, Bozic KJ, Berry DJ, Parvizi J. Prosthetic joint infection risk after total hip arthroplasty in the Medicare population. J Arthroplasty. 2009;24 Suppl 6:105–9.

119. Ridgeway S, Wilson J, Charlet A, Kafatos G, Pearson A, Coello R. Infection of the surgical site after arthroplasty of the hip. J Bone Joint Surg Br. 2005;87:844–50.
120. Willis-Owen CA, Konyves A, Martin DK. Factors affecting the incidence of infection in hip and knee replacement: an analysis of 5277 cases. J Bone Joint Surg Br. 2010;92:1128–33.
121. Tustanowski J. Effect of dressing choice on outcomes after hip and knee arthroplasty: a literature review. J Wound Care. 2009;18:449–450, 452, 454.
122. Lipp C, Kirker K, Agostinho A, James G, Stewart P. Testing wound dressings using an in vitro wound model. J Wound Care. 2010;19:220–6.
123. Cho CY, Lo JS. Dressing the part. Dermatol Clin. 1998;16:25–47.

Chapter 10
Pathogenesis of Prosthetic Joint Infections

Rihard Trebše and Jurij Štalc

Abstract Every wound is contaminated, but not all wounds end with a prosthetic joint infection (PJI). The pathogenic process involves bacterial adhesion steps that are fundamental in the early stage of PJI development and the consecutive biofilm formation. Biofilm development is an essential step in establishment of a chronic PJI. Due to its physical and chemical proprieties, it serves as a basic structure that protects bacteria from environmental influences like host immune defenses and antibiotics. To understand the diagnostic principles and treatment modes, it is imperative to understand the basics of the pathogenesis of PJI.

Keywords Pathogenesis • Interactions • Biofilm • Bacteria • Host

10.1 Introduction

Prosthetic joint infections (PJI) can be difficult to diagnose in some cases and are difficult to treat in most instances. To understand the value of diagnostic tools and treatment modalities and to recognize their inherent limitations, it is important to understand the mechanisms of the pathogenic processes that govern the initiation and development of PJI. The condition may evolve into a steady state, death of the host, or cure depending on the dynamic interplay between host defenses, implant biocompatibility, virulence factors, and medical actions (Table 10.1)

R. Trebše, M.D., Ph.D. (✉) • J. Štalc, M.D.
Department for Bone infections and Adult reconstructions, Orthopaedic Hospital Valdoltra,
Jadranska cesta 31, Ankaran SI-6286, Slovenia
e-mail: rihard.trebse@ob-valdoltra.si; jurij.stalc@ob-valdoltra.si

R. Trebše (ed.), *Infected Total Joint Arthroplasty*,
DOI 10.1007/978-1-4471-2482-5_10, © Springer-Verlag London 2012

Table 10.1 Difference between minimal infectious dose in the presence of foreign material and without

Study (subjects)	Type of foreign material	Minimal infectious dose		Bacteria
		No FM	FM	
Elek 1857 (human)	Suture 8	6×10^6	$\mathbf{3 \times 10^1}$	*Staphylococcus aureus*
Jame 8 1881 (mice)	Suture 8	10^6	$\mathbf{<10^2}$	*Staphylococcus aureus*
Zimmerli 1832 (guinea pig 3)	Tissue cage 3	$>10^7$	$\mathbf{10^2}$	*Staphylococcus aureus*
Widmer 1833 (guinea pig 3)	Tissue cage 3	$>10^7$	$\mathbf{10^3}$	*Staphylococcus epidermidis*

10.2 Bacterial Adhesion

Bacterial microorganisms tend to adhere to surfaces since growing on a solid surface is a preferred form of living for majority of them [27]. Bacteria can reach the surface of an implant in different ways: with direct inoculation during surgical procedure, hematogenously in case of bacteremia, or with dissemination from a proximate septic focus [26]. All surgical wounds can be considered contaminated since there are always some bacteria present in skin glands independently of means of surgical field preparation and disinfection. In spite of this, not all wounds get infected. Clinical infection results from the interaction of microbial invasion and host organism's defense. There are three elements important for the development of an infection: dose of inoculated bacteria (normally $>10^5$ CFU/g of tissue), virulence of the invading microorganisms, and defensive capability of contaminated organism. The dose of bacteria needed for development of infection is greatly diminished in presence of a foreign body. The presence of a foreign body can therefore be added to the classic triad of factors that determine the potential for development of a wound infection [25, 26] (Fig. 10.1).

As soon as a new device gets implanted in a surgical site, a process notoriously called "race for the surface" begins [10]. According to this concept, there is a competition for colonizing the surface between extracellular matrix proteins (fibrinogen, fibronectin, vitronectin, trombospondin, bone sialoprotein) and eukaryotic cells (fibroblasts, osteoblasts, endothelial cells) on one hand and prokaryotic bacterial cells on the other. Matrix proteins are known to cover foreign material as soon as it appears in the human body. In the next step, fibroblasts interact with a layer of matrix proteins using specific receptors called integrins. In such a way, the implant becomes covered by a viable barrier, capable of defense functions against bacteria. In case there are bacteria present at the time of implantation, they enter the competition for the surface, and the outcome largely depends on their number and features.

Bacterial adhesion is a complex well-governed process influenced by multiple environmental factors: type of host surface, presence of protein film on an adhering surface, presence of serum proteins, presence of toxic substances (antibiotics and disinfectants [17]), duration of exposure, number of pathogens, temperature, and pH. Bacterial adhesion to biomaterial surfaces can be described as a two-stage process starting with

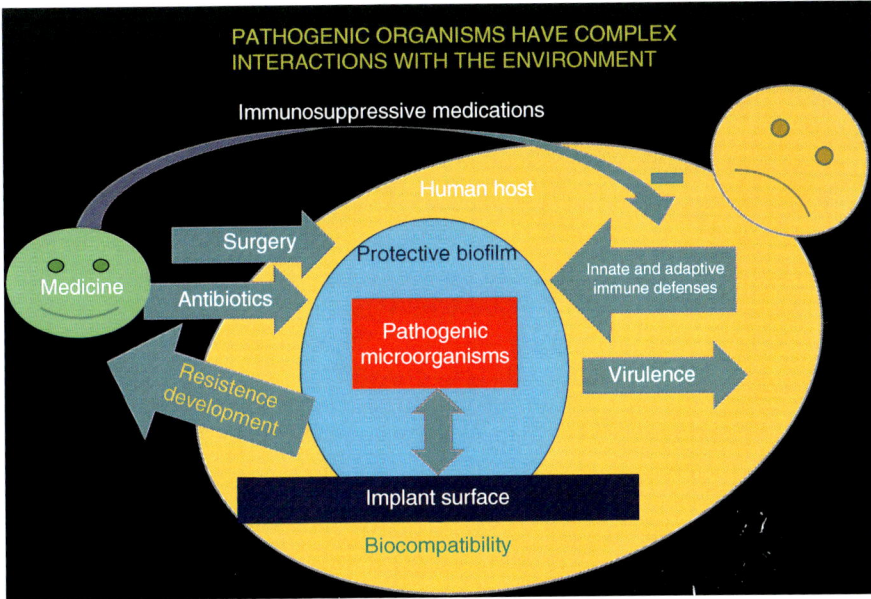

Fig. 10.1 Graphic depiction of the interactions between host, implant, and pathogenic organism

a physical reversible first phase (phase I) continuing into time-dependent irreversible active energy-dependent molecular and cellular second phase (phase II) [14].

10.2.1   Phase I

Inoculated bacteria in planktonic form diffuse through fluids propelled by nonspecific physical factors like gravity, Braun's movement, surface tension, and van der Waals bonds. Eventually, they come into proximity of an implant. At distances smaller than 3 nm, they start interacting with biomaterial by means of hydrogen, ionic, and hydrophobic bonds. Energy needed for disruption of these bonds is small; therefore, the process can be reversed [5, 13]. This represents the first phase of bacterial adhesion.

10.2.2   Phase II

The second phase of bacterial adhesion is characterized by events on molecular level. Macromolecules capable of adhering are called adhesins. This is a general name for any molecular structure which has an active site being able to bond with a receptive structure on an implant surface. Microorganisms appear to have different adhesins for different surface materials [12]. On their surface, bacteria form special polymeric structures which help them adhere to surfaces, namely, capsule, fimbriae, fibrillae, and flagella. Bacterial capsule contains proteins which function as adhesives [22]. Although there is always some negative charge on a protein surface in aqueous solution, the hydrophobicity varies among species. More hydrophobic capsule has stronger adhering capability. Fimbriae are polymeric structures of pillin monomers. They have a filamentary shape and are present in vast numbers scattered across whole surface of bacteria. Normally, fimbriae measure 7 nm in diameter but can sometimes reach up to a mm in length. Even bacteria that do not form fimbriae are capable of adhering, but their virulence is lower [11]. *Pseudomonas aeruginosa*, *Escherichia coli*, and other mainly Gram-negative bacteria connect to implant surface using flagella [4]. Flagella are protein hooks sized 20 nm used for grabbing the surroundings [1]. Some bacterial species adhere to implant surface using more specific means, e.g., *S. aureus* uses MSCRAMM adhesive molecule (microbial surface components recognizing adhesive matrix molecules) to connect with extracellular matrix proteins covering the implant [18].

Adhesion to a surface leads to important changes in many aspects of bacterial metabolism. Genes needed for biofilm development become activated. There are also other prerequisites for induction of this process like availability of nutrients, temperature, pH, osmolality, availability of iron, and presence of different signal molecules from other bacteria.

10.3 Biofilm

Adhesion of bacteria is followed by biofilm formation. Biofilm forms on a solid surface and is composed of bacterial biomass and an extracellular slime (Fig. 10.2). It is a very common form of bacterial cohabitation in nature, and its presence is not limited to implant infections within living systems. Besides bacteria, some fungi

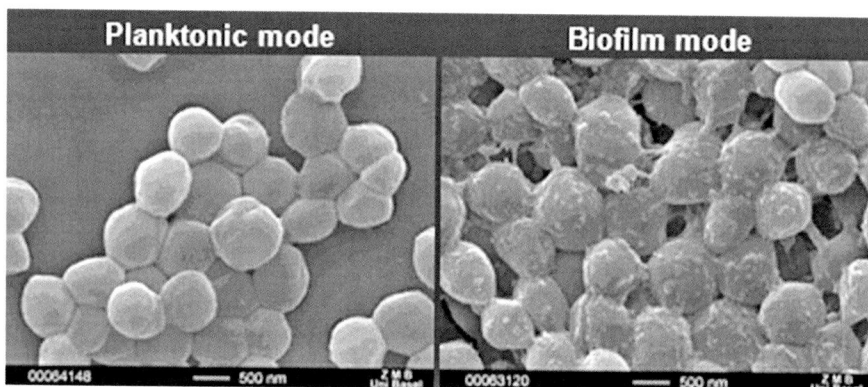

Fig. 10.2 Biofilm formation in the extracellular space around a bacterial cluster (Photomicrograph courtesy of Andrej Trampuž)

(e.g., *Candida albicans*) are also capable of biofilm formation. Biofilm can be produced by one species of bacteria, but coexistence of different species within the same extracellular matrix is more common [5].

Biofilm formation starts with bacterial excretion of slimy material that envelops them (Fig. 10.2). Its main components are exopolymers – polysaccharides of glucose, galactose, mannose, fructose, rhamnose, amino sugars, polyols, and uronic acid [1]. Secretion of bioslime is followed by other changes in bacterial phenotype, probably resulting from oxygen and nutrient shortage and/or higher concentration of waste products. Through maturation of biofilm, an organized society is formed characterized by structural and functional specialization of individual cells. This society is tightly bonded to underlying surface. With time, biofilm becomes funneled with water channels that allow for flow of nutrients and signal molecules [3].

Bacteria have developed a mechanism of mutual interaction inside biofilm which allows for functional and morphological structuring of the colony. They communicate within themselves using signal molecules. The phenomenon of inter-bacterial signaling is called "quorum sensing" [21, 24]. The concentration of signal molecules rises with increasing number of adhered cells. Certain concentration of signal molecules is required to induce changes in gene transcription that result in phenotype alteration. The signal molecule in Gram-negative bacteria is acyl-homoserine lactone, in Gram-positive species, different oligopeptides.

Development of biofilm is a basic bacterial survival mechanism in a hostile environment [1, 7]. Bacterial cells inside the biofilm are well protected from complement system, neutrophilic granulocytes, killer cells, antibiotic peptides, antibodies, phagocytosis, oxidative stress, antibiotics, and disinfectants. Ceri needed a 500-times increase in minimal inhibitory concentration (MIC) of ampicillin to reduce the number of *E. coli* for 3 log inside biofilm compared to bacteria in the planktonic form [2]. Other authors have found even 1,000 times higher resistance of bacteria in the biofilm compared to their planktonic counterparts. [5, 20]. Reasons for poor effect of antibiotics are numerous. They poorly penetrate the bioslime, chemically interact with biofilm molecules, and have lower activity in an acid and hypoxic environment. Changes that influence resistance to antimicrobials are determined also by bacteria which slow their metabolism, lower the transport rate over the cell wall, and prolong the reproductive cycle.

Inside biofilm, the antibiotic activity differs considerably. Ciprofloxacin acts more efficiently on *P. aeruginosa* biofilm compared to many other antibiotics including piperacillin/imipenem combination or ceftazidime [2]. In the staphylococcal biofilm, there is frequently no increase in resistance for ciprofloxacin [19]. Similarly, gentamycin has bigger effect on *S. aureus* biofilm compared to oxacillin or vancomycin [2] and is more efficient than cefamandole, ciprofloxacin, and vancomycin in *Propionibacterium acnes* biofilm [19].

Resistance to antibiotics grows with age of a biofilm. Plasmid interchange is largely facilitated inside biofilm. The reason is the close proximity of bacteria. Reduction of shear forces by the slime also eases conjugating process [6]. Authors have shown plasmid acquired resistance against beta-lactams, erythromycin, aminoglycosides, tetracyclines, glycopeptides, and sulfonamides [8, 9, 15–17, 23].

Well protected from noxious agents, microorganisms can live inside the biofilm for a long period of time. If host immunity weakens for some reason, some of the colony members can change back to planktonic form of living leading into local and systemic spread and reactivation of clinical manifestation of infection [8].

References

1. An HY, Friedman R. Concise review of mechanisms of bacterial adhesion to biomaterial surface. J Biomed Mater Res. 1997;43:338–48.
2. Ceri H, Olson ME, Stremick C. The Calgary biofilm device: new technology for rapid determination of antibiotic susceptibility of bacterial biofilms. J Clin Microbiol. 1999;37:1771–6.
3. Costerton JW, Stewart PS, Greenberg EP. Bacterial biofilms: a common cause of persistent infections. Science. 1999;284:1318–22.
4. Darouiche RO. Device-associated infections: a macroproblem that starts with microadherence. Clin Infect Dis. 2001;33:1567–72.
5. Donlan RM. Biofilms: microbial life on surfaces. Emerg Infect Dis. 2002;8:881–90.
6. Ehlers LJ, Bouwer EJ. RP4 plasmid transfer among species of *Pseudomonas* in a biofilm reactor. Water Sci Technol. 1999;7:163–71.
7. Gray ED, Peters G. Effect of extracellular slime substance from *Staphylococcus epidermidis* on the human cellular immune response. Lancet. 1984;1:365–7.
8. Gristina AG, Hobgood CD, Webb LX. Adhesive colonisation of biomaterials and antibiotic resistance. Biomaterials. 1987;8:423–6.
9. Gristina AG, Jennings RA, Naylor PT, Myrvik QN, Webb LX. Comparative in vitro antibiotic resistance of surface-colonizing coagulase-negative *staphylococci*. Antimicrob Agents Chemother. 1989;33:813–6.
10. Gristina AG, Oga M, Webb LX, Hobgood CD. Adherent bacterial colonization in the pathogenesis of osteomyelitis. Science. 1985;228:990–3.
11. Hacker J. Role of fimbrial adhesin in the pathogenesis of *Escherichia coli* infections. Can J Microbiol. 1992;38:720–7.
12. Hasty DL, Ofek I, Courtney HS, Doyle RJ. Multiple adhesins for *streptococci*. Infect Immunol. 1992;60:2147–52.
13. Krekeler C, Ziehr H, Klein J. Physical methods for characterization of microbial cell surfaces. Experientia. 1989;45:1047–54.
14. Marshall KC. Mechanisms of bacterial adhesions at solid water interfaces. In: Savage DC, Fletcher M, editors. Bacterial adhesion. Mechanisms and physiological significance. New York: Plenum Press; 1985.
15. Nylor PT, Jennings R, Webb LX, Gristina AG. Antibiotic sensitivity of biomaterial adherent *Staphylococcus epidermidis* and *Staphylococcus aureus*. Trans Orthop Res Soc. 1989;14:108.
16. Nylor PT, Myrvik QN, Gristina AG. Antibiotic resistance of coagulase-negative and coagulase positive *staphylococci*. Clin Orthop Relat Res. 1990;261:126–33.
17. Pascual A, de Arellano ER, Martinez LM, Parea EJ. Effect of polyurethane catheters and bacterial biofilm on the in-vitro activity of antimicrobials agents *Staphylococcus epidermidis*. J Hosp Infect. 1993;24:211–8.
18. Patti JM, Allen BL, McGavin MJ, Hook M. MSCRAMM-mediated adherence of microorganisms to host tissues. Annu Rev Microbiol. 1994;48:585–617.
19. Ramage G, Tunney MM, Patrick S, Gorman SP, Nixon JR. Formation of *Propionibacterium acnes* biofilms on orthopaedic biomaterials and their susceptibility to antimicrobials. Biomaterials. 2003;24:3221–7.
20. Stewart PS, Costerton JW. Antibiotic resistance of bacteria in biofilms. Lancet. 2001;358: 135–8.

21. Steyer A. Interakcije med mikrobi. Med Razgl. 2004;43:37–44.
22. Sutherland IW. Microbial exopolysaccharides. Their role in microbial adhesion in aqueous systems. CRC Crit Rev Microbiol. 1983;10:173–201.
23. Tenover FC, Schaberg DR. Molecular biology of resistance. In: Bennett JV, Brachman PS, editors. Hospital infections. 4th ed. Philadelphia: Lippincott-Raven; 1998.
24. Vuong C, Gerke C, Somerville GA, Fischer ER, Otto M. Quorum-sensing control of biofilm factors in *Staphylococcus epidermidis*. J Infect Dis. 2003;188:706–18.
25. Zimmerli W, Waldvogel FA, Vaudaux P, Nydegger UE. Pathogenesis of foreign body infection: description and characteristics of an animal model. J Infect Dis. 1982;146:487–97.
26. Zimmerli W, Zak O, Vosbeck K. Experimental hematogenous infection of subcutaneously implanted foreign bodies. Scand J Infect Dis. 1985;17:303–10.
27. Zobell CE. The effect of solid surfaces upon bacterial activity. J Bacteriol. 1943;46:39–56.

Chapter 11
Bacteria–Biomaterial Interactions

**Antti Soininen, Emilia Kaivosoja, Jaime Esteban,
Riina Rautemaa-Richardson, Alberto Ortiz-Pérez, Gonçalo Barretto,
and Yrjö T. Konttinen**

Abstract The prevalence of orthopedic implant-related (deep) infections is approximately 0.5–1.5 %. They are divided to early (<1 months after the implantation) and delayed (1 months–2 years after the implantation) infections, which are somewhat overlapping with late infections (over 1–2 years after the implantation). Early and delayed infections are usually caused by direct contamination during the operation by more or less virulent microbes in patients with lowered local and/or systemic

A. Soininen
ORTON Research Institute, ORTON Orthopaedic Hospital,
Tenholantie 14, Helsinki 00280, Finland
e-mail: antti.soininen@orton.fi

E. Kaivosoja • G. Barretto
Department of Medicine, Institute of Clinical Medicine, Biomedicum 1 Hus,
Haartmaninkatu 8, P.O. Box 700, Helsinki 00029, Finland
e-mail: emilia.kaivosoja@helsinki.fi; goncaloalmeidabarreto@gmail.com

J. Esteban, M.D., Ph.D. • A. Ortiz-Pérez, Ph.D.
Bone and Joint Infectious Unit, Department of Clinical Microbiology,
IIS-Fundación Jiménez Díaz,
Av. Reyes Católicos 2, Madrid 28040, Spain
e-mail: jestebanmoreno@gmail.com; aortizp@gmail.com

R. Rautemaa-Richardson, DDS
School of Translational Medicine, Manchester Academic Health Science Centre,
University Hospital of South Manchester,
Southmoor Road, Manchester M23 9LT, UK
e-mail: riina.richardson@manchester.ac.uk

Y.T. Konttinen, M.D., Ph.D.(✉)
ORTON Research Institute, ORTON Orthopaedic Hospital,
Tenholantie 14, Helsinki 00280, Finland

Department of Medicine, Institute of Clinical Medicine, Biomedicum 1 Hus,
Haartmaninkatu 8, P.O. Box 700, Helsinki 00029, Finland

Department of Medicine, COXA Hospital for Joint Replacement,
Tampere 33101, Finland
e-mail: yrjo.konttinen@helsinki.fi

R. Trebše (ed.), *Infected Total Joint Arthroplasty*,
DOI 10.1007/978-1-4471-2482-5_11, © Springer-Verlag London 2012

bacterial resistance, but late infections are usually hematogenous. Microbes in the body are usually fought back in healthy living tissues, but implantation-associated hemorrhage and the abiotic implants form an unprotected surface, *locus minoris resistentiae*. Here, planktonic bacteria easily adhere and soon form a protective extracellular polymeric substance (EPS, biofilm, "bacterial slime") and transform to dormant but intercommunicating and even polymicrobial colonies. Embedded in the biofilm, antibiotics cannot by diffusion reach high enough (therapeutic concentrations), and suboptimal concentrations only select for resistant strains. Leukocytes, antibodies, and complement have poor access to biofilms. Further, using quorum sensing, biofilm bacteria behave very intelligently, adjusting the colonies to various threats to their existence, by adjusting the bacterial population to a size which realistically can survive, by developing antibiotic resistance and exchanging resistance between themselves, and by developing organized structures so that the microbes at every layer and depth have adjusted to their local micromilieu, e.g., oxygen tension, nutrients, EPS composition, antibiotics, and antifungals. If the in vivo "culture conditions" are favorable for the microbes, e.g., due to developing immunosuppression of the host, colonies can activate and start to send metastatic satellites to invade adjacent and remote new sites (foci). Removal of the infected implant is often the only effective therapy but happens at the cost of the implant, with antibiotics only playing an adjunct role. Diagnosis can be verified by detaching biofilm hidden bacteria by ultrasonication from the retrieved implant contained in fluid in a plastic bag and by combining routine microbial diagnosis, such as culture and staining, with more modern polymerase chain reaction analysis of the microbial DNA. The race between evolutionary antimicrobial resistance development and the drug companies developing new antibiotics seems to be tipping in favor of microbes. Therefore, intelligent use of systemic and local antibiotic prophylaxis, disinfection, aseptic techniques, testing of eventual carriers of resistant but asymptomatic strains, and separating carriers from clean but infection-prone patients are important principles. The development of implants and implant coatings able to resist bacterial adhesion and colonization is important, and new antimicrobial drugs working using new modes of action, e.g., based on the use of bacteriophages, should get more scientific attention.

Keywords Bacteria • Cytokine • Biomaterial • Adhesion • Coatings

11.1   Introduction

The use of surgically implanted devices and endoprosthetic joints has increased as a result of their beneficial effect on the quality of life and in some instances, even on the patient survival rates. Use of implants, however, can be associated with a variety of complications, one of the most dreaded being implant-related infections. Biomaterial-associated infection (BAI) is one of the most common complications of implantation of any abiotic biomaterial, regardless of its form or function. Treatment of BAIs is difficult mainly due to biofilm formation. Therefore, inhibition of bacterial adhesion to material surface, the first step of biofilm formation (via which the implant surface at the implant-body interface interacts with its surrounding), is an important strategy in the prevention of surface colonization, biofilm formation and BAI. Most nosocomial implant-related infections are caused by a spectrum of Staphylococci instead of epidemic strains [1–3]. Aspects contributing to BAIs are important to understand because of the high morbidity and mortality, which are associated with them. Development of BAIs begins with colonization of the surface of the implant material, followed by a complex metamorphosis, quorum sensing and biofilm formation and maturation. There has been an increasing recognition of the role that microbial biofilms play in human medicine and it has been estimated that more than 80 % of all human microbial infections involve biofilms [4, 5].

Biomaterial infections are difficult to treat by use of antibiotics alone, due to the presence of the biofilm and the dormant and intercommunicating nature of the bacterial flora in the biofilm. Biofilm renders the infection impervious to antimicrobial agents and host defenses and the dormant state of bacteria in the biofilm renders them less susceptible to antibiotics, which usually are most effective against rapidly dividing and growing bacteria [6–8]. Even though the causative agents were susceptible to the commonly used antimicrobials when tested *in vitro*, their biofilm forms are highly resistant to most agents. Further, a common problem with the long-term treatment with potent antibiotics is the development and continuous expansion of bacterial strains resistant to the commonly used antibiotics [9, 10]. As a result, surgical removal and replacement of the implants in one- (e.g. artificial heart valves) or two-stage (e.g. artificial joints) revision operations is often the only effective treatment, followed by an adjuvant treatment with systemic antimicrobial therapies, which naturally causes morbidity and increases cost of the treatment [11].

11.2 Staphylococcal Interactions

Cluster-forming Gram-positive *Staphylococcus epidermidis* and *Staphylococcus aureus* are the two most common pathogens involved in BAIs. *S. epidermidis* is a common skin commensal and can also be found on mucous membranes. Its ability to adhere derives in part from its ability to produce extracellular polymeric substance (ESP, "bacterial slime"), which together with the intricate staphylococcal cell wall protect it against drying, mechanical rubbing off, osmotic rupture, antimicrobials and other threats. Most *S. epidermidis* are thus inherently resistant to a number of antibiotics. ESP also protects *S. epidermidis* against naive and adaptive immunity so their presence on normal skin and mucosal surface is not normally associated with any signs of inflammatory or immune reactions in form of e.g. redness, swelling, pain, increased temperature or functional impairment of the body surface.

However, the host-staphylococcal balance becomes disrupted if the bacterium gains entry into the tissues. Normally the keratinized surface layer of the skin or the superficial mucosal epithelium forms a passive physical barrier keeping

S. epidermidis out and away from e.g. bloodstream. Although the immune mechanisms in blood are a threat to bacteria, blood also forms a rich source of nutrients for S. epidermidis (which can be cultured on blood agar plates), activating it up from the dormant biofilm-associated "resistant state". During implantation of the prosthetic joint, Staphylococci can get direct access to subcutaneous tissues, to the deeper lying muscle and fascial tissues, or even to the joint cavity and implant surface. These can cause superficial surgical site infections, deep surgical site infections and implant-related (organ/space) infections, respectively. Later on, if the blood gate is opened e.g. due to a wound, S. epidermidis can be seeded to blood and via bacteremia can cause a late hemotogenic implant-related infection. This together with its resistance to commonly used antibiotics has contributed to S. epidermidis emergence in recent years as a major nosocomial pathogen associated with infections of implanted medical devices. Staphylococci adhere to the abiotic and relatively defenseless implant surface and can form biofilms, which constitutes an important virulence factor and probably the most relevant pathogenic mechanism of staphylococcal infection [12, 13]. After adhering to the implant surface S. epidermidis secretes a layer of slime, making the bacterium less accessible to the host defense systems and decreases its antibiotic susceptibility significantly [14].

S. aureus infections are also common, severe and associated with significant morbidity and mortality. S. aureus is more virulent than S. epidermidis and causes relatively more often infections of the joint implants occurring (manifesting) early after the joint replacement arthroplasty. Therefore, perioperative antibiotic prophylaxis is mainly targeted to S. aureus which has had a major impact on the prevalence of BAIs caused by it. Nevertheless, S. aureus is the most common cause of purulent arthritis and infective endocarditis worldwide. These tissues are relatively poorly vascularized and therefore the host response is less effective than in better vascularized tissues; in this respect, articular cartilage and valvular tissue in the heart resemble biomaterials as revealed by their susceptibility to Staphylococci [15]. Further, due to its virulence, S. aureus is the most common cause of skin and soft tissue infections and is a frequent cause of serious infections such as health care-associated bloodstream infections, device-associated infections and osteomyelitis. Biofilm-producing S. aureus displays greater adhesive abilities in comparison to nonproducing ones [16, 17].

Most bacterial in vitro adhesion studies have been done under static conditions for practical reasons. However, in vivo bacteria and biofilms are usually subjected to shear forces of the human body fluid flow. The best primary prophylaxis against infections would be to use biomaterials or coatings able to inhibit or resist bacterial adhesion.

Some research has been done on adhesion of different Staphylococcal strains to most common biomaterials and to diamond-like carbon (DLC) and diamond-like carbon polymer hybrid (DLC-p-h) coatings. These tests evaluated which materials would present best antifouling properties to prevent or diminish Staphylococcus adherence and thus reduce implant-related infections. Under static condition, biomaterial samples are allowed to interact directly with bacterial solution at body temperature for different times (normally done without protein treatment of the sample). Static adhesion results indicated that S. epidermidis (ATCC 35984) adhered significantly ($p<0.05$) more to DLC coating than to titanium or silicon, but diamond-like carbon polytetrafluoroethylene hybrid (DLC-PTFE-h) showed better antifouling ability than other tested materials. No other significant differences were observed between the materials tested. *S. aureus* (ATCC 25923) showed significantly lower adherence to DLC-PTFE-h coating ($p<0.05$) compared to other material surfaces tested (DLC, Ti and Si) [18]. The above-mentioned results suggest that applying DLC-PTFE-h coating on the surface of implants could inhibit bacterial adhesion on it and thus reduce the risk of implant infection.

It can be debated if such static models and fluids without proteins adequately mimic the situation *in vivo*. After surgery, the implant surface is always instantly but dynamically coated by a monolayer of adsorbed interstitial or serum proteins, regulated also by the biomaterial surface properties, such as the chemical composition and phase, topography, hydrophobicity/-philicity, zeta potential etc. Microbial attachment process on the material depends on the composition of this protein coating. It is hypothesized that by surface treatment with proteins, an adhesion environment which is somewhat more reminiscent to that prevailing in the human body can be achieved [12, 19]. In static conditions, to achieve this, tested biomaterial samples are first treated with protein to implement proteins on the surface before immersion in bacterial solution. Kinnari *et al.* showed that by coating titanium surface with a protein, such as albumin (human serum albumin, HSA), antifouling surface properties were achieved, which reduced adhesion of *S. aureus* (ATCC 25923) to the titanium surface [20]. In *S. aureus* (S-15981), adhesion tests samples were first treated with fetal calf serum. DLC, Cr, Ta, and Ti surfaces showed the following adhesion rank order (% of surface area covered by adhered bacteria): titanium (22.69 %), tantalum (14.34 %), chromium (1.41 %) and DLC (0.38 %) [19]. These results in static adhesion conditions show that protein coating changes the adhesion of *S. aureus* and that much less bacteria adhered to DLC surfaces than to titanium surfaces compared to tests performed in the absence of proteins.

Implant or coating designed for clinical use will be subjected to continuously flowing body fluids and shear forces. This suggests that bacterial adhesion should be studied under dynamic rather than under static conditions to mimic more precisely the conditions prevailing *in vivo*. The dynamic bacterial adhesion tests can be done in flow chambers which allow bacterial solution to flow (with the desired shear rate) on the surface of the tested material. Dynamic bacterial adhesion tests with different *S. epidermidis* (HBH276, 236, 3294) strains to DLC and surgical steel (AISI316L) did not show significant differences ($p<0.05$) in bacterial adherence to these surfaces. Similar results were obtained with *S. aureus* (7323) to DLC and surgical steel. This suggested that DLC coating could be applied to implant surfaces without increasing the risk of implant-related infections compared to surgical steel, the most commonly used biomaterial. These tests were done using the shear rate of 15.7 1/s, but also without proteins, using phosphate-buffered saline to suspend bacteria [21].

Dynamic adhesions tests have been reported using the shear rate of 200 1/s and three commonly used biomaterial metals (Ta, Ti, Cr) and three different DLC coatings, which all showed similar results when *S. epidermidis* (ATCC 35984) was used for testing. No significant ($p<0.05$) difference between the tested materials was observed. *S. aureus* (S-15981) adhered to DLC, DLC-PDMS-h, DLC-PTFE-h, Ta, Ti and Cr, showing slightly more adherence to DLC *vs.* DLC-PDMS-h and tantalum. With all other tested materials, no significant differences were observed; however, also these studies were done using phosphate-buffered saline, without proteins [22].

Bacterial adhesion is a complicated process that is affected by many factors, including some characteristics of the bacteria, the target material surface and the environmental factors, such as flow rate and the presence of serum proteins or bactericidal substances. This makes comparison of *in vitro* and *in vivo* results difficult. For example, when van der Mei *et al.* did bacterial adhesion tests (both *in vivo* and *in vitro*) with *S. epidermidis* (3399) and *S. aureus* (ATCC12600) to poly(ethylene glycol) PEG (OptiChem®), no correlation between biofilms formed *in vitro* and *in vivo* conditions was found [12].

11.3 Mycobacterial Interactions

The genus *Mycobacterium* is a special group among microorganisms. The type species (*Mycobacterium tuberculosis*) is the primary human pathogen and is one of the leading causes of death throughout history, but almost all other mycobacterial species are environmental organisms that only rarely cause disease in humans. Biofilms are extremely important for these organisms because they may be considered reservoirs for the survival of mycobacteria in water distribution systems and contributors to the continuous bacteriological contamination of the water via an erosion process [23]. Some of the most often isolated species in environmental biofilms are commonly isolated also as human pathogens, like *Mycobacterium avium* complex (MAC) species, *Mycobacterium lentiflavum* or nonpigmented rapidly growing mycobacteria (NPRGM) [24–26]. These species also have the ability to form biofilms *in vitro*, where the composition of the media and the temperature significantly influence the development of biofilms [27]. All these findings suggest that water could form a potential source of human infections caused by these microorganisms.

Biofilm formation by mycobacteria requires steps rather similar to other microorganisms. First mycobacteria must adhere to the surface. The initial bond strength is due to weak hydrophobic or van der Waals forces. Later, stronger covalent bonds are formed. Finally, the microorganisms begin to multiply [28, 29]. Adherence studies showed that there are intra- and interspecies differences in mycobacterial attachment to polymers. After adherence, biofilm development follows a sigmoid growth curve until the doubling time of cells becomes shorter than that of planktonic bacteria [27, 30].

Molecular mechanisms and environmental factors involved in biofilm formation have been described for different species of mycobacteria [31]. Presence of ions, such as magnesium, calcium and zinc, in the medium affects the biofilm formation by MAC species. Moreover, several carbon sources, such as glucose or peptone, improve the development of the biofilm [32].

Several reports have linked the ability of mycobacteria to perform sliding movements with the development of biofilms. Both characteristics are linked to the presence of glycopeptidolipids (GPLs) in the mycobacterial cell wall. These molecules are integrated in the complex wall structure, where they expose their hydrophobic tails to the outer environment. Thus, the cell becomes hydrophobic and creates links with hydrophilic surfaces, facilitating motility and biofilm formation [33]. The different expressions of genes involved in GPLs biosynthesis influence the development of biofilm, which indicates that the outer surface of the bacterium is important for this property [34]. The absence of GPLs in the outermost layer of the cell wall abolishes the ability of mycobacteria to form biofilm on polyvinyl chloride (PVC) [35]. Likewise, the role of other genes has been analyzed in the development of the biofilm. The *lsr2* gene, identified in several species of mycobacteria, is one of them. Although its function is not clarified, mutant strains for this gene develop nonpolar lipid disorders affecting biofilm formation by Mycobacteria [36]. Another study linked the presence of *GroEL* gene with the biofilms produced by *Mycobacterium smegmatis*, an environmental NPRGM. This gene encodes the Hsp60 chaperone. Mycobacteria contain two forms of Hsp60-related chaperone regulated by heat shock, oxidative stress or immune response. Other properties of this chaperone are its ability to participate in intercellular signaling and transcriptional regulation. Mutant strains for this gene showed altered biofilm formation [37]. The GroEL1 chaperone is also involved in the metabolism of short-chain mycolates, which indicates their involvement in biofilm development. Other genes are currently under research to evaluate their actual role in biofilm development by NPRGM [38–42].

From the clinical point of view, the importance of biofilm relates to implant-related infections but also to chronic diseases characterized by the presence of biofilms, such as respiratory infections in patients with chronic obstructive lung diseases [43]. A relationship has been demonstrated between the ability to develop biofilm *in vitro* and the clinical significance of the NPRGM strains [44]. Biofilm-defective *Mycobacterium abscessus* cannot cause disease in an animal model [45]. Biofilm growth also leads to development of antibiotic resistance and helps to escape from host defense [46]. Mycobacteria in biofilms show diminished susceptibility to antibiotics which are active against planktonic mycobacteria due to differences in the metabolic state of biofilm and planktonic bacteria [47, 48]. Fortunately, diseases caused by environmental mycobacteria are relatively rarely seen in clinical practice. However, tuberculosis is one of the leading causes of mortality among humans and some reports suggest that biofilms could have a role also in the pathogenesis of disease caused by *M. tuberculosis* [49, 50]. *In vitro* studies showed that *M. tuberculosis* can develop biofilm and that biofilm development affects the antibiotic susceptibility of these strains. These studies also demonstrated the importance of mycolic acids as part of the extracellular matrix of the biofilm [50]. Clinical data also supports that prosthesis infected by *M. tuberculosis* is extremely rare but in these cases of implant-related tuberculosis it normally cannot be treated without implant removal, so the importance of biofilm in some types of human tuberculosis seems to be clear [51–53]. In industrialized nations tuberculous arthritis has become rare but throughout the rest of the world still cripples many patients. Even in developed countries joint replacement arthroplasties have been done in old cases of tuberculosis of the hip and the knee. Reactivation of the old tuberculous arthritis is threatening upon revision operations of the replaced joints and anti-tuberculotic prophylaxis is recommended [54–56].

11.4   Candidal Interactions

Candidal, in particular *Candida albicans*, biofilms are usually found on the oral mucosal membranes in medically compromised patients. Candida participates often in mixed candidal-bacterial biofilm infections. As with other biofilm-forming strains, *C. albicans* is usually reasonably sensitive to antifungal agents *in vitro* but shows resistance to then in *in vivo* biofilms. Use of azol antifungals in such cases also leads to formation and enrichment of resistant species. Medical treatment and supportive antifungal treatment is based on the disruption of the biofilm and use of a combination medication [57]. Although better known for its involvement in endocarditis, candidal species have also been described in infections of replaced joints [58, 59].

11.5   Microbial Interactions with Quaternary Ammonium Compounds

One option to diminish the risk for implant-related infection is to use coating with materials with antimicrobial effects. Quaternary ammonium compounds (QACs) have such activity and they are widely employed in industrial applications, water treatment, in pharmaceutical, and everyday consumer products as preserving agents, foam boosters, and detergents. QACs are lethal to vegetative bacteria, yeasts, mould, algae and lipophilic viruses but not to bacterial spores, mycobacteria or hydrophilic viruses. There are reports on bacterial resistance to QAC, which cause a concern that extensive use of QACs could lead to the selection of bacteria that show resistance to both antibiotics and biocides [60].

The antimicrobial activity of QACs is mainly caused by their cationic characteristics, which exert a strong adhesive force on negatively charged bacteria. The membranes of the contacting microbes are disrupted and become leaky and consequently the involved microbe dies. There are concerns that similar reactions could occur with host cells, and thus the *in vivo* use of QACs surfaces is limited, although QACs can be used in contact with the skin or for materials that are used in the hospital like textiles, floors and ceilings in the operating room etc.

Recently, more attention has been paid to the effects of QACs on the host cells. For example, poly(vinyl pyridinium bromide) did not show to induce significant membrane damage to mouse fibroblasts, but increased the average number of cationic charges per monomer unit in partially quaternized polymers correlated with cytotoxicity [61].

Biocompatibility of copolymers of 4-vinyl-*N*-hexylpyridinium bromide (HBVP) and poly(ethylene glycol) methyl ether methacrylate (PEGMA) was studied using human intestinal epithelial Caco-2 cells [62]. Homopolymer of PEGMA and its copolymer containing 10 % HBVP did not cause cell death, whereas the copolymers containing 50 % or more HBVP were less biocompatible. Insoluble cross-linked quaternary ammonium polyethylenimine was biocompatible and exerted long-lasting antimicrobial effects against a wide range of bacteria [63]. Future research will determine if QAC surfaces can be used as antimicrobial surface coatings for medical implants.

11.6 Microbial Interactions with Silver- or Copper-Containing Biomaterials

Silver has been used as an antimicrobial agent for over 6,000 years [64]. In addition to silver, also non-tarnishing copper is being developed to e.g. hospital door handles and other applications. In a moist electrolyte environment, metallic silver releases silver ions. Ionic silver is the most potent antimicrobial form of silver, but it is difficult to use in combination with medical devices because the poor solubility of most silver salts does not allow effective antimicrobial activity. The use of silver as nanoparticles is a novel approach. This increases the active surface and silver ion production. Antimicrobial activity can be regulated by modulating fixation of the silver particles to the surface layers of the implant. Silicon disks impregnated with silver nanoparticles efficiently prevent bacterial adhesion and growth, but when the sliver nanoparticles are gradually washed out of the elastomer, also their antimicrobial effect decreases with time [65].

Silver nanoparticle coatings are successfully applied to some medical devices. For example, external ventricular drains (EVD) coated with silver nanoparticles are now being tested in patients. Colonization of these drains was reduced by a factor of four and the infection of the central spinal fluid by a factor of 2 [66]. Another small-scale study with 20 patients showed that none of the coated drains became infected, whereas the control group (without silver nanoparticle coating) shoved five cases of infection leading to ventriculitis [67]. Silver coating also significantly reduces catheter-associated urinary tract infections [68–70]. Silver coating of venous catheters reduces surface colonization and catheter-related bloodstream infections (CBSI) [71–73]. However, some studies report the reduction of surface colonization without a direct significant effect on CBSI [74], and some report no significant reduction of surface colonization or CBSI [75].

It is not yet understood how silver kills bacteria. A number of possible targets for silver inside the (bacterial) cell have been identified [76]. Silver ions (and silver nanoparticles) bind directly to the cell membrane. Accumulation of silver in negatively charged parts of the cellular membrane leads to rupture of the membrane, leakage of the cellular compounds out of the cell and cell death. Silver ion binds to sulfhydryl and phosphor groups of proteins, rendering them inactive and causing aggregation of these denatured proteins. Because apparently many different processes are affected by silver, resistance to silver is not widespread and has not been a major concern in clinical practice.

The extended use of silver and silver solutions can lead to a number of disorders [77], of which the most common condition is argyria, in which silver is stored in the skin, which assumes a grayish tinge [78]. Argyria is considered a harmless condition except for its cosmetic consequences. Reports of silver-induced organ toxicity or organ damage are rare, even though silver accumulates in some organs and tissues [77]. As always when nanosize biomaterials are discussed, the concern of biosafety has to be brought up. Currently, the biocompatibility of silver nanoparticle containing coatings *in vivo* is not clear. Silver nanoparticles are not specifically damaging cells (reviewed by Johnston *et al.* [79]). The bacterial- and fungicidal mechanisms of action of silver nanoparticles are not specific and can affect also other living cells. Therefore, host cells are at risk when exposed to high concentration of silver nanoparticles. Nanoparticles bind to and migrate into cells, damaging proteins, genetic material and membranes, which can lead to cell death [80–82]. However, if the silver nanoparticles are tightly embedded in the coating, extensive release of free silver nanoparticles is avoided. Tight embedding could also improve the efficiency and longevity of the antimicrobial surface, as nanoparticles are not flushed away.

It remains unclear, how surface-bound nanoparticles exert their antimicrobial activity, but at least surface-to-volume ratio is important for the antimicrobial efficiency [79]. The bactericidal activity of silver nanoparticles is dependent on the size and shape of the particles [83–85]. Smaller sized silver nanoparticles (<10 nm) have higher antibiotic activity than larger particles. In addition, triangular shaped silver particles kill more bacterial than rods and spherical particles [83].

References

1. Lew DP, Waldvogel FA. Osteomyelitis. N Engl J Med. 1997;336(14):999–1007.
2. Lowy FD. Medical progress – *Staphylococcus aureus* infections. N Engl J Med. 1998; 339(8):520–32.
3. Sanderson PJ. Infection in orthopedic implants. J Hosp Infect. 1991;18:367–75.
4. Romero R, Schaudinn C, Kusanovic JP, Gorur A, Gotsch F, Webster P, Nhan-Chang CL, Erez O, Kim CJ, Espinoza J, Goncalves LF, Vaisbuch E, Mazaki-Tovi S, Hassan SS, Costerton JW. Detection of a microbial biofilm in intraamniotic infection. Am J Obstet Gynecol. 2008;198(1): 135. doi:10.1016/j.ajog.2007.11.026.
5. Ghannoum M, O'Toole GA. Microbial biofilms. Washington, DC: ASM Press; 2004.
6. Knobloch JKM, von Osten H, Horstkotte MA, Rohde H, Mack D. Minimal attachment killing (MAK): a versatile method for susceptibility testing of attached biofilm-positive and -negative *Staphylococcus epidermidis*. Med Microbiol Immunol. 2002;191(2):107–14. doi:10.1007/ s00430-002-0125-2.
7. Otto M, Kong KF, Vuong C. Staphylococcus quorum sensing in biofilm formation and infection. Int J Med Microbiol. 2006;296(2–3):133–9. doi:10.1016/j.ijmm.2006.01.042.
8. Otto M. Quorum-sensing control in *Staphylococci* – a target for antimicrobial drug therapy? FEMS Microbiol Lett. 2004;241(2):135–41. doi:10.1016/j.femsle.2004.11.016.
9. Hench LL, Thompson I. Twenty-first century challenges for biomaterials. J R Soc Interface. 2010;7:S379–91. doi:10.1098/rsif.2010.0151.focus.

10. Wenzel RP. Health care-associated infections: major issues in the early years of the 21st century. Clin Infect Dis. 2007;45:85–8. doi:10.1086/518136.

11. Klevens RM, Edwards JR, Richards CL, Horan TC, Gaynes RP, Pollock DA, Cardo DM. Estimating health care-associated infections and deaths in US hospitals, 2002. Public Health Rep. 2007;122(2):160–6.

12. van der Mei HC, Fernandez ICS, Metzger S, Grainger DW, Engelsman AF, Nejadnik MR, Busscher HJ. In vitro and in vivo comparisons of staphylococcal biofilm formation on a cross-linked poly(ethylene glycol)-based polymer coating. Acta Biomater. 2010;6(3):1119–24. doi:10.1016/j.actbio.2009.08.040.

13. Sousa C. Staphylococcus epidermidis: adhesion and biofilm formation onto biomaterials. Saarbrücken: LAP LAMBERT Academic Publishing; 2011.

14. An YH, Friedman RJ. Concise review of mechanisms of bacterial adhesion to biomaterial surfaces. J Biomed Mater Res. 1998;43(3):338–48.

15. Miller LG, Perlroth J, Kuo M, Tan J, Bayer AS. Adjunctive use of rifampin for the treatment of Staphylococcus aureus infections. Arch Intern Med. 2008;168(8):805–19.

16. Svensater G, Welin J, Wilkins JC, Beighton D, Hamilton IR. Protein expression by planktonic and biofilm cells of Streptococcus mutans. FEMS Microbiol Lett. 2001;205(1):139–46.

17. Gal L, Rollet C, Guzzo J. Biofilm-detached cells, a transition from a sessile to a planktonic phenotype: a comparative study of adhesion and physiological characteristics in Pseudomonas aeruginosa. FEMS Microbiol Lett. 2009;290(2):135–42. doi:10.1111/j.1574-6968.2008. 01415.x.

18. Kinnari TJ, Soininen A, Esteban J, Zamora N, Alakoski E, Kouri VP, Lappalainen R, Konttinen YT, Gomez-Barrena E, Tiainen VM. Adhesion of staphylococcal and Caco-2 cells on diamond-like carbon polymer hybrid coating. J Biomed Mater Res A. 2008;86A(3):760–8. doi:10.1002/jbm.a.31643.

19. Konttinen YT, Levon J, Myllymaa K, Kouri VP, Rautemaa R, Kinnari T, Myllymaa S, Lappalainen R. Patterned macroarray plates in comparison of bacterial adhesion inhibition of tantalum, titanium, and chromium compared with diamond-like carbon. J Biomed Mater Res A. 2010;92A(4):1606–13. doi:10.1002/jbm.a.32486.

20. Kinnari TJ, Peltonen LI, Kuusela T, Kivilahti J, Kononen M, Jero J. Bacterial adherence to titanium surface coated with human serum albumin. Otol Neurotol. 2005;26(3):380–4.

21. Soininen A, Tiainen VM, Konttinen YT, van der Mei HC, Busscher HJ, Sharma PK. Bacterial adhesion to diamond-like carbon as compared to stainless steel. J Biomed Mater Res B Appl Biomater. 2009;90B(2):882–5. doi:10.1002/jbm.b.31359.

22. Soininen A, Levon J, Katsikogianni M, Myllymaa K, Lappalainen R, Konttinen YT, Kinnari TJ, Tiainen VM, Missirlis Y. In vitro adhesion of staphylococci to diamond-like carbon polymer hybrids under dynamic flow conditions. J Mater Sci Mater Med. 2011;22(3):629–36. doi:10.1007/s10856-011-4231-9.

23. Dailloux M, Albert M, Laurain C, Andolfatto S, Lozniewski A, Hartemann P, Mathieu L. Mycobacterium xenopi and drinking water biofilms. Appl Environ Microbiol. 2003;69(11): 6946–8.

24. September SM, Brozel VS, Venter SN. Diversity of nontuberculoid Mycobacterium species in biofilms of urban and semiurban drinking water distribution systems. Appl Environ Microbiol. 2004;70(12):7571–3. doi:10.1128/AEM.70.12.7571-7573.2004. PII:70/12/7571.

25. Falkinham 3rd JO, Norton CD, LeChevallier MW. Factors influencing numbers of Mycobacterium avium, Mycobacterium intracellulare, and other Mycobacteria in drinking water distribution systems. Appl Environ Microbiol. 2001;67(3):1225–31. doi:10.1128/ AEM.67.3.1225-1231.2001.

26. Marshall HM, Carter R, Torbey MJ, Minion S, Tolson C, Sidjabat HE, Huygens F, Hargreaves M, Thomson RM. Mycobacterium lentiflavum in drinking water supplies, Australia. Emerg Infect Dis. 2011;17(3):395–402.

27. Esteban J, Martin-de-Hijas NZ, Kinnari TJ, Ayala G, Fernandez-Roblas R, Gadea I. Biofilm development by potentially pathogenic non-pigmented rapidly growing mycobacteria. BMC Microbiol. 2008;8:184. doi:10.1186/1471-2180-8-184. PII:1471-2180-8-184.

28. Costerton JW. Biofilm theory can guide the treatment of device-related orthopaedic infections. Clin Orthop Relat Res. 2005;437:7–11. PII:00003086-200508000-00003.
29. Donlan RM, Costerton JW. Biofilms: survival mechanisms of clinically relevant microorganisms. Clin Microbiol Rev. 2002;15(2):167–93.
30. Hall-Stoodley L, Lappin-Scott H. Biofilm formation by the rapidly growing mycobacterial species *Mycobacterium fortuitum*. FEMS Microbiol Lett. 1998;168(1):77–84. PII:S0378-1097(98)00422-4.
31. Martinez A, Torello S, Kolter R. Sliding motility in mycobacteria. J Bacteriol. 1999;181(23): 7331–8.
32. Carter G, Wu M, Drummond DC, Bermudez LE. Characterization of biofilm formation by clinical isolates of *Mycobacterium avium*. J Med Microbiol. 2003;52(Pt 9):747–52.
33. Recht J, Martinez A, Torello S, Kolter R. Genetic analysis of sliding motility in *Mycobacterium smegmatis*. J Bacteriol. 2000;182(15):4348–51.
34. Yamazaki Y, Danelishvili L, Wu M, Macnab M, Bermudez LE. Mycobacterium avium genes associated with the ability to form a biofilm. Appl Environ Microbiol. 2006;72(1):819–25. doi:10.1128/AEM.72.1.819-825.2006. PII:72/1/819.
35. Recht J, Kolter R. Glycopeptidolipid acetylation affects sliding motility and biofilm formation in *Mycobacterium smegmatis*. J Bacteriol. 2001;183(19):5718–24. doi:10.1128/JB.183.19.5718-5724.2001.
36. Arora K, Whiteford DC, Lau-Bonilla D, Davitt CM, Dahl JL. Inactivation of lsr2 results in a hypermotile phenotype in *Mycobacterium smegmatis*. J Bacteriol. 2008;190(12):4291–300. doi:10.1128/JB.00023-08. PII:JB.00023-08.
37. Ojha A, Anand M, Bhatt A, Kremer L, Jacobs Jr WR, Hatfull GF. GroEL1: a dedicated chaperone involved in mycolic acid biosynthesis during biofilm formation in mycobacteria. Cell. 2005;123(5):861–73. doi:10.1016/j.cell.2005.09.012. PII:S0092-8674(05)00965-7.
38. Nessar R, Reyrat JM, Davidson LB, Byrd TF. Deletion of the mmpL4b gene in the *Mycobacterium abscessus* glycopeptidolipid biosynthetic pathway results in loss of surface colonization capability, but enhanced ability to replicate in human macrophages and stimulate their innate immune response. Microbiology. 2011. doi:10.1099/mic.0.046557-0. PII: mic.0.046557-0.
39. Deshayes C, Bach H, Euphrasie D, Attarian R, Coureuil M, Sougakoff W, Laval F, Av-Gay Y, Daffe M, Etienne G, Reyrat JM. MmpS4 promotes glycopeptidolipids biosynthesis and export in *Mycobacterium smegmatis*. Mol Microbiol. 2010;78(4):989–1003. doi:10.1111/j.1365-2958. 2010.07385.x.
40. Deshayes C, Laval F, Montrozier H, Daffe M, Etienne G, Reyrat JM. A glycosyltransferase involved in biosynthesis of triglycosylated glycopeptidolipids in *Mycobacterium smegmatis*: impact on surface properties. J Bacteriol. 2005;187(21):7283–91. doi:10.1128/JB.187.21.7283-7291.2005. PII:187/21/7283.
41. Kocincova D, Singh AK, Beretti JL, Ren H, Euphrasie D, Liu J, Daffe M, Etienne G, Reyrat JM. Spontaneous transposition of IS1096 or ISMsm3 leads to glycopeptidolipid overproduction and affects surface properties in *Mycobacterium smegmatis*. Tuberculosis (Edinb). 2008;88(5):390–8. doi:10.1016/j.tube.2008.02.005. PII:S1472-9792(08)00021-8.
42. Kocincova D, Winter N, Euphrasie D, Daffe M, Reyrat JM, Etienne G. The cell surface-exposed glycopeptidolipids confer a selective advantage to the smooth variants of *Mycobacterium smegmatis* in vitro. FEMS Microbiol Lett. 2009;290(1):39–44. doi:10.1111/j.1574-6968.2008.01396.x. PII:FML1396.
43. Esteban J, Martin-de-Hijas NZ, Fernandez AI, Fernandez-Roblas R, Gadea I. Epidemiology of infections due to nonpigmented rapidly growing mycobacteria diagnosed in an urban area. Eur J Clin Microbiol Infect Dis. 2008;27(10):951–7. doi:10.1007/s10096-008-0521-7.
44. Martin-de-Hijas NZ, Garcia-Almeida D, Ayala G, Fernandez-Roblas R, Gadea I, Celdran A, Gomez-Barrena E, Esteban J. Biofilm development by clinical strains of non-pigmented rapidly growing mycobacteria. Clin Microbiol Infect. 2009;15(10):931–6. doi:10.1111/j.1469-0691.2009.02882.x. PII:CLM2882.

45. Byrd TF, Lyons CR. Preliminary characterization of a *Mycobacterium abscessus* mutant in human and murine models of infection. Infect Immun. 1999;67(9):4700–7.
46. Falkinham 3rd JO. Growth in catheter biofilms and antibiotic resistance of *Mycobacterium avium*. J Med Microbiol. 2007;56(Pt 2):250–4. doi:10.1099/jmm.0.46935-0. PII:56/2/250.
47. Greendyke R, Byrd TF. Differential antibiotic susceptibility of *Mycobacterium abscessus* variants in biofilms and macrophages compared to that of planktonic bacteria. Antimicrob Agents Chemother. 2008;52(6):2019–26. doi:10.1128/AAC.00986-07. PII:AAC.00986-07.
48. Ortiz-Perez A, Martin-de-Hijas N, Alonso-Rodriguez N, Molina-Manso D, Fernandez-Roblas R, Esteban J. Importance of antibiotic penetration in the antimicrobial resistance of biofilm formed by non-pigmented rapidly growing mycobacteria against amikacin, ciprofloxacin and clarithromycin. Enferm Infecc Microbiol Clin. 2011;29(2):79–84. doi:10.1016/j.eimc.2010.08.016. PII:S0213-005X(10)00451-9.
49. Ha KY, Chung YG, Ryoo SJ. Adherence and biofilm formation of *Staphylococcus epidermidis* and *Mycobacterium tuberculosis* on various spinal implants. Spine (Phila Pa 1976). 2005;30(1):38–43. PII:00007632-200501010-00008.
50. Ojha AK, Baughn AD, Sambandan D, Hsu T, Trivelli X, Guerardel Y, Alahari A, Kremer L, Jacobs Jr WR, Hatfull GF. Growth of *Mycobacterium tuberculosis* biofilms containing free mycolic acids and harbouring drug-tolerant bacteria. Mol Microbiol. 2008;69(1):164–74. doi:10.1111/j.1365-2958.2008.06274.x. PII:MMI6274.
51. Brown A, Grubbs P, Mongey AB. Infection of total hip prosthesis by *Mycobacterium tuberculosis* and *Mycobacterium chelonae* in a patient with rheumatoid arthritis. Clin Rheumatol. 2008;27(4):543–5. doi:10.1007/s10067-007-0788-6.
52. Fernandez-Valencia JA, Garcia S, Riba J. Presumptive infection of a total hip prosthesis by *Mycobacterium tuberculosis*: a case report. Acta Orthop Belg. 2003;69(2):193–6.
53. Wright RA, Yang F, Moore WS. Tuberculous infection in a vascular prosthesis: a case of aortic graft infection resulting from disseminated tuberculosis. Arch Surg. 1977;112(1):79–81.
54. Eskola A, Santavirta S, Konttinen YT, Tallroth K, Hoikka V, Lindholm ST. Cementless total replacement for old tuberculosis of the hip. J Bone Joint Surg Br. 1988;70(4):603–6.
55. Santavirta S, Eskola A, Konttinen YT, Tallroth K, Lindholm ST. Total hip-replacement in old tuberculosis - a report of 14 cases. Acta Orthop Scand. 1988;59(4):391–5.
56. Eskola A, Santavirta S, Konttinen YT, Tallroth K, Lindholm ST. Arthroplasty for old tuberculosis of the knee. J Bone Joint Surg Br. 1988;70(5):767–9.
57. Rautemaa R, Ramage G. Oral candidiasis – clinical challenges of a biofilm disease. Crit Rev Microbiol. 2011;37(4):328–36.
58. Younkin S, Evarts CM, Steigbigel RT. Candida-parapsilosis infection of a total hip-joint replacement – successful reimplantation after treatment with amphotericin-B and 5-fluorocytosine – a case-report. J Bone Joint Surg Am. 1984;66A(1):142–3.
59. Koch AE. Candida-albicans infection of a prosthetic knee replacement – a report and review of the literature. J Rheumatol. 1988;15(2):362–5.
60. Russell AD, Tattawasart U, Maillard JY, Furr JR. Possible link between bacterial resistance and use of antibiotics and biocides. Antimicrob Agents Chemother. 1998;42(8):2151–1.
61. Fischer D, Li YX, Ahlemeyer B, Krieglstein J, Kissel T. In vitro cytotoxicity testing of polycations: influence of polymer structure on cell viability and hemolysis. Biomaterials. 2003;24(7):1121–31.
62. Youngblood JP, Stratton TR, Rickus JL. In vitro biocompatibility studies of antibacterial quaternary polymers. Biomacromolecules. 2009;10(9):2550–5. doi:10.1021/bm9005003.
63. Domb AJ, Beyth N, Houri-Haddad Y, Baraness-Hadar L, Yudovin-Farber I, Weiss EI. Surface antimicrobial activity and biocompatibility of incorporated polyethylenimine nanoparticles. Biomaterials. 2008;29(31):4157–63. doi:10.1016/j.biomaterials.2008.07.003.
64. Alexander JW. History of the medical use of silver. Surg Infect. 2009;10(3):289–92. doi:10.1089/sur.2008.9941.
65. Bayston R, Furno F, Morley KS, Wong B, Sharp BL, Arnold PL, Howdle SM, Brown PD, Winship PD, Reid HJ. Silver nanoparticles and polymeric medical devices: a new approach to

prevention of infection? J Antimicrob Chemother. 2004;54(6):1019–24. doi:10.1093/jac/dkh478.

66. Raabe A, Fichtner J, Guresir E, Seifert V. Efficacy of silver-bearing external ventricular drainage catheters: a retrospective analysis clinical article. J Neurosurg. 2010;112(4):840–6. doi:10.3171/2009.8.JNS091297.

67. Lackner P, Beer R, Broessner G, Helbok R, Galiano K, Pleifer C, Pfausler B, Brenneis C, Huck C, Engelhardt K, Obwegeser AA, Schmutzhard E. Efficacy of silver nanoparticles-impregnated external ventricular drain catheters in patients with acute occlusive hydrocephalus. Neurocrit Care. 2008;8(3):360–5. doi:10.1007/s12028-008-9071-1.

68. Johnson JR, Kuskowski MA, Wilt TJ. Systematic review: Antimicrobial urinary catheters to prevent catheter-associated urinary tract infection in hospitalized patients. Ann Intern Med. 2006;144(2):116–26.

69. Trautner BW. Management of catheter-associated urinary tract infection. Curr Opin Infect Dis. 2010;23(1):76–82. doi:10.1097/QCO.0b013e328334dda8.

70. Gray M, Willson M, Wilde M, Webb ML, Thompson D, Parker D, Harwood J, Callan L. Nursing interventions to reduce the risk of catheter-associated urinary tract infection part 2: staff education, monitoring, and care techniques. J Wound Ostomy Continence Nurs. 2009;36(2):137–54.

71. Gilbert RE, Harden M. Effectiveness of impregnated central venous catheters for catheter related blood stream infection: a systematic review. Curr Opin Infect Dis. 2008;21(3):235–45.

72. Karthaus M, Jaeger K, Zenz S, Juttner B, Ruschulte H, Kuse E, Heine J, Piepenbrock S, Ganser A. Reduction of catheter-related infections in neutropenic patients: a prospective controlled randomized trial using a chlorhexidine and silver sulfadiazine-impregnated central venous catheter. Ann Hematol. 2005;84(4):258–62. doi:10.1007/s00277-004-0972-6.

73. Rupp ME, Lisco SJ, Lipsett PA, Ped TM, Keating K, Civetta JM, Mermel LA, Lee D, Dellinger EP, Donahoe M, Giles D, Pfaller MA, Maki DG, Sherertz R. Effect of a second-generation venous catheter impregnated with chlorhexidine and silver sulfadiazine on central catheter – related infections – a randomized, controlled trial. Ann Intern Med. 2005;143(8):570–80.

74. Bukhari SS, Khare MD, Swann A, Spiers P, McLaren L, Myers J. Reduction of catheter-related colonisation by the use of a silver zeolite-impregnated central vascular catheter in adult critical care. J Infect. 2007;54(2):146–50. doi:10.1016/j.jinf.2006.03.002.

75. Kalfon P, De Vaumas C, Samba D, Boulet E, Lefrant JY, Eyraud D, Lherm T, Santoli F, Naija W, Riou B. Comparison of silver-impregnated with standard multi-lumen central venous catheters in critically ill patients. Crit Care Med. 2007;35(4):1032–9. doi:10.1097/01.Ccm.0000259378.53166.1b.

76. Landmann R, Gordon O, Slenters TV, Brunetto PS, Villaruz AE, Sturdevant DE, Otto M, Fromm KM. Silver coordination polymers for prevention of implant infection: thiol interaction, impact on respiratory chain enzymes, and hydroxyl radical induction. Antimicrob Agents Chemother. 2010;54(10):4208–18. doi:10.1128/Aac.01830-09.

77. Drake PL, Hazelwood KJ. Exposure-related health effects of silver and silver compounds: a review. Ann Occup Hyg. 2005;49(7):575–85.

78. Aberer W, Tomi NS, Kranke B. A silver man. Lancet. 2004;363(9408):532–2.

79. Johnston HJ, Hutchison G, Christensen FM, Peters S, Hankin S, Stone V. A review of the in vivo and in vitro toxicity of silver and gold particulates: particle attributes and biological mechanisms responsible for the observed toxicity. Crit Rev Toxicol. 2010;40(4):328–46. doi:10.3109/10408440903453074.

80. Sondi I, Salopek-Sondi B. Silver nanoparticles as antimicrobial agent: a case study on *E-coli* as a model for Gram-negative bacteria. J Colloid Interface Sci. 2004;275(1):177–82. doi:10.1016/j.jcis.2004.02.012.

81. Mayr M, Kim MJ, Wanner D, Helmut H, Schroeder J, Mihatsch MJ. Argyria and decreased kidney function: are silver compounds toxic to the kidney? Am J Kidney Dis. 2009;53(5):890–4. doi:10.1053/j.ajkd.2008.08.028.

82. Valiyaveettil S, AshaRani PV, Mun GLK, Hande MP. Cytotoxicity and genotoxicity of silver nanoparticles in human cells. ACS Nano. 2009;3(2):279–90. doi:10.1021/nn800596w.

83. Song JM, Pal S, Tak YK. Does the antibacterial activity of silver nanoparticles depend on the shape of the nanoparticle? A study of the gram-negative bacterium *Escherichia coli*. Appl Environ Microbiol. 2007;73(6):1712–20. doi:10.1128/Aem.02218-06.

84. Sharma VK, Panacek A, Kvitek L, Prucek R, Kolar M, Vecerova R, Pizurova N, Nevecna T, Zboril R. Silver colloid nanoparticles: synthesis, characterization, and their antibacterial activity. J Phys Chem B. 2006;110(33):16248–53. doi:10.1021/jp063826h.

85. Pratsinis SE, Sotiriou GA. Antibacterial activity of nanosilver ions and particles. Environ Sci Technol. 2010;44(14):5649–54. doi:10.1021/es101072s.

Chapter 12
Biomaterial–Host Interactions in Aseptic and Septic Conditions

Jukka Pajarinen, Yuya Takakubo, Zygmunt Mackiewicz, Michiaki Takagi, Eemeli Jämsen, Puyi Sheng, and Yrjö T. Konttinen

Abstract Implanted total joint replacement is initially osteointegrated via successive steps of inflammation, resorption of necrotic bone, bone matrix production and ultimately bone remodeling, and is largely mediated by the coordinated action of

J. Pajarinen, M.D.
Department of Anatomy, Institute of Biomedicine, University of Helsinki,
Haartmaninkatu 8, 63, Helsinki FI-00014, Finland
e-mail: jukka.s.pajarinen@helsinki.fi

Y. Takakubo, M.D., Ph.D.
Department of Medicine, Biomedicum Helsinki C402b, University of Helsinki,
Haartmaninkatu 8, 700, Helsinki 00029, Finland
e-mail: takakubo-y@med.id.yamagata-u.ac.jp

Z. Mackiewicz, Ph.D.
Department of Histology and Embryology, Medical University in Bialystok,
G. Washington 13, Bialystok 15-269, Poland
e-mail: zmzm.ackiewicz@gmail.com

M. Takagi, M.D., Ph.D.
Department of Orthopaedics, Yamagata University,
Iida-Nishi, Yamagata 990-9585, Japan
e-mail: mtakagi@med.id.yamagata-u.ac.jp

E. Jämsen
Department of Medicine, University of Helsinki,
Haartmaninkatu 8, Helsinki 00029, Finland
e-mail: eemeli.jamsen@helsinki.fi

P. Sheng, M.D., Ph.D.
Department of Joints, The First Affiliated Hospital,
Zhong Shan 2 Road #58, Guangzhou 510080, China
e-mail: shengpuyi@hotmail.com

Y.T. Konttinen, M.D., Ph.D.(✉)
Department of Medicine, Institute of Clinical Medicine, Biomedicum 1 Hus,
Haartmaninkatu 8, 700, Helsinki 00029, Finland
e-mail: yrjo.konttinen@helsinki.fi

osteoclasts and osteoblasts. Years later, a total joint replacement that has previously been well osteointergrated, can become loosened necessitating technically difficult and costly revision operations. Two different modes of prosthesis loosening have traditionally been distinguished, namely prosthesis infection, also known as septic loosening, and aseptic prosthesis loosening. Septic and aseptic prosthesis loosening have long been considered as two separate entities where septic loosening is due to chronic inflammation and accompanied osteolysis caused by bacterial infection of prosthesis components while aseptic loosening is driven by macrophages inflammatory foreign body reaction against biomaterial wear particles that are generated due to unavoidable abrasion between prosthesis components. During last decade this strict dichotomy between septic and aseptic prosthesis loosening has been questioned by observations that subclinical bacterial biofilms are present at last in some cases of aseptic prosthesis loosening and that the pro-inflammatory and osteolytic properties of wear particles are largely dependent on the presence of bacterial structural components adhering to their surfaces. The recognition of such bacterial product coated wear particles and subsequent activation of macrophages to inflammatory phenotype is possibly mediated by Toll-like receptors expressed in the interface tissues. Further studies are warranted to better characterize the role of subclinical bacterial biofilms in the aseptic prosthesis loosening. Peri-implant B lymphocyte and plasma cell infiltrates might provide additional diagnostic tools to detect such, low-grade, biofilm hidden implant infections.

Keywords Osseointegration • Host • Cytokine • Loosening • Receptors

12.1 Initial Prosthesis Integration

Initial stable fixation and correct prosthesis alignment are considered essential for long-term prosthesis survival, and thus in the primary surgery, firm contact with the surrounding bone tissue and prosthesis is sought. The early events in total hip replacement tissue integration are, however, relatively poorly understood as most of the research has focused on the pathophysiology of prosthesis loosening and not so much on the initial tissue integration.

When a foreign body object is implanted into bone tissue, it is rapidly and dynamically covered by proteins derived from plasma or tissue fluid, and it is thought that this protein coating mediates the initial interaction between the host and the prosthesis. Some proteins remain attached to the prosthesis while some are later detached: the factors governing the ultimate composition of the protein layer are not fully understood. If conditions are favorable, host cells adhere to this protein coating and start to produce their own extracellular matrix (ECM) that later calcifies to mature bone tissue. The gap between the prosthesis and surrounding bone is bridged from all sides. Micromotion during this stage is considered to be deleterious to initial osseointegration. This is why, according to the original Brånemark principle, dental root implants (fixtures, covered with the cover screw) are first left unloaded below the mucosal membrane, until they have been osseointegrated. This is not so easily applicable for joint replacement implants. Micromotion early on leads to formation of thick fibrotic interface tissue (see below) instead of bone tissue. It is often stated that bone formation surrounding implanted prosthesis is typically intramembranous ossification, while cartilage tissue and endochondral ossification is not typically seen in the periprosthetic tissue. In later stages of osseointegration, active bone remodeling is observed most likely to accommodate the mechanical forces transmitted to the bone-prosthesis interface [30]. However, early works by Willert and Semlitsch [43] and Jasty et al. [16] suggest a different three-phase process (see below).

There is evidence that cemented and uncemented prostheses are initially integrated in a different way. In cemented prosthesis, it seems that the surgical trauma and the toxic effects as well as exodermal reaction of bone cement cause an initial rim of bone necrosis into the implant bed and that the prosthesis is integrated by active remodeling of this necrotic bone. Necrotic bone is resorbed and replaced by bone trabeculae that grow into the immediate proximity of relatively smooth bone cement surface [43]. These bone trabeculae are further remodeled, most likely to better accommodate mechanical forces transmitted to the interface, into a secondary dense neocortex that surrounds the cement mantle and is connected to the primary outer femoral cortex via trabecular bone struts [16]. In uncemented prosthesis, on- and ingrowth of bone into porous osteoconductive coatings is typically observed [9]. In both instances a marginal rim of damaged and necrotic bone is initially formed around the implant (necrotic phase). This local bone necrosis and associated inflammation induces production of macrophage-colony stimulating factor (M-CSF) and receptor activator of nuclear factor kappa B ligand (RANKL) from local osteoblasts and fibroblasts. Together these mediators induce osteoclast differentiation and stimulate their activation, leading in to the resorption of damaged bone during the weeks following the surgery. This removal of damaged bone by osteoclast is closely followed by production of new bone matrix by osteoblasts (repair phase). The differentiation and function of osteoblasts is tightly coupled to and regulated by osteoclast function, e.g. by various factors released both from the resorbed bone matrix e.g. transforming growth factor beta (TGF-β) or produced by activated osteoclasts e.g. sphingosine-1-phosphate (S1P) (Matsuo and Irie 2008, Pederson et al. 2008). Later on, after 1-2 years, peri-implant bone starts to undergo remodeling as induced by the forces mediated to the peri-implant bone tissue (remodeling phase) [24, 29].

Earlier attempts to improve osseointegration have focused on production of osteoconductive surfaces, like porous titanium oxide, calcium phosphate, or hydroxyapatite [41]. Appreciation of the above-mentioned osteoclast and osteoblast functional coupling, the paradigm should perhaps be reevaluated: maybe the most osteoattractive surface would first stimulate osteoclastogenesis and activity, which then upon activation of the activation-reversal-formation cycle (ARF) in a natural way would stimulate peri-implant bone formation.

The extent to which bone directly attaches to the prosthesis or bone cement varies, and often more or less thin layer of connective tissue termed interface tissue separates bone from prosthesis or bone cement's surface. This thin layer of interface tissue is composed of fibrous loose connective tissue in which mostly fibroblasts and occasional macrophages are seen. The thickness of the interface tissue is considered to be a function of initial prosthesis micromotion, and especially in well-osseointegrated uncemented prosthesis, only a very thin layer of noncollagenous acellular connective tissue, consisting of, e.g., osteopontin and bone sialoprotein, is observed [30].

The artificial joint cavity is enclosed by fibrous pseudocapsule which closely resembles joint capsule surrounding normal joints. Pseudocapsule is on the internal side (joint cavity) lined by a synovial membrane-like tissue (pseudosynovial membrane), the lining of which is, like the actual synovial lining, composed of type A macrophage-like cells and type B fibroblasts-like cells, which take normally care of the apoptotic cell rests as part of the reticuloendothelial system (RES) of the body and produce and regulate the composition of pseudosynovial fluid (e.g., by synthesizing hyaluronan).

12.2   Septic Loosening

Postoperative prosthesis infection is a severe complication of total hip replacement surgery that necessitates large-scale, typically two-stage, revision operations and long-term antibiotic treatments. Extensive pre-, intra-, and postoperative measures are undertaken to prevent this devastating postoperative complication [17], and currently, the risk of developing a deep prosthetic joint infection after total hip replacement operation is considered to be less than 1 % [46].

Postoperative prosthesis infections are typically classified by using the time of onset into three groups: early postoperative infections (<1 month postoperatively), late chronic infections (usually 6–24 months postoperatively), and hematogenous infections (usually occurring 2 years after arthroplasty or later) [6]. Most of the purulent prosthesis infections that develop early after the operation are caused by virulent bacteria (e.g., *Staphylococcus aureus*) that particularly in the early postoperative infections may have gained access to the prosthetic joint already during the primary operation. Similarly high virulent bacteria may colonize the prosthesis via hematogenous route and cause purulent prosthesis infections several years after the original implantation. These infections are usually accompanied by symptoms and signs of systemic inflammation as well as elevated C-reactive protein (CRP) and erythrocyte sedimentation rates (ESR) and typically do not cause diagnostic problems.

A key characteristic of the prosthesis infections is the formation of a so-called biofilm [40, 46]. Relatively low-virulent bacteria (e.g., coagulase-negative staphylococci, *Staphylococcus epidermidis*) gain access to the prosthesis most often during the primary surgery or more rarely later via circulation, adhere to the prosthesis surfaces, multiply, and produce mucous extracellular polymeric substance (EPS, "bacterial slime") or matrix that effectively protects them from host defense mechanisms as well as antibiotics. Bacteria in biofilm may also set themselves into quiescent nondividing and intercommunicating (quorum sensing) state and thereby survive extended periods of time.

According to the "race for the surface" model, the fate of the implant and ultimate tissue integration depends on how rapidly after the initial implantation it is covered by host cells: there is a competition between microbial and host cell adhesion [13]. If the race is won by the cells of the host, then the surface is covered by protective host tissue and is in the future less vulnerable to bacterial colonization than the abiotic ("dead") implant surface. Alternatively, if the race is won by bacteria, the implant surface is rapidly covered by a biofilm. As the foreign-body-related bacterial biofilms are exceedingly difficult to eradicate and often require the removal of an implant, great effort is put into the development of biomaterials that would resist bacterial adhesion and biofilm formation while at the same time, the same material should support the growth of host cells, thereby giving them a head start in the race for the surface. Thus far, the most promising results utilizing this theory have been acquired by using antibiotic-loaded bone cement and perioperative antibiotic prophylaxis which seems to improve prosthesis survival rates, probably by diminishing initial growth of planktonic bacteria during the early phases and possibly preventing the colonization of the implant surface [8].

The natural course and prognosis of low-grade, biofilm-hidden prosthesis infection is variable and currently poorly understood. It can be, however, postulated that the outcome is determined by both the bacterial virulence factors and immunecompetence of the host. Such an infection may remain quiescent for years but can also become activated to purulent prosthesis infection after the host immune system is compromised. Recent evidence also indicates that quiescent prosthesis infections may produce a clinical picture indistinguishable from aseptic loosening, even more so because biofilm-hidden bacteria are difficult to demonstrate using conventional bacterial culture methods [25].

Accordingly also, the diagnostic criteria for prosthesis infection are somewhat controversial and vary between studies. Generally used diagnostic criteria require that purulent bacterial culture-positive infection can be demonstrated, e.g., open surgical wound infection or sinus communicating to the joint, purulence of the synovial fluid, growth of the same microorganism in two or more deep samples (to avoid false-positive culture results due to contamination), or acute inflammation in histological intraoperative frozen sections, often defined as more than five neutrophils per high-power field [15, 38]. As subclinical prosthesis infections are difficult to demonstrate using conventional bacterial cultures and, furthermore, biofilm residing infection be largely concealed also from the innate immune system as bacteria are released from biofilm only sporadically (so that short-lived neutrophils are not necessarily continuously present in the interface tissue), it is possible that these diagnostic criteria might underestimate the prevalence of implant related infection.

The osteolytic lesions in late chronic and hematogenous septic states, characterized by positive bacterial cultures and prosthesis loosening, are composed largely of hypertrophied lining tissue covering loose connective tissue infiltrated by various inflammatory cell populations, while also large areas of necrosis and fibrosis are seen. In cell-rich areas, typically sheet-like macrophage infiltrates and occasional giant cell formation is seen, and it likely represents underlying foreign body reaction and developing aseptic osteolysis (see below). In purulent prosthesis infections, large neutrophil infiltrates are typically seen, as well as large lymphocyte infiltrates consisting of CD4+ T-helper lymphocytes and CD20+ B lymphocytes, as well as plasma cells. Thus, in contrast to the aseptic loosening in which osteolysis seems to be driven primarily by the activation of the innate immunity and macrophages (see below), the activation of both the innate (including also neutrophils) and adaptive immune system (lymphocytes, plasma cells) is typically observed in septic loosening. Accordingly, we have proposed that especially the presence of dividing B lymphocytes and mature antibody-producing plasma cells in the peri-implant tissues might be an additional useful histopathological marker for the biofilm-hidden prosthesis infections as their role in purely aseptic loosening seems unlikely [28] and metal hypersensitivity in metal-on-metal joint replacements has different histological characteristics, e.g., perivascular infiltrates of T and B lymphocytes and plasma cells, high endothelial venules, massive fibrin exudation, accumulation of macrophages with drop-like inclusions, and infiltrates of eosinophilic granulocytes and necrosis [42].

12.3 Aseptic Loosening

Aseptic prosthesis loosening is the most common reason for total replacement failure and leading cause of revision total hip replacement operations [19]. Aseptic loosening is a late complication of total hip replacement, which typically develops after 15–20 years of service. Prosthesis loosening is called aseptic when there are no clinical signs of infection and the diagnostic criteria presented above for septic loosening are not fulfilled, and thus traditionally, the involvement of microbes to the pathogenesis of aseptic loosening has been excluded by its definition. Several theories of aseptic loosening have been suggested but currently best established of these is the so-called particle disease theory [14, 31, 34], which however may represent a consequence rather than the reasons of loosening. It is also difficult to explain why many patients with apparently numerous implant-derived wear particles do not develop aseptic loosening. As a result of abrasion between prosthesis components, depending on the biomaterials used, high numbers of bone cement, high molecular weight, or highly cross-linked polyethylene, metal, or ceramic particles are generated through the course of prosthesis life span at the various gliding surfaces of the often modular implants and at the bone/bone cement interfaces. It is generally accepted that it is this wear particle load that causes chronic peri-implant foreign body reaction and inflammation and at least contributes to osteolysis. The pumping action and the pressure waves generated in the pseudosynovial fluid dissect the host-implant interface, increase the effective joint size, and effectively drive wear particles to the peri-implant tissues. The synovial lining is extended from its original location from the pseudojoint, to cover also the interface membrane with surface contact with synovial fluid until the so-called effective joint space surrounds more or less the whole prosthesis [33] so that, e.g., x-ray contrast medium injected into the pseudojoint can be seen to surround almost all of the perimetry of the joint implants.

The osteolytic lesions in aseptic loosening are composed of hypertrophied interface tissue covered by synovial lining and containing chronic foreign body inflammation, including chronic foreign body giant cells and granulomas, with activated osteoclasts but also osteoblasts lining the host bone, which discloses a high metabolic turnover rate [35]. Underlying well-vascularized loose connective tissue is heavily infiltrated by monocyte/macrophages organized into sheet-like formations. High amounts of metal or high molecular weight polyethylene wear particles are phagocytosed by these macrophages. Some of the macrophages have fused to form multinucleated foreign body giant cells that often surround larger foreign bodies. At the bone interface, tissue interface increased osteoclast formation, and active bone resorption is typically seen, coupled to a high bone formation rate (but with a negative net balance). Tissue fibroblasts, which form the second most prevalent cell type in the aseptic interface tissue, are squeezed between the sheets of macrophages. Increased numbers of mast cells are also detected. Some scattered CD4+ T-helper lymphocytes are observed, whereas, in sharp contrast to the septic interface, B cells, plasma cells, and neutrophils are only rarely, if at all, seen. Typically more quiescent areas are also seen surrounding the loosened prosthesis, and these are mostly composed of relatively dense fibrotic tissue, the fibroblast being the most prevalent cell type (implant capsule). Again, cemented and uncemented prostheses seem to somewhat differ in this regard, the osteolytic lesions characterized by massive monocyte/macrophage infiltrates being somewhat more prominent in cemented prosthesis, whereas more fibrotic tissue scar with fibroblasts is observed surrounding uncemented prosthesis [10]. As the survival rates of cemented and uncemented prostheses are about the same, the clinical meaning of these findings remains unclear.

Retrieval studies using several methodologies have demonstrated that a chronic inflammation reaction is ongoing in these periprosthetic osteolytic lesions. Increased production of a vast array of pro-inflammatory chemokines, cytokines, and growth factors including MCP-1, MIP-1α, TNFα, IL-1β, IL-6, IL-8, M-CSF, GM-CSF, and VEGF are observed both in the peri-implant tissues as well as in pseudosynovial fluid [11, 14, 31, 45]. The osteoclast and foreign body giant cell formation is most likely driven by the locally increased RANKL/OPG ratio [22].

As the monocyte/macrophage and foreign body giant cells are by far the most dominant cell type in the periprosthetic tissue, the wear-particle-activated macrophage has long been considered to play a pivotal role in the development of aseptic loosening. This purely histopathological notion is supported by the observed peri-implant pro-inflammatory chemokine and cytokine profile indicating primarily the involvement of innate immunity, whereas cytokine characteristics for adaptive immunity are rarely seen. Indeed, several studies have demonstrated that monocyte/macrophages challenged in vitro with wear particles are activated to produce a wide variety of chemokines (e.g., IL-8, MCP-1, and MIP-1α/β), pro-inflammatory cytokines (e.g., TNFα, IL-1β, IL-6), and growth factors (VEGF, M-CSF, GM-CSF), all of which are also seen in the periprosthetic tissue [11, 14, 31, 44]. This chronic inflammation reaction leads to the further recruitment of monocytes and osteoclast precursors to the periprosthetic tissue. Furthermore, pro-inflammatory cytokines, and to some extent also wear particles directly, drive the production of RANKL in mesenchymal cells and at the same time suppress the production of OPG and bone formation, which, together with the pro-inflammatory cytokines, create an environment which favors ostoclastogenesis, bone resorption, and finally prosthesis loosening [18, 21].

12.4 Toll-Like Receptors in Prosthesis Loosening

It is generally accepted that aseptic osteolysis is primarily driven by the wear particles that cause macrophage activation and chronic inflammatory reaction that shift the balance from bone formation to bone destruction. The exact molecular mechanisms by which wear particles are recognized by the host cells and how they cause macrophage activation have, however, remained elusive.

The strict distinction between the septic and aseptic loosening has been questioned as it has become increasingly clear that bacterial products or biofilms can often be detected from the seemingly aseptic interface tissues and explanted prosthesis if special sampling methods (e.g., polymerase chain reaction, lipopolysaccharide/LPS detection, sonication of the explanted implants) are applied [25, 25, 38, 39]. The role of subclinical biofilms in the aseptic loosening is further supported by observations showing that antibiotic-loaded bone cement effectively reduced the occurrence of so-called aseptic loosenings [8]. Likewise, several in vitro and in vivo studies have demonstrated that wear particles of various natures as such are, in fact, relatively inert in in vitro experiments and that several of their previously observed pro-inflammatory and osteoclastogenic properties can be better explained by hydrophobic bacterial structural products (e.g., LPS) effectively adhering to their foreign body surfaces, owning to the high-surface area of the small wear debris particles [3–5, 7].

Toll-like receptors (TLRs) are a family of ten different germ-line-encoded, transmembrane pattern recognition receptor proteins of the innate immunity that enable the immune system to recognize numerous evolutionary well-conserved bacterial-, viral-, and fungal-derived structures, so-called pathogen-associated molecular patterns (PAMPs) [1, 2, 23]. TLR stimulation with an appropriate ligand causes cell activation and, e.g., via activation of pro-inflammatory transcription factor, nuclear factor kappa beta (NFκB) production of several pro-inflammatory cytokines, which then further activates the innate and also adaptive immunity.

We and others have suggested that microbial product-coated wear particles are in the peri-implant tissues initially recognized by macrophages via their TLRs and that TLRs mediate the particle-induced cell activation [20, 36, 37]. Numerous studies have furthermore demonstrated that the shape, size, number, and biomaterial composition of wear particles seem to have an effect on the quantity and quality of the cytokines produced by the activated macrophage. These effects of particle size and biomaterial composition are likely, at least in part, to be mediated by the different binding of PAMP molecules on the implant and wear debris surface.

Our studies indicate that TLRs are extensively expressed in the macrophages of the peri-implant tissues, and thus the prosthesis interface is very reactive to any TLR ligand present [20]. Especially noteworthy is the presence of TLR2, TLR4, TLR6, and TLR9 in the peri-implant tissues as these are the TLRs that recognize structural products of those gram-positive and gram-negative bacteria that are most prevalent in aseptic loosening.

The high expression of TLRs in the periprosthetic tissue is potentially very interesting as, in addition to traditional exogenous, foreign ligands, also several endogenous TLR ligands have recently been identified [32]. These molecules, called alarmins, are typically released from necrotic cells (e.g., heat shock proteins and high-mobility group box 1, HMGB1) or fragmented extracellular matrix (e.g., heparan sulfate, versican, biglycan, low molecular weight hyaluronic acid, fibrinogen), and they are recognized by TLR2 and TLR4. Alarmins might be released due to biomechanical loading, low-grade chronic inflammation, and tissue necrosis in the interface tissues. They may be concentrated locally and preserved extended periods protected from degradation perhaps in part by binding to the surface of wear particles, but at the same time opsonizing them for TLR2- and TLR4-expressing monocyte/macrophages. They would exert pro-inflammatory effects in the absence of bacteria or PAMPs. Internalization would then be dependent on both the opsonins and the physical size of the particle, which via the multiplicity of the ligand-receptor binding strengthen the interaction and facilitate endocytosis.

Direct evidence that TLRs are involved in the wear particle recognition is emerging. In a study conducted by Pearl et al., it was shown that knockout mice lacking MyD88, an important adaptor molecule in the TLR intracellular signaling machinery, did not develop PMMA particle induced osteolysis whereas wild-type mice did. Similarly, in macrophages isolated from these MyD88$^{-/-}$ knockouts, PMMA particle induced production of TNF-α was clearly reduced. These observations demonstrate that TLR signaling pathways are involved in to the pro-inflammatory response and accompanied osteolysis elicited by PMMA particles (Pearl et al. 2011). Greenfield et al. investigated the role of TLR2 and TLR4 in the recognition and osteolysis caused by PAMP contaminated titanium particles (Greenfield at al. 2010). Using mice model of particle induced osteolysis and TLR2$^{-/-}$, TLR4$^{-/-}$ and TLR2$^{-/-}$/TLR4$^{-/-}$ double knockout mice, as well as wild type control mice, Greenfield et al. show that the magnitude of osteolysis caused by titanium particles was greater if particles where contaminated with PAMPs (either with gram positive bacterial lipoteichoic acid or gram negative bacteria lipopolysaccharide) and that this effect was dependent on the existence of corresponding PAMP receptors TLR2 or TLR4. Corresponding results were obtained from in vitro experiments in which bone marrow macrophages isolated from these mice strains and subsequently challenged with titanium particles up-regulated TNF-α mRNA expression if LTA or LPS contaminated particles and their corresponding receptors TLR2 and TLR4 were also present on the macrophages.

These results indicate that TLRs are directly involved in titanium particle mediated inflammation and accompanied osteolysis, especially if particles are contaminated with PAMPs.

Particle coating by danger signals or danger-associated molecular patterns/ DAMPS (exogenous PAMPs or endogenous alarmins) and subsequent TLR stimulation is probably crucial in inducing a shift in macrophage activation state. Our recent findings indicate that M1 macrophage polarization (or so-called classical activation), induced among others by TLR signaling, greatly enhances, while M2a macrophage polarization (or alternative activation) suppresses the pro-inflammatory response provoked by wear particles. Interestingly, however, the phagocytotic activity and the cell mobility of the M2 cells were far greater than that of the M1 cells, and it thus seems that M2-polarized macrophages constrain wear particles into the intracellular compartment without inflammatory and osteolytic reactions, while M1-polarized macrophages are easily irritated to produce great amounts of pro-inflammatory cytokines stimulating osteolysis, possibly due to their increased TLR expression and enhancement of TLR signaling.

Thus, the development of aseptic osteolysis is likely, not only a function of wear particle load or the exact physicochemical properties of the particles, but is also crucially determined by the balance of pro- and anti-inflammatory factors prevailing in the peri-implant tissues. It has become increasingly clear that using special sampling methods, subclinical bacterial biofilms or bacterial structural components can be found from seemingly aseptic interface tissues, together with endogenous TLR ligands. Together, locally, before being diluted by diffusion, these factors could shift the local tissue homeostasis from an anti-inflammatory scavenging state to a pro-inflammatory osteolytic state, thus creating a vicious circle that in the end leads to aseptic loosening of the implant.

Acknowledgment   This study was supported by the Sigrid Juselius Foundation, by the Helsinki University Central Hospital evo funds, Finska Läkaresällskapet, Wilhelm och Else Stockmanns Stiftelse, ORTON Orthopaedic Hospital of the Invalid Foundation, National Doctoral Programme of Musculoskeletal Disorders and Biomaterials, Danish Council for Strategic Research, and European Science Foundation "Regenerative Medicine" RNP.

References

1. Aderem A, Ulevitch RJ. Toll-like receptors in the induction of the innate immune response. Nature. 2000;406(6797):782–7.
2. Akira S, Takeda K, Kaisho T. Toll-like receptors: critical proteins linking innate and acquired immunity. Nat Immunol. 2001;2(8):675–80.
3. Bi Y, Collier TO, Goldberg VM, Anderson JM, Greenfield EM. Adherent endotoxin mediates biological responses of titanium particles without stimulating their phagocytosis. J Orthop Res. 2002;20:696–703.
4. Bi Y, Seabold JM, Kaar SG, Ragab AA, Goldberg VM, Anderson JM, Greenfield EM. Adherent endotosin on orthopedic wear particles stimulates cytokine production and osteoclast differentiation. J Bone Miner Res. 2001;16(11):2082–91.

5. Cho DR, Shanbhag AS, Hong CY, Baran GR, Goldring SR. The role of adsorbed endotoxin in particle-induced stimulation of cytokine release. J Orthop Res. 2002;20:704–13.
6. Coventry MB. Treatment of infections occurring in total hip surgery. Orthop Clin North Am. 1975;6(4):991–1003.
7. Daniels AU, Barnes FH, Charlebois SJ, Smith RA. Macrophage cytokine response to particles and lipopolysaccharide in vitro. J Biomed Mater Res. 2000;49:469–78.
8. Engesaeter LB, Lie SA, Espehaug B, Furnes O, Vollset SE, Havelin LI. Antibiotic prophylaxis in total hip arthroplasty: effects of antibiotic prophylaxis systemically and in bone cement on the revision rate of 22,170 primary hip replacements followed 0–14 years in the Norwegian Arthroplasty Register. Acta Orthop Scand. 2003;74(6):644–51.
9. Engh CA, Hooten Jr JP, Zettl-Schaffer KF, Ghaffarpour M, McGovern TF, Bobyn JD. Evaluation of bone ingrowth in proximally and extensively porous-coated anatomic medullary locking prostheses retrieved at autopsy. J Bone Joint Surg Am. 1995;77(6):903–10.
10. Goodman SB, Huie P, Song Y, Schurman D, Maloney W, Woolson S, Sibley R. Cellular profile and cytokine production at prosthetic interfaces. Study of tissues retrieved from revised hip and knee replacements. J Bone Joint Surg Br. 1998;80(3):531–9.
11. Goodman SB, Ma T. Cellular chemotaxis induced by wear particles from joint replacements. Biomaterials. 2010;31(19):5045–50.
12. Greenfield EM, Beidelschies MA, Tatro JM, Goldberg VM, Hise AG. Bacterial pathogen-associated molecular patterns stimulate biological activity of orthopaedic wear particles by activating cognate Toll-like receptors. J Biol Chem. 2010;285(42):32378–84.
13. Gristina AG. Biomaterial-centered infection: microbial adhesion versus tissue integration. Science. 1987;237:1588–95.
14. Holt G, Murnaghan C, Reilly J, Meek RM. The biology of aseptic osteolysis. Clin Orthop Relat Res. 2007;460:240–52.
15. Horan TC, Gaynes RP, Martone WJ, Jarvis WR, Emori TG. CDC definitions of nosocomial surgical site infections, 1992: a modification of CDC definitions of surgical wound infections. Infect Control Hosp Epidemiol. 1992;13(10):606–8.
16. Jasty M, Maloney WJ, Bragdon CR, Haire T, Harris WH. Histomorphological studies of the long-term skeletal responses to well fixed cemented femoral components. J Bone Joint Surg Am. 1990;72(8):1220–9.
17. Jämsen E, Furnes O, Engesaeter LB, Konttinen YT, Odgaard A, Stefánsdóttir A, Lidgren L. Prevention of deep infection in joint replacement surgery. Acta Orthop. 2010;81: 660–6.
18. Koreny T, Tunyogi-Csapó M, Gál I, Vermes C, Jacobs JJ, Glant TT. The role of fibroblasts and fibroblast-derived factors in periprosthetic osteolysis. Arthritis Rheum. 2006;54(10): 3221–32.
19. Kurtz S, Mowat F, Ong K, Chan N, Lau E, Halpern M. Prevalence of primary and revision total hip and knee arthroplasty in the United States from 1990 through 2002. J Bone Joint Surg Am. 2005;87:1487–97.
20. Lähdeoja T, Pajarinen J, Kouri VP, Sillat T, Salo J, Konttinen YT. Toll-like receptors and aseptic loosening of hip endoprosthesis-a potential to respond against danger signals? J Orthop Res. 2010;28(2):184–90.
21. Mandelin J, Li TF, Hukkanen M, Liljeström M, Salo J, Santavirta S, Konttinen YT. Interface tissue fibroblasts from loose total hip replacement prosthesis produce receptor activator of nuclear factor-kappaB ligand, osteoprotegerin, and cathepsin K. J Rheumatol. 2005;32(4): 713–20.
22. Mandelin J, Li TF, Liljeström M, Kroon ME, Hanemaaijer R, Santavirta S, Konttinen YT. Imbalance of RANKL/RANK/OPG system in interface tissue in loosening of total hip replacement. J Bone Joint Surg Br. 2003;85(8):1196–201.
23. Miyake K. Innate immune sensing of pathogens and danger signals by cell surface Toll-like receptors. Semin Immunol. 2007;19:3–10.
24. Matsuo K, Irie N. Osteoclast-osteoblast communication. Arch Biochem Biophys. 2008 May 15;473(2):201–9.

25. Nalepka JL, Lee MJ, Kraay MJ, Marcus RE, Goldberg VM, Chen X, Greenfield EM. Lipopolysaccharide found in aseptic loosening of patients with inflammatory arthritis. Clin Orthop Relat Res. 2006;451:229–35.

26. Nelson CL, McLaren AC, McLaren SG, Johnson JW, Smeltzer MS. Is aseptic loosening truly aseptic? Clin Orthop Relat Res. 2005;437:25–30.

27. Pajarinen J, Cenni E, Savarino L, Gomez-Barrena E, Tamaki Y, Takagi M, Salo J, Konttinen YT. Profile of toll-like receptor-positive cells in septic and aseptic loosening of total hip arthroplasty implants. J Biomed Mater Res. 2010;94(1):84–92.

28. Pearl JI, Ma T, Irani AR, Huang Z, Robinson WH, Smith RL, Goodman SB. Role of the Toll-like receptor pathway in the recognition of orthopedic implant wear-debris particles. Biomaterials. 2011;32(24):5535–42.

29. Pederson L, Ruan M, Westendorf JJ, Khosla S, Oursler MJ. Regulation of bone formation by osteoclasts involves Wnt/BMP signaling and the chemokine sphingosine-1-phosphate. Proc Natl Acad Sci U S A. 2008 Dec 30;105(52):20764–9.

30. Puleo DA, Nanci A. Understanding and controlling the bone-implant interface. Biomaterials. 1999;20(23–24):2311–21.

31. Purdue PE, Koulouvaris P, Potter HG, Nestor BJ, Sculco TP. The cellular and molecular biology of periprosthetic osteolysis. Clin Orthop Relat Res. 2007;454:251–61.

32. Rifkin IR, Leadbetter EA, Busconi L, Viglianti G, Marshak-Rothstein A. Toll-like receptors, endogenous ligands, and systemic autoimmune disease. Immunol Rev. 2005;204:27–42.

33. Schmalzried TP, Jasty M, Harris WH. Periprosthetic bone loss in total hip arthroplasty. Polyethylene wear debris and the concept of the effective joint space. J Bone Joint Surg Am. 1992;74(6):849–63.

34. Sundfeldt M, Carlsson LV, Johansson CB, Thomsen P, Gretzer C. Aseptic loosening, not only a question of wear: a review of different theories. Acta Orthop. 2006;77:177–97.

35. Takagi M, Santavirta S, Ida H, Ishii M, Takei I, Niissalo S, Ogino T, Konttinen YT. High-turnover periprosthetic bone remodeling and immature bone formation around loose cemented total hip joints. J Bone Miner Res. 2001;16:79–88.

36. Takagi M, Tamaki Y, Hasegawa H, Takakubo Y, Konttinen L, Tiainen VM, Lappalainen R, Konttinen YT, Salo J. Toll-like receptors in the interface membrane around loosening total hip replacement implants. J Biomed Mater Res. 2007;81(4):1017–26.

37. Tamaki Y, Takakubo Y, Goto K, Hirayama T, Sasaki K, Konttinen YT, Goodman SB, Takagi M. Increased expression of Toll-like receptors in aseptic loose periprosthetic tissues and septic synovial membranes around total hip implants. J Rheumatol. 2009;36(3):598–608.

38. Trampuz A, Piper KE, Jacobson MJ, Hanssen AD, Unni KK, Osmon DR, Mandrekar JN, Cockerill FR, Steckelberg JM, Greenleaf JF, Patel R. Sonication of removed hip and knee prostheses for diagnosis of infection. N Engl J Med. 2007;357(7):654–63.

39. Tunney MM, Patrick S, Curran MD, Ramage G, Hanna D, Nixon JR, Gorman SP, Davis RI, Anderson N. Detection of prosthetic hip infection at revision arthroplasty by immunofluorescence microscopy and PCR amplification of the bacterial 16S rRNA gene. J Clin Microbiol. 1999;37:3281–90.

40. van de Belt H, Neut D, Schenk W, van Horn JR, van der Mei HC, Busscher HJ. Infection of orthopedic implants and the use of antibiotic-loaded bone cements. A review. Acta Orthop Scand. 2001;72(6):557–71.

41. Voigt JD, Mosier M. Hydroxyapatite (HA) coating appears to be of benefit for implant durability of tibial components in primary total knee arthroplasty. A systematic review of the literature and meta-analysis of 14 trials and 926 evaluable total knee arthroplasties. Acta Orthop. 2011;82:448–59.

42. Willert HG, Buchhorn GH, Fayyazi A, Flury R, Windler M, Köster G, Lohmann CH. Metal-on-metal bearings and hypersensitivity in patients with artificial hip joints. A clinical and histomorphological study. J Bone Joint Surg Am. 2005;87:28–36.

43. Willert HG, Semlitsch M. Reactions of the articular capsule to wear products of artificial joint prostheses. J Biomed Mater Res. 1977;11(2):157–64.

44. Xu JW, Konttinen YT, Lassus J, Natah S, Ceponis A, Solovieva S, Aspenberg P, Santavirta S. Tumor necrosis factor-alpha (TNF-alpha) in loosening of total hip replacement (THR). Clin Exp Rheumatol. 1996;14:643–8.
45. Xu JW, Konttinen YT, Waris V, Pätiälä H, Sorsa T, Santavirta S. Macrophage-colony stimulating factor (M-CSF) is increased in the synovial-like membrane of the periprosthetic tissues in the aseptic loosening of total hip replacement (THR). Clin Rheumatol. 1997;16:243–8.
46. Zimmerli W, Trampuz A, Ochsner PE. Prosthetic-joint infections. N Engl J Med. 2004; 351(16):1645–54.

Chapter 13
Influence of Wear Particles on Local and Systemic Immune System

Emmanuel Gibon and Stuart B. Goodman

Abstract Decreasing periprosthetic osteolysis due to wear particles is a current challenge and an on-going research endeavor to prolong the longevity of joint replacements. The aim of this chapter is to provide the reader keys to the understanding of how the immune system interacts with metallic and non metallic wear particles and other byproducts from joint replacements. The local and systemic immune system is involved in a complex network of chemokines, cytokines, and different cell types which in the end leads to inflammation and a foreign body reaction.

Keywords Wear debris • Immune reactions • Cytokines • Cells

13.1 Wear Particles

Wear particles are produced by different types of bearing surfaces. Bozic et al. [1] have shown that metal-on-polyethylene is the most commonly used bearing surface, followed by metal-on-metal, and then ceramic-on-ceramic. Related to this fact, the same author has shown that metal-on-metal bearing surfaces are associated with a higher risk of periprosthetic joint infection for total hip arthroplasty (THA) [2]. Aseptic loosening is the most common cause of failure for THA, accounting for up to two-thirds of hip revisions [3], and is the second most common reason for total knee arthroplasty (THA) revisions [4]. Given the fact

E. Gibon, M.D. (✉)
Department of Orthopaedic Surgery, Stanford University School of Medicine,
300 Pasteur Dr, Edwards Bldg. R116, Stanford, CA 94305, USA

Department of Orthopaedic Surgery, Bichat Teaching Hospital,
Paris School of Medicine, Paris VII University, Paris, France
e-mail: egibon@stanford.edu

S.B. Goodman, M.D., Ph.D.
Department of Orthopaedic Surgery, Stanford University School of Medicine,
450 Broadway Street M/C 6342, Redwood City, CA 94063, USA
e-mail: goodbone@stanford.edu

R. Trebše (ed.), *Infected Total Joint Arthroplasty*,
DOI 10.1007/978-1-4471-2482-5_13, © Springer-Verlag London 2012

Table 13.1 Characteristics of wear debris from different bearing surfaces

Bearing surface	Particles size	Wear rate (mm³/10⁶ cycles)	References
UHMWPE-on-CoCr	<1.0 μm	≈ 15–80	[5, 6]
HXLPE-on-CoCr		≈ 2	
Metal-on-metal	20–90 nm	0.02–0.32	[7, 8, 10, 43]
Alumina-on-alumina	Bimodal size distribution	0.09–0.15	[9, 11]

UHMWPE ultra high molecular weight polyethylene, *HXLPE* highly cross-linked polyethylene, *CoCr* cobalt-chrome

that the number of THA and TKA revisions will increase 137 and 601 %, respectively, over the next 25 years, increasing the lifetime of joint replacements is a current challenge.

The size of wear particles is dependent on the bearing surface from which they come: polyethylene particles (conventional and highly cross-linked) are submicron [5, 6], metal particles are nanometer [7, 8] (20–90 nm), and ceramic wear particles have a bimodal size distribution [9] with nanometer-sized (5–20 nm) and larger particles (0.2–10 μm). Characteristics of wear debris are summarized in Table 13.1.

13.2 Orthopedic Wear Debris and the Immune System

13.2.1 The Immune System

The immune response to orthopedic wear debris involves either the innate or the adaptive immune system. Their features are summarized in Table 13.2.

13.2.2 Local Immune Response

13.2.2.1 Nonmetallic Particles

Production of polyethylene (PE) particles leads to a nonspecific macrophage-mediated foreign body reaction [10]. Locally, PE particles produced from joint replacements are able to move within the whole prosthetic bed [11] (the effective joint space) and to interact with surrounding tissues, resident phagocytic macrophages, and osteoblasts and finally mediate local paracrine and autocrine events. Macrophages become activated either by phagocytosis [12] of PE particles or simply by cell membrane contact without phagocytosis. Activation occurs through receptors present in the outer cell membrane (CD11b, CD14, Toll-like receptors, etc.). The Toll-like receptors (TLRS)

Table 13.2 Features of innate and adaptive immune systems

| Innate | | Acquired = adaptive = specific | | | |
		Type I	Type II	Type III	Type IV
Synonym	Nonspecific, natural	Anaphylaxis	Cytotoxic	Immune-complex	Cell-mediated
Time elapsed	Minutes to hours	Seconds to minutes	Hours to a day	Hours to a day	2–3 days
Specific immune	TLRs	IgE	IgG, IgM	IgG, IgM	T-cell reactant
Memory	No memory	Memory	Memory	Memory	Memory
Cells	Macrophages, dendritic cells, NK cells	Neutrophils, eosinophils	Cytotoxic T-cell activity	Neutrophils, macrophages	Lymphocytes
Wear particle response	Polymers, ceramics, and in some cases metals	Non-involved	Non-involved	Non-involved	In some cases, metals

are known to function in the innate immune response [13]. TLRs are activated by different types of stimuli and act through an adapter protein called myeloid differentiation primary response gene 88 (MyD88) to induce activation of nuclear factor such as nuclear factor kappa B (NFκB). In in vitro and in vivo studies, Pearl et al. have shown a main role played by MyD88 for TLR signaling when macrophages were challenged with PMMA particles [14]. Macrophages are the key cells involved in the local reaction and act as a trigger for the local and systemic response. Indeed, macrophages are the most abundant cells found in histological studies from retrieval tissues [15–17]. Activation of macrophages occurs through different intracellular pathways. Among them, p38 mitogen-activated protein kinase (MAP kinase) and JNK MAP kinase are important [18]. The next step is the local release of pro-inflammatory mediators such as cytokines, chemokines, growth factors, and others. Basically, release of pro-inflammatory cytokines is mediated by the activation of NFκB through the intracellular MAP-kinase pathway in activated macrophages. Therefore, high levels of pro-inflammatory factors are released in the surrounding tissues, as shown in a retrieval study comparing cemented and cementless implant groups [19]. Using submicron clinically relevant UHMWPE particles, Green et al. found the same results: increases of both TNF-α, IL-1β, IL-6, and prostaglandin E$_2$ (PGE$_2$) [20]. Locally, chemokines are also released by activated macrophages. Monocyte chemoattractant protein-1 belongs to the γ chemokine subfamily (C–C chemokines) and is an immediate early stress-responsive factor [21]. Epstein et al. have shown an increase of mononuclear cell pro-inflammatory gene (MCP-1, TNF-α, IL-1β, IL-6) in an in vivo murine model. Another relevant chemokine locally released is macrophage inhibitory molecule-1 (two main isoforms: MIP-1α and MIP-1β). MIP-1 is released by activated macrophages and T lymphocytes; Nakashima et al. have shown high levels of MIP-1α and MCP-1 when macrophages from retrieved periprosthetic tissues have been challenged with PMMA particles in vitro. MIP-1α will enhance the release of IL-1 and IL-6 affecting neighboring cells in a paracrine manner [22].

Locally, other resident cells take part in the immune response:

a. Osteoblasts

TNF-α released by locally activated macrophages [23] will stimulate osteoblasts to release granulocyte macrophage colony-stimulating factor (GM-CSF), IL-6, and PGE$_2$. GM-CSF will enhance the release of reactive oxygen species (ROS) such as nitric oxide (NO) which, in turn, activates osteoclastic bone resorption [24]. High levels of inducible NO synthase (iNOS) have been found in retrieval study by Moilanen et al. [25]. Macrophages challenged with zirconia or PMMA particles are also able to enhance release of NO [26, 27]. Locally, NO will promote osteolysis through pro-inflammatory factor pathway such as AP-1 and NFκB. Osteoblasts also express receptor activator of nuclear factor κB ligand (RANKL) which belongs to the tumor necrosis factor (TNF) superfamily. RANKL will bind its receptor (RANK) expressed by bone-marrow-derived osteoclast progenitors and mature osteoclasts which enhance local osteoclastogenesis supporting the differentiation, activation, and survival of osteoclasts. When retrieved tissues from primary total hip arthroplasty (THA) were compared to revision tissues, higher levels of RANKL were found in revision group [28, 29].

b. Osteoclasts

Locally osteoclast-like cell growth and differentiation [30] is enhanced by TGF-α and osteoclastic bone resorption [31] as well. PMMA particles increase the number of osteoclasts as shown by Clohisy et al. in an in vitro study in which bone-marrow-derived murine osteoclasts were challenged with PMMA particles [32]. Osteoclasts mobility is increased by local release of IL-8 from activated macrophages, mesenchymal stem cells, and osteoblasts [33].

c. Mesenchymal stem cells (MSCs)

MSCs are very abundant within bone marrow stroma [34, 35]. Proliferation and differentiation of bone-marrow-derived MSCs is decreased by PMMA particles as shown by Chiu et al. in an in vitro study. Likewise, in a similar study, Huang et al. have shown a decrease of chemotaxis of human MSCs (hMSCs) when cultured in a condition media from UHMWPE particle-exposed macrophages [36].

d. Multinucleated giant cells (MGCs)

Also called polykaryons, foreign body giant cells have been widely found within the bone-implant interface [37, 38]. MGCs come from fusion of multiple macrophages in response to hematopoietic growth factors [39] (GM-CSF) and interleukins (IL-3, IL-4) [40, 41]. Adhesion molecules have also been reported to be involved in the MGCs development: intercellular adhesion molecule-1 (ICAM-1/CD54) and the receptor CR3 (CD11b/CD18) expressed by multinucleated giant cells [42]. Locally, the presence of MGCs increases both osteoclastic bone resorption and osteoclast-like cell growth and differentiation by their ability to release TGF-α and other factors.

13.2.2.2   Metallic Particles

Metallic particles are smaller by a factor 10 compared to the PE particles: most metal particles are less than 50 nm in diameter [7], and wear rate of metal-on-metal (MOM) implants ranges from 0.02 to 0.32 $mm^3/10^6$ cycles [43]. Retrieval studies have exhibited differences in the tissues surrounding MOM articulations compared to metal-on-polyethylene (MOP) bearing surfaces. Willert et al. [44] first described perivascular lymphocytic cuffing with accumulation of T lymphocytes around MOM implants. Park et al. [45] studied retrieved tissues from early osteolysis in MOM hip replacements. They found perivascular accumulation of CD63-positive T cells, CD68 macrophages, and high levels of IL-1β and TNF-α. They also performed skin-patch tests to assess hypersensitivity to metal which were positive (higher rate of hypersensitivity) for patients with early osteolysis. Davies et al. [46] had more "ulcerated" retrieved tissue from MOM hip replacements compared to MOP. Locally, metal particles are phagocytized by CD68 macrophages [47] which will act as antigen-presenting cells to T lymphocytes leading to a cell-mediated type IV immunological reaction. This hypothesis has been confirmed by Hallab et al. [48] in a study assessing lymphocytic responses to implant metal particles and by Lalor and Revell [49]. Both found high levels of IL-2 receptor expression (a sign of T-lymphocyte activation) when tissues (retrieved tissues or blood cells) were challenged with metal particles. Following activation, T-lymphocyte responses are increased by co-stimulation with CD28/CD86 between antigen-presenting cells and activated T cells [50]. Metal particles have effect on all relevant bone cells:

a. Osteoblasts

  Metal ions have important effects on cellular functions of osteoblasts. When cultured with chromium (Cr) ions, alkaline phosphatase (ALP) activity from osteoblasts is markedly decreased, especially with Cr (IV) [51]. Cobalt (Co) ions have adverse effects as well. As shown by Fleury et al., Co ions induce oxidized and nitrated proteins released from osteoblasts [52]. Metal ions also dramatically affect osteoblast proliferation. When cultured with Co ions, human osteoblast-like cells have shown a decrease in proliferation in a dose-dependent manner. Furthermore, Co ions also increased the production of IL-6, whereas collagen type I and osteocalcin release decreased [53]. Stainless steel (SS) ions also affect osteoblast as shown by Morais et al. In presence of SS ions, expression of ALP was altered and tissue mineralization retarded [54, 55].

b. Osteoclasts

  RANKL is a critical factor for osteoclast differentiation and proliferation. High levels of RANKL have been reported when osteoclasts and stromal cells have been cultured in the presence of titanium (Ti) particles. However, no increase in the number of osteoclast was found. Addition of a mechanical stimulation increased RANKL release even more [56]. Interestingly, when rat marrow cells were cultured with devitalized bone, a decrease in size and number of resorption pits in presence of Ti^{4+} and Cr^{6+} ions was observed [57].

c. Fibroblasts and macrophages

Fibroblasts take part in the local immune reaction, releasing pro-inflammatory mediators. Manlapaz et al. [58] challenged fibroblasts with titanium-aluminum-vanadium (Ti-Al-V) particles and found an increase of IL-6, PGE_2, and fibroblast growth factor (FGF), promoting fibrosis and scar formation locally. Fibroblasts are responsible for synthesis and deposition of type 1 collagen [59]. Metal ions also increase the production of free radicals: ROS and reactive nitrogen species (RNS). Interestingly, Shanbhag et al. [27] have found that the release of ROS by macrophages is dependent upon the type of particles: Ti-Al-V particles are the most stimulatory, followed by commercially pure titanium (CpTi) and PMMA. Generation of free radicals is due to a series of intracellular steps transforming Cr^{6+} ions into Cr^{3+} ions by oxidation. Thereafter, free radicals react with DNA inducing cross-links and damage to purine and pyrimidine bases [60]. Wolf et al. demonstrated the direct binding of Cr^{3+} to DNA, as well [61]. Moreover, in addition to DNA damage caused by free radicals, repair mechanisms are also affected by cobalt ions, namely, Co^{2+} and chrome ions Cr^{6+} [62].

13.2.3 Systemic Immune Response

13.2.3.1 Nonmetallic Particles

The foreign body reaction induced by nonmetallic particles, leading to a periprosthetic granulomatous lesion, is due to an accumulation of local macrophages and fibroblasts but also due to a systemic recruitment of cells from the bloodstream. As highlighted above, high levels of chemokines have been found in periprosthetic tissues. Recent studies have established a direct link between chemokines and systemic recruitment of cells. Using a murine particle infusion model into bone and clinically relevant particles, Ren et al. have demonstrated the systemic migration of macrophages induced by UHMWPE particles, PMMA particles accompanied by increased osteolysis [63, 64]. Such recruitment occurs through different chemokine-receptor axes: MCP-1 locally released by activated macrophages acts through its receptor CCR2 expressed by monocytes and activated NK cells [65], MIP-1α increases the systemic recruitment of macrophages [66] through several receptors (CCR1, CCR5), and IL-8 induces the chemotaxis of neutrophils and monocytes/macrophages through CXCR1 and CXCR2. Huang et al., using conditioned media from macrophages RAW 264.7 challenged by PMMA particles, have shown an increase of human MSCs (hMSCs) recruitment, which was markedly blocked by MCP-1α-neutralizing antibody [36].

13.2.3.2 Metallic Particles

The main systemic immune response to metallic particles is an emergence of a type IV delayed immune response. This hypersensitivity, as an extreme complication, has been estimated by Hallab et al. to be less than 1 % of patients undergoing a joint replacement [67]. T lymphocytes are the key cells for the type IV immunological response. As mentioned above, T lymphocytes may be activated through antigen-presenting cells (CD68+ macrophages or by other cells). Indeed, metal-protein complexes may be formed through a binding between metal ions and specific serum proteins (e.g., albumin, chromodulin, nickel/cobalt transporters – NiCo Ts) [68–70]. Thereafter, these new metal-protein complexes may act as antigens. Moreover, T cells may be activated only by metal ions, without any metal-protein complexes, by tyrosine kinase activation induced by cross-linking of thiols of cell surface proteins [67].

13.3   Summary

Wear particles from joint replacements took a significant place in orthopedic basic research and remain a topic of current interest. Recent studies highlighted that immune reactions to wear particles are not only local but systemic as well. Improvement of bearing surfaces with new generation of polyethylene and ceramic helps to mitigate the granulomatous response to material by-products. For metal particles, modulation of the immune reactions by improving our knowledge will lead to increase the lifetime of MOM arthroplasties.

References

1. Bozic KJ, Kurtz S, Lau E, et al. The epidemiology of bearing surface usage in total hip arthroplasty in the United States. J Bone Joint Surg Am. 2009;91:1614–20.
2. Bozic KJ, Ong K, Lau E, et al. Risk of complication and revision total hip arthroplasty among Medicare patients with different bearing surfaces. Clin Orthop Relat Res. 2010;468:2357–62.
3. Sundfeldt M, Carlsson LV, Johansson CB, et al. Aseptic loosening, not only a question of wear: a review of different theories. Acta Orthop. 2006;77:177–97.
4. Bozic KJ, Kurtz SM, Lau E, et al. The epidemiology of revision total knee arthroplasty in the United States. Clin Orthop Relat Res. 2009;468:45–51.
5. Ries MD, Scott ML, Jani S. Relationship between gravimetric wear and particle generation in hip simulators: conventional compared with cross-linked polyethylene. J Bone Joint Surg Am. 2001;83-A(Suppl 2 Pt 2):116–22.
6. Campbell P, Ma S, Yeom B, et al. Isolation of predominantly submicron-sized UHMWPE wear particles from periprosthetic tissues. J Biomed Mater Res. 1995;29:127–31.
7. Doorn PF, Campbell PA, Worrall J, et al. Metal wear particle characterization from metal on metal total hip replacements: transmission electron microscopy study of periprosthetic tissues and isolated particles. J Biomed Mater Res. 1998;42:103–11.
8. Ingham E, Fisher J. The role of macrophages in osteolysis of total joint replacement. Biomaterials. 2005;26:1271–86.
9. Hatton A, Nevelos JE, Nevelos AA, et al. Alumina-alumina artificial hip joints. Part I: a histological analysis and characterisation of wear debris by laser capture microdissection of tissues retrieved at revision. Biomaterials. 2002;23:3429–40.
10. Goodman SB. Wear particles, periprosthetic osteolysis and the immune system. Biomaterials. 2007;28:5044–8.

11. Schmalzried TP, Jasty M, Harris WH. Periprosthetic bone loss in total hip arthroplasty. Polyethylene wear debris and the concept of the effective joint space. J Bone Joint Surg Am. 1992;74:849–63.

12. Xing S, Waddell JE, Boynton EL. Changes in macrophage morphology and prolonged cell viability following exposure to polyethylene particulate in vitro. Microsc Res Tech. 2002;57:523–9.

13. Tuan RS, Lee FY, T Konttinen Y, et al. What are the local and systemic biologic reactions and mediators to wear debris, and what host factors determine or modulate the biologic response to wear particles? J Am Acad Orthop Surg. 2008;16 Suppl 1:S42–8.

14. Pearl JI, Ma T, Irani AR, et al. Role of the Toll-like receptor pathway in the recognition of orthopedic implant wear-debris particles. Biomaterials. 2011;32:5535–42.

15. Willert HG, Semlitsch M. Reactions of the articular capsule to wear products of artificial joint prostheses. J Biomed Mater Res. 1977;11:157–64.

16. Goodman SB, Lind M, Song Y, Smith RL. In vitro, in vivo, and tissue retrieval studies on particulate debris. Clin Orthop Relat Res. 1998;352:25–34.

17. Santavirta S, Konttinen YT, Bergroth V, et al. Aggressive granulomatous lesions associated with hip arthroplasty. Immunopathological studies. J Bone Joint Surg Am. 1990;72:252–8.

18. Rakshit DS, Ly K, Sengupta TK, et al. Wear debris inhibition of anti-osteoclastogenic signaling by interleukin-6 and interferon-gamma. Mechanistic insights and implications for periprosthetic osteolysis. J Bone Joint Surg Am. 2006;88:788–99.

19. Goodman SB, Huie P, Song Y, et al. Cellular profile and cytokine production at prosthetic interfaces. Study of tissues retrieved from revised hip and knee replacements. J Bone Joint Surg Br. 1998;80:531–9.

20. Green TR, Fisher J, Matthews JB, et al. Effect of size and dose on bone resorption activity of macrophages by in vitro clinically relevant ultra high molecular weight polyethylene particles. J Biomed Mater Res. 2000;53:490–7.

21. Goodman SB, Trindade M, Ma T, et al. Pharmacologic modulation of periprosthetic osteolysis. Clin Orthop Relat Res. 2005;430:39–45.

22. Cook DN. The role of MIP-1 alpha in inflammation and hematopoiesis. J Leukoc Biol. 1996;59:61–6.

23. Horowitz SM, Gonzales JB. Effects of polyethylene on macrophages. J Orthop Res. 1997;15:50–6.

24. Archibeck MJ, Jacobs JJ, Roebuck KA, Glant TT. The basic science of periprosthetic osteolysis. Instr Course Lect. 2001;50:185–95.

25. Moilanen E, Moilanen T, Knowles R, et al. Nitric oxide synthase is expressed in human macrophages during foreign body inflammation. Am J Pathol. 1997;150:881–7.

26. Wang ML, Hauschka PV, Tuan RS, Steinbeck MJ. Exposure to particles stimulates superoxide production by human THP-1 macrophages and avian HD-11EM osteoclasts activated by tumor necrosis factor-alpha and PMA. J Arthroplasty. 2002;17:335–46.

27. Shanbhag AS, Macaulay W, Stefanovic-Racic M, Rubash HE. Nitric oxide release by macrophages in response to particulate wear debris. J Biomed Mater Res. 1998;41:497–503.

28. Horiki M, Nakase T, Myoui A, et al. Localization of RANKL in osteolytic tissue around a loosened joint prosthesis. J Bone Miner Metab. 2004;22:346–51.

29. Wang C-T, Lin Y-T, Chiang B-L, et al. Over-expression of receptor activator of nuclear factor-kappaB ligand (RANKL), inflammatory cytokines, and chemokines in periprosthetic osteolysis of loosened total hip arthroplasty. Biomaterials. 2010;31:77–82.

30. Stern PH, Krieger NS, Nissenson RA, et al. Human transforming growth factor-alpha stimulates bone resorption in vitro. J Clin Invest. 1985;76:2016–9.

31. Takahashi N, MacDonald BR, Hon J, et al. Recombinant human transforming growth factor-alpha stimulates the formation of osteoclast-like cells in long-term human marrow cultures. J Clin Invest. 1986;78:894–8.

32. Clohisy JC, Frazier E, Hirayama T, Abu-Amer Y. RANKL is an essential cytokine mediator of polymethylmethacrylate particle-induced osteoclastogenesis. J Orthop Res. 2003;21:202–12.

33. Baggiolini M, Clark-Lewis I. Interleukin-8, a chemotactic and inflammatory cytokine. FEBS Lett. 1992;307:97–101.

34. Tuan RS, Boland G, Tuli R. Adult mesenchymal stem cells and cell-based tissue engineering. Arthritis Res Ther. 2003;5:32–45.
35. Chen FH, Rousche KT, Tuan RS. Technology Insight: adult stem cells in cartilage regeneration and tissue engineering. Nat Clin Pract Rheumatol. 2006;2:373–82.
36. Huang Z, Ma T, Ren P-G, et al. Effects of orthopedic polymer particles on chemotaxis of macrophages and mesenchymal stem cells. J Biomed Mater Res A. 2010;94:1264–9.
37. Goldring SR, Jasty M, Roelke MS, et al. Formation of a synovial-like membrane at the bone-cement interface. Its role in bone resorption and implant loosening after total hip replacement. Arthritis Rheum. 1986;29:836–42.
38. Goodman SB, Chin RC, Chiou SS, et al. A clinical-pathologic-biochemical study of the membrane surrounding loosened and nonloosened total hip arthroplasties. Clin Orthop Relat Res. 1989;244:182–7.
39. Elliott MJ, Vadas MA, Cleland LG, et al. IL-3 and granulocyte-macrophage colony-stimulating factor stimulate two distinct phases of adhesion in human monocytes. J Immunol (Baltimore, Md: 1950). 1990;145:167–76.
40. McInnes A, Rennick DM. Interleukin 4 induces cultured monocytes/macrophages to form giant multinucleated cells. J Exp Med. 1988;167:598–611.
41. McNally AK, Anderson JM. Interleukin-4 induces foreign body giant cells from human monocytes/macrophages. Differential lymphokine regulation of macrophage fusion leads to morphological variants of multinucleated giant cells. Am J Pathol. 1995;147:1487–99.
42. al-Saffar N, Mah JT, Kadoya Y, Revell PA. Neovascularisation and the induction of cell adhesion molecules in response to degradation products from orthopaedic implants. Ann Rheum Dis. 1995;54:201–8.
43. Firkins PJ, Tipper JL, Saadatzadeh MR, et al. Quantitative analysis of wear and wear debris from metal-on-metal hip prostheses tested in a physiological hip joint simulator. Biomed Mater Eng. 2001;11:143–57.
44. Willert H-G, Buchhorn GH, Fayyazi A, et al. Metal-on-metal bearings and hypersensitivity in patients with artificial hip joints. A clinical and histomorphological study. J Bone Joint Surg Am. 2005;87:28–36.
45. Park Y-S, Moon Y-W, Lim S-J, et al. Early osteolysis following second-generation metal-on-metal hip replacement. J Bone Joint Surg Am. 2005;87:1515–21.
46. Davies AP, Willert HG, Campbell PA, et al. An unusual lymphocytic perivascular infiltration in tissues around contemporary metal-on-metal joint replacements. J Bone Joint Surg Am. 2005;87:18–27.
47. Witzleb W-C, Hanisch U, Kolar N, et al. Neo-capsule tissue reactions in metal-on-metal hip arthroplasty. Acta Orthop. 2007;78:211–20.
48. Hallab NJ, Anderson S, Stafford T, et al. Lymphocyte responses in patients with total hip arthroplasty. J Orthop Res. 2005;23:384–91.
49. Lalor PA, Revell PA. T-lymphocytes and titanium aluminium vanadium (TiAlV) alloy: evidence for immunological events associated with debris deposition. Clin Mater. 1993;12:57–62.
50. Bainbridge JA, Revell PA, Al-Saffar N. Costimulatory molecule expression following exposure to orthopaedic implants wear debris. J Biomed Mater Res. 2001;54:328–34.
51. McKay GC, Macnair R, MacDonald C, Grant MH. Interactions of orthopaedic metals with an immortalized rat osteoblast cell line. Biomaterials. 1996;17:1339–44.
52. Fleury C, Petit A, Mwale F, et al. Effect of cobalt and chromium ions on human MG-63 osteoblasts in vitro: morphology, cytotoxicity, and oxidative stress. Biomaterials. 2006;27:3351–60.
53. Anissian L, Stark A, Dahlstrand H, et al. Cobalt ions influence proliferation and function of human osteoblast-like cells. Acta Orthop Scand. 2002;73:369–74.
54. Morais S, Sousa JP, Fernandes MH, Carvalho GS. In vitro biomineralization by osteoblast-like cells. I. Retardation of tissue mineralization by metal salts. Biomaterials. 1998;19:13–21.
55. Fernandes MH. Effect of stainless steel corrosion products on in vitro biomineralization. J Biomater Appl. 1999;14:113–68.

56. MacQuarrie RA, Fang Chen Y, Coles C, Anderson GI. Wear-particle-induced osteoclast osteolysis: the role of particulates and mechanical strain. J Biomed Mater Res B Appl Biomater. 2004;69:104–12.

57. Nichols KG, Puleo DA. Effect of metal ions on the formation and function of osteoclastic cells in vitro. J Biomed Mater Res. 1997;35:265–71.

58. Manlapaz M, Maloney WJ, Smith RL. In vitro activation of human fibroblasts by retrieved titanium alloy wear debris. J Orthop Res. 1996;14:465–72.

59. Kovacs EJ, DiPietro LA. Fibrogenic cytokines and connective tissue production. FASEB J. 1994;8:854–61.

60. Dizdaroglu M, Jaruga P, Birincioglu M, Rodriguez H. Free radical-induced damage to DNA: mechanisms and measurement. Free Radic Biol Med. 2002;32:1102–15.

61. Wolf T, Kasemann R, Ottenwälder H. Molecular interaction of different chromium species with nucleotides and nucleic acids. Carcinogenesis. 1989;10:655–9.

62. Witkiewicz-Kucharczyk A, Bal W. Damage of zinc fingers in DNA repair proteins, a novel molecular mechanism in carcinogenesis. Toxicol Lett. 2006;162:29–42.

63. Ren PG, Irani A, Huang Z, et al. Continuous infusion of UHMWPE particles induces increased bone macrophages and osteolysis. Clin Orthop Relat Res. 2011;469:113–22.

64. Ren PG, Lee SW, Biswal S, Goodman SB. Systemic trafficking of macrophages induced by bone cement particles in nude mice. Biomaterials. 2008;29:4760–5.

65. Deshmane SL, Kremlev S, Amini S, Sawaya BE. Monocyte chemoattractant protein-1 (MCP-1): an overview. J Interferon Cytokine Res. 2009;29:313–26.

66. Menten P, Wuyts A, Van Damme J. Macrophage inflammatory protein-1. Cytokine Growth Factor Rev. 2002;13:455–81.

67. Hallab N, Merritt K, Jacobs JJ. Metal sensitivity in patients with orthopaedic implants. J Bone Joint Surg Am. 2001;83-A:428–36.

68. Bar-Or D, Curtis G, Rao N, et al. Characterization of the Co(2+) and Ni(2+) binding amino-acid residues of the N-terminus of human albumin. An insight into the mechanism of a new assay for myocardial ischemia. Eur J Biochem/FEBS. 2001;268:42–7.

69. Clodfelder BJ, Emamaullee J, Hepburn DD, et al. The trail of chromium(III) in vivo from the blood to the urine: the roles of transferrin and chromodulin. J Biol Inorg Chem. 2001;6:608–17.

70. Eitinger T, Suhr J, Moore L, Smith JAC. Secondary transporters for nickel and cobalt ions: theme and variations. Biometals. 2005;18:399–405.

Chapter 14
Diagnostic Evaluations

Rihard Trebše

Abstract Laboratory investigations are always performed during PJI workout, but the interpretation of the results is not always simple. If properly interpreted, they give a lot of information in the diagnostic evaluation of PJI suspicion and in the follow-up of treated patients. The diagnostic evaluation of PJI always includes imaging. There are plenty of possibilities from simple plain radiography to the most sophisticated PET-NMR scans. This chapter discusses the advantages and strengths of various imaging studies in PJI assessment.

Keywords Serology • Radiography • Bone scans • Computed tomography • Magnetic resonance

14.1 Laboratory Investigations

14.1.1 Serology

By laboratory investigations, we can measure systemic parameters that present an indirect, nonspecific response of the organism to infection of any type. It is not surprising that in low-grade infections or in well-drained infective processes, the serological parameters may be normal or nearly normal. More than a tool for diagnosing infection, serological investigations are instruments for measuring infection activity and severity. With clinical suspicion of PJI, normal parameters suggest a more thorough and direct diagnostic investigation like synovial cytology and microbiological sampling. Serial investigations are more informative. They can demonstrate the progress of the healing process, the progress in the infection activity, or a relapse.

R. Trebše, M.D., Ph.D.
Department for Bone Infections and Adult Reconstructions,
Orthopaedic Hospital Valdoltra,
Jadranska cesta 31, Ankaran SI-6286, Slovenia
e-mail: rihard.trebse@ob-valdoltra.si

R. Trebše (ed.), *Infected Total Joint Arthroplasty*,
DOI 10.1007/978-1-4471-2482-5_14, © Springer-Verlag London 2012

Since serology is a systemic and indirect tool, we must always be cautious to find the real reason for elevated serologic parameters. It is thus very likely that sudden increase of inflammatory markers, a week after gradual improving after surgical treatment of a PJI is not caused by reactivation of the primary infection but rather by a collateral process.

Peripheral-blood leukocyte count has a low sensitivity for detecting PJI, and it is not of a great value in diagnosis of PJI [1].

Erythrocyte sedimentation rate (ESR) is usually elevated in PJI. The investigation is however very nonspecific and obsolete and not useful in the evaluation of PJI.

C-reactive protein (CRP) measurement is the most useful blood test for diagnostic evaluation of the suspicious PJI in the absence of underlying inflammatory condition. It has a specificity of 81–86 % and sensitivity between 73 and 91 % for the diagnosis of TKR infection with the cutoff point set at 13.5 mg/L [4, 6]. Similarly, it has a specificity of 62 % and a sensitivity of 96 % in THA infection with the cutoff point at 5.0 mg/L [12]. In our series, 25 % out of 140 patients with microbiologically proven PJI patients have had the CRP value below 5 mg/L. Negative CRP value has very limited role in ruling out infection.

In uncomplicated arthroplasty surgery, the CRP value is elevated after surgery with the peak during the second day after TKR and the third day after THR. The CRP value typically normalizes within 3 weeks to 2 months [21]. The dynamics of serial measurements is important. The stagnation or sudden increase of the postoperative CRP values needs evaluation to rule out unsuccessful treatment. The main cause to a sudden increase in CRP is usually not a periprosthetic infection relapse, but other reasons, including viral disease, enteritis, urinary tract infection, i.v. line-associated infection, and pneumonia. In the case of a concomitant inflammatory disease such as rheumatoid arthritis and psoriatic arthritis, the CRP levels usually do not normalize completely [9].

Procalcitonin has a low sensitivity for detecting PJI. Levels can be elevated in acute infections.

14.2 Imaging

14.2.1 Plain Radiography

Plain radiography is the most important tool for evaluation of patients with failed TJA. It has an important role for diagnosing subsidence, shifting of the implant and loosening, for detecting osteolytic zones, and for diagnosing various other conditions related to prosthetic joints. Particularly useful are serial radiographs. It has only limited role in discriminating between a septic and an aseptic prosthetic joint failure due to low sensitivity and specificity [10]. Chronic PJI can cause periosteal and/or endosteal reactions and osteopenia with osteolyses. The most discriminating is serial dynamic because septic processes are evolving faster than aseptic on plain radiographs [19].

Fig. 14.1 Fistulography
showing the fistula extending
to the femoral component of
the hip prosthesis

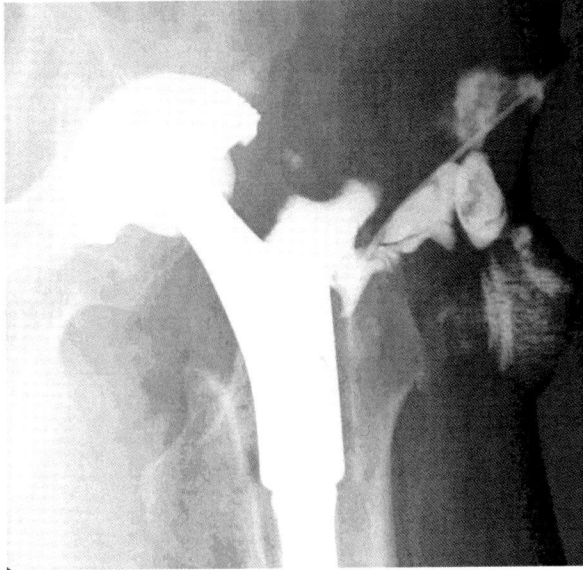

14.2.2   Arthrography

Arthrography is an x-ray imaging study which includes application of contrast and occasionally air in the joint. It is important for evaluation of failed prosthetic joint because it is more sensitive for detecting loosening than plain radiography. Arthrography enables the clinician to see the contrast trapped within the interface between a loosened prosthesis (or cement) and bone. It is also valid for viewing sinuses and abscesses where contrast accumulates. It also reliably confirms correct intra-articular placement of the needle for pseudosynovial sampling [16, 19].

14.2.3   Fistulography

Fistulography is an x-ray imaging study with application of the contrast into the fistular opening (see Fig. 14.1). The investigation demonstrates the depth and the morphology of the fistular canal which may influence surgical planning. It is important for determination of communication between discharging sinus and the prosthetic joint.

14.2.4   Ultrasound Imaging

Ultrasound is a noninvasive study important for demonstrating fluid collection (pus, synovial fluid, and haemathoma). It is mainly useful for evaluation of hip joint because of difficult clinical assessment of swelling and liquid accumulation due to its deep location. It is also useful for guiding needles for diagnostic and therapeutic aspirations.

14.2.5 Computer Tomography (CT)

Computer tomography is more sensitive than plain imaging studies for discerning septic from aseptic prosthetic joint failure because it may discriminate between normal and inflamed tissues (see Fig. 14.2). Artifacts caused by metal implants limit considerably its value. Novel CT technology (dual energy) allows for excellent morphological evaluation even in the presence of massive metal implants by adopting a subtraction method. CT allows for precise needle placement for aspiration and surgical planning in particular cases [7].

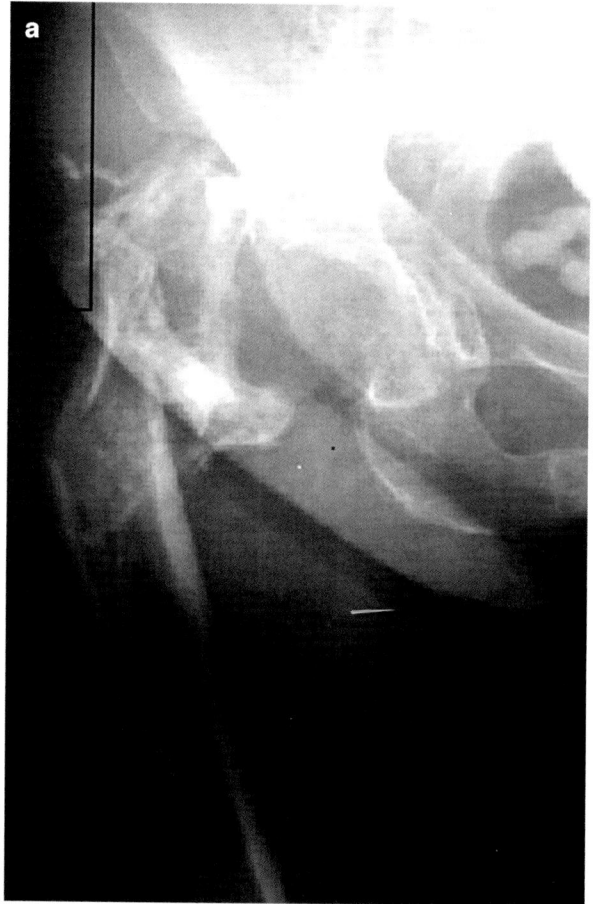

Fig. 14.2 (a) Showing a plain radiograph of a complex proximal femoral deformation after a septic complication of an osteosynthesis presenting for a prosthetic reconstruction. (b) A 3-D CT reconstruction helps planning the surgical procedure. (c) Plain radiography at 10-year follow-up after the reconstruction

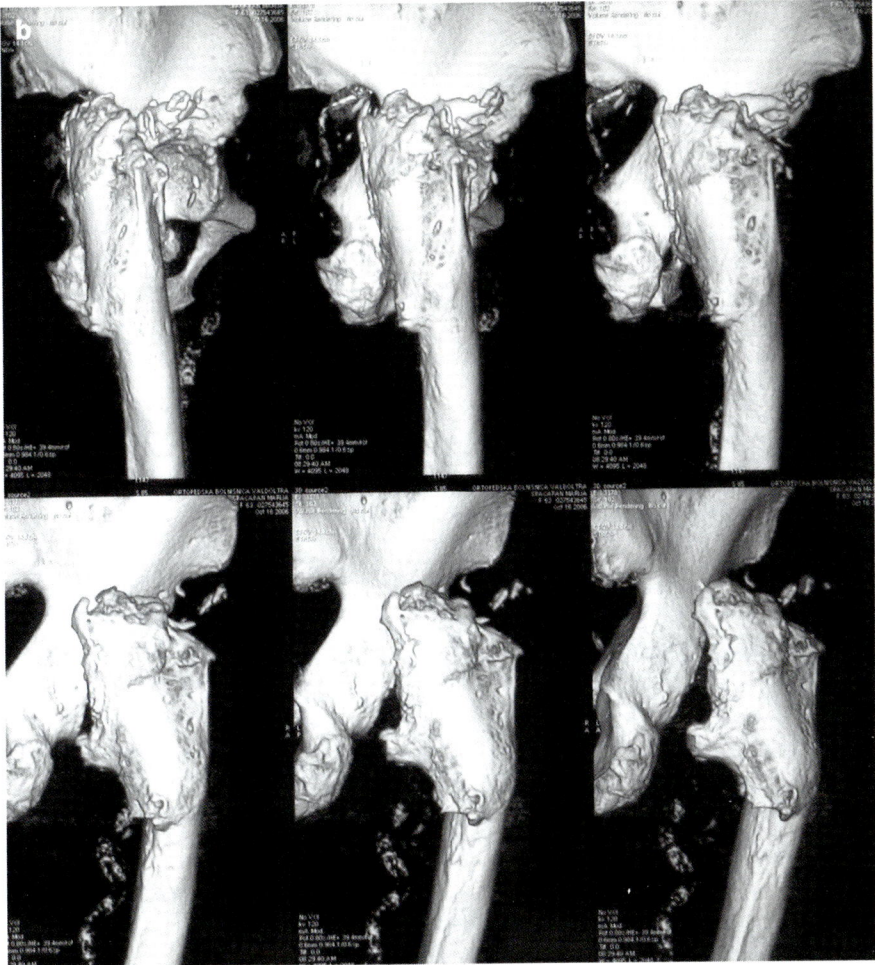

Fig. 14.2 (continued)

Fig. 14.2 (continued)

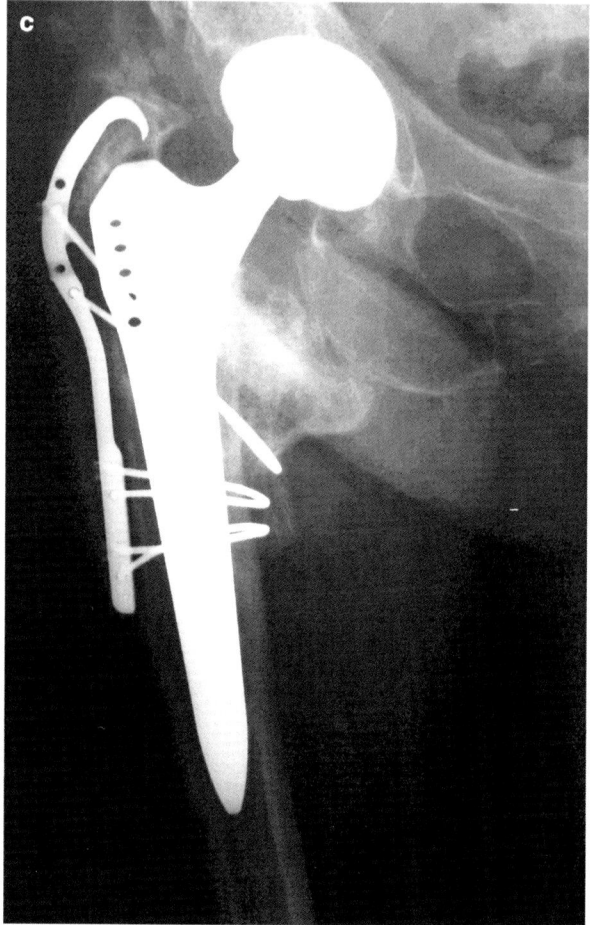

14.2.6   Magnetic Resonance Imaging (MRI)

MRI safe implants are not a contraindication for MR evaluation of a failed prosthetic joint. MRI study is hampered by artifacts produced by implants [7, 22]. Non-
ferromagnetic implants like those made of tantalum or titanium are, however,
associated with minimal artifacts, and good resolution for detecting soft tissue
pathology around implants is possible. Modified MRI techniques allow for precise
analysis of osteolysis, periprosthetic tissues, and especially bone-implant interface.
These information can be valuable in diagnostic workout of a PJI [14].

14.2.7   Nuclear Bone Scans

Bone scans are frequently used for evaluation of a presumably septic failed
prosthetic joint as well as in suspicious aseptic failure not evident on plain

radiography. Bone scans obtained after administration of technetium-99m-labeled methylene diphosphonate are nonspecific for infection but very sensitive for detecting failed septic or aseptic prosthetic joints [3, 15, 18]. The scan is abnormal up to a year after a successful arthroplasty procedure due to bone remodeling around the implant. Labeled-leukocyte imaging (indium-111) and gallium citrate scan are more important for detection of infection. For the former, the specificity is 86 %, sensitivity 77 %, positive predictive value 54 %, and 95 % negative predictive value [17]. Combined bone and Ga^{67} scans are more specific than bone scans alone [13]. Positive Tc^{99} and negative Ga^{67} scans are suggesting more a mechanical problem, while vice versa more an inflammation [20]. The most accurate seems to be a combination of indium-111-labeled leukocyte scan and bone marrow imaging with the use of technetium-99m-labeled sulfur colloid [11].

14.2.8 Positron-Emission Tomography (PET)

PET is a nuclear medicine study that visualizes in 2- or 3-D the desired functional biochemical processes within the body. The device detects pairs of gamma rays that are released during positron emission. The method bases on application of radioactive isotopes which emit positrons through disintegration. There are various positron emitters available like 11C, 13N, 15O, 18F, 68Ga, and 82Rb. The most frequently used is fluorine (18F) bound to glucose molecule to form 18FDG-fluorodeoxyglucose. The advantage of this particular isotope is a relatively slow breakdown process with the longest half-life so that it does not need to be synthesized just before the application. Metabolic pathways of 18FDG are similar as for glucose. 18FDG is thus accumulating in cells that use glucose as their primary source of energy through glycolysis. It has its role in diagnosing inflammatory processes because inflammation increases the rate of glucose metabolism.

Contemporary PET cameras are linked with a CT or NMR scanners (signal co-acquisition) which allow for spatial anatomic biochemical process imaging.

The accuracy of the method for diagnosing PJI stands between 81 and 100 % depending on type of implant [2, 5, 8].

References

1. Berbari E, Mabry T, Tsaras G, Spangehl M, Erwin PJ, Murad MH, Steckelberg J, Osmon D. Inflammatory blood laboratory levels as markers of prosthetic joint infection: a systematic review and meta-analysis. J Bone Joint Surg Am. 2010;92(11):2102–9.
2. Chacko TK, Zhuang H, Nakhoda KZ, Moussavian B, Alavi A. Applications of fluorodeoxyglucose positron emission tomography in the diagnosis of infection. Nucl Med Commun. 2003;24:615–24.
3. Corstens FH, van der Meer JW. Nuclear medicine's role in infection and inflammation. Lancet. 1999;354:765–70.

4. Fink B, Makowiak C, Fuerst M, Berger I, Schafer P, Frommelt L. The value of synovial biopsy, joint aspiration and C-reactive protein in the diagnosis of late periprosthetic infection of total knee replacements. J Bone Joint Surg Br. 2008;90:874–8.
5. Gravius S, Gebhard M, Ackermann D, Bohll U, Hermanns-Sachweh B, Mumme T. Analysis of 18F-FDG uptake pattern in PET for diagnosis of aseptic loosening versus prosthesis infection after total knee arthroplasty. A prospective pilot study. Nuklearmedizin. 2010;49:115–23.
6. Greidanus NV, Masri BA, Garbut DS, et al. Use of erythrocyte sedimentation rate and C-reactive protein level to diagnose infection before revision total knee arthroplasty: a prospective evaluation. J Bone Joint Surg Am. 2007;89:1409–16.
7. Hain SF, O'Doherty MJ, Smith MA. Functional imaging and the orthopaedic surgeon. J Bone Joint Surg Br. 2002;84:315–21.
8. Kwee TC, Kwee RM, Alawi A. FDG PET for diagnosing prosthetic joint infection: systematic review and metaanalysis. Eur J Nucl Med Mol Imaging. 2008;35:2122–32.
9. Laiho K, Maenpaa H, Kautiainen H. Rise in serum C reactive protein after hip and knee arthroplasties in patients with rheumatoid arthritis. Ann Rheum Dis. 2001;60:275–7.
10. Love C, Marwin SE, Palestro CJ. Nuclear medicine and the infected joint replacement. Semin Nucl Med. 2008;39:66–78.
11. Love C, Marwin SE, Palestro CJ. Nuclear medicine and the infected joint replacement. Semin Nucl Med. 2009;39(1):66–78.
12. Muller M, Moravietz L, Hassart O, Strube P, Perka C, Tothz S. Diagnosis of periprosthetic infection following total hip arthroplasty – evaluation of the diagnostic values of pre- and intraoperative parameters and the associated strategy to preoperatively select patients with high probability of joint infection. J Orthop Surg. 2008;3:31.
13. Palestro CJ. Radionuclide imaging after skeletal interventional procedures. Semin Nucl Med. 1995;25:3–14.
14. Potter HG, Nestor BJ, Sofka CM. Magnetic resonance imaging after total hip arthroplasty: evaluation of periprosthetic soft tissue. J Bone Joint Surg Am. 2004;86:1947–54.
15. Reing CM, Richin PF, Kemnore PI. Differential bone scanning in the evaluation in the painful total joint replacement. J Bone Joint Surg Am. 1979;61(6A):933–6.
16. Schafroth M, Zimmerli W, Brunazzi M, Ochsner PE. Infections. In: Ochsner PE, editor. Total hip replacement. Berlin: Springer; 2003.
17. Scher DM, Pak K, Lonner JH. The predictive value of indium-111 leucocyte scan in the diagnosis of infected total hip, knee, or resection arthroplasties. J Arthroplasty. 2000;15:295–300.
18. Smith SL, Wastie ML, Forster I. Radionuclide bone scintigraphy in the detection of significant complications after total knee joint replacement. Clin Radiol. 2001;56:221–4.
19. Tigges S, Stiles RG, Robertson JR. Appearance of septic hip prostheses on plain radiographs. Am J Roentgenol. 1994;163:377–80.
20. van der Bruggen W, Bleeker-Rovers CP, Boerman OC, Gotthardt M, Oyen WJ. PET and SPECT in osteomyelitis and prosthetic bone and joint infections: a systematic review. Semin Nucl Med. 2010;40:3–15.
21. White J, Kelly M, Dunsmuir R. C-reactive protein after total hip and total knee replacement. J Bone Joint Surg Br. 1998;80:909–11.
22. White LM, Kim JK, Mehta M. Complications of total hip arthroplasty: MR imaging-initial experience. Radiology. 2000;215:254–62.

Chapter 15
Synovial Fluid Cytology

René Mihalič and Dunja Terčič

Abstract In the evaluation of artificial joint disorders, synovial fluid analysis can become a very efficient diagnostic tool. This chapter explains the role of synovial fluid cytological analysis in diagnosing prosthetic joint infection (PJI). Recommended cutoff values for diagnosing PJI for leukocyte count are 1,700 cells/μL and for neutrophils 65 %. Considering those cutoff values for diagnosing PJI, the specificity is very high, exceeding 90 %, which means that negative cytological result of synovial fluid analysis indicates absence of infection. The results are comparable to intraoperative tissue cultures and histopathology, which are frequently used as reference standard diagnostic markers in diagnosing prosthetic joint infection.

Keywords Synovial fluid • Leukocytes • Neutrophils • Cytology • Diagnosis

15.1 Introduction

In the last decade, there was a remarkable increase in implantations of prosthetic joints. The procedure is a very efficient solution for solving problems related to degenerative and other derangements of major joints. According to the trends from the past, by year 2030, the projected demand for primary total hip arthroplasties will grow by 174 %, and the demand for primary total knee arthroplasties is projected to grow by 673 %. In the same period, the increase is also expected in revision arthroplasty procedures. Total hip and total knee revisions are projected to grow by 137 and 601 %, respectively [1]. Prosthetic joints improve the quality of life, but they may fail. Causes of failure include, but are not limited to, aseptic loosening, dislocation, fracture of the implant or bone, and infection. The last one is probably

R. Mihalič, M.D. (✉) • D. Terčič
Orthopaedic Hospital Valdoltra,
Jadranska cesta 31, Ankaran 6280, Slovenia
e-mail: rene.mihalic@ob-valdoltra.si

R. Trebše (ed.), *Infected Total Joint Arthroplasty*,
DOI 10.1007/978-1-4471-2482-5_15, © Springer-Verlag London 2012

the most serious complication and is related to significant morbidity and substantial health-care costs [2, 3]. In many cases, it is difficult to distinguish between septic and aseptic loosening of an implant. Since treatment strategies are different, it is very important to establish the correct cause of failure. Before planning the surgery, different tests and imaging studies have to be performed to determine the accurate diagnosis. This is especially important in cases of low-grade implant infections and chronic implant infections without a sinus tract. In these circumstances, the clinical presentation is discreet.

The laboratory criteria and imaging findings for diagnosing infection are different in patients with native joint infections than for prosthetic joint infections (PJI). This is why the former are not suitable for diagnosing PJI [3]. Laboratory tests include measurements of leukocyte count in blood and the C-reactive protein (CRP). Imaging studies include plain radiography, labeled-leukocyte scanning, and positron-emission tomography (PET). None of this tests and imaging studies, alone, can provide a definitive diagnosis of septic loosening because their sensitivity and specificity are too low. In the last few years, another efficient and economical diagnostic test is getting widely accepted. This is pre- or intraoperative aspiration of the synovial fluid for leukocyte count and differential [2–4]. The test has become important after leukocyte count and differential cutoffs for PJI were established. In cases of PJI, cutoffs are dramatically lower than those used to diagnose native joint infection. In the past, the use of improper, native joint infection cutoffs were the main reason for misdiagnosing PJI as aseptic.

Another important advantage of synovial cytology in diagnosing low-grade and chronic PJI is that the method is not affected by prior antimicrobial therapy [5].

15.2 Synovial Fluid

Synovial fluid fills the space within joint cavities. It lubricates articular cartilage and provides its nourishment through diffusion. Joint cavities are covered with synovial tissue which is composed of vascularized connective tissue that lacks a basement membrane. With histological analysis of synovial tissue, three types of cells with different function were identified. Type A cells are important in phagocytosis, type B cells (fibroblast-like cells) produce components of synovial fluid and are a source of glycoproteins and hyaluronic acid, and type C cells exist as an intermediate type. Additional mechanism for synovial fluid production is ultrafiltration of blood plasma through capillaries in synovial tissue. In fact synovial fluid is a mixture of components produced by type B cells and blood plasma ultrafiltrate [6–8]. Large joints contain up to 3.5 mL of synovial fluid. Since it is an ultrafiltrate of blood plasma, its composition is similar to that, but concentration of protein components and blood cells is lower, except for some components produced by B-type cells (e.g., lubricin, glycoproteins, and hyaluronic acid). The amount of erythrocytes (RBC) is lower than 2×10^9/L, the amount of leukocytes (WBC) is lower than 0.2×10^9/L, and the amount of polymorphonuclear granulocytes (PMN) is lower than 10 % [6]. Other

components of synovial fluid are hyaluronic acid, lubricin (key lubricating component), proteinases, collagenases, prostaglandins, glucose, uric acid, lactate, lactate
dehydrogenase, acid phosphatase, and immunoglobulins. In healthy native joints,
synovial fluid contains no crystals and no fibrinogen, and it is sterile [6, 8]. The
analysis of synovial fluid is a fundamental diagnostic tool in the evaluation of native
joint disorders by which we can point to etiologic causes of inflammation. Main
etiologic causes of inflammation include [9]:

- Infectious arthritis
- Crystal-induced arthritis
- Trauma
- Avascular bone necrosis
- Osteoarthritis
- Tumors and metastases
- Reactive arthritis
- Intra-articular hemorrhage

In infected native joints, synovial fluid cytological diagnostic criteria are well
defined. If the amount of WBC is higher than $50 \times 10^9/L$ and the share of PMN is
higher than 90 %, then the native joint is infected [10]. These cytological criteria are
not applicable for prosthetic joints [5].

15.3   Synovial Fluid Cytology in Presence of Implants

The pathogenesis of infection associated with a prosthetic joint involves interaction
among the implant, the host's immune system, and the involved microorganism.
Microorganisms are capable to adhere to the implant surface, where they form
biofilm an extracellular structure in which microorganisms are enclosed in a polymeric matrix and develop into organized, complex communities with functional and
structural specialization. Enclosed in biofilm, microorganisms are protected from
antimicrobial agents and the host immune system [2, 3, 11, 12]. Biofilm microorganisms have higher resistance to antimicrobials than do their planktonic counterparts [13]. As long as bacteria are mainly concealed in the biofilm, the host's local
and systemic immune system response is discreet. Biofilm is thus probably the main
reason why the cutoff values of synovial fluid leukocyte count and differential are
much lower in presence of foreign material than in cases of native joints.

The first prospective study, aimed to determine synovial fluid leukocyte count
and PMN differential (%PMN) cutoff values for infected total knee joints, was
designed by Trampuz et al. in 2004 [5]. Prior to revision, he analyzed synovial fluid
aspirates from failed total knee replacements, where the reason for arthroplasty was
osteoarthritis. Patients with underlying inflammatory joint disease, crystal-induced
arthropathy, or connective tissue disease were excluded from the study. PJI was
diagnosed if at least one of the following criteria was met [2, 3, 14, 15]: growth of
the same microorganism in at least two cultures of synovial fluid or periprosthetic

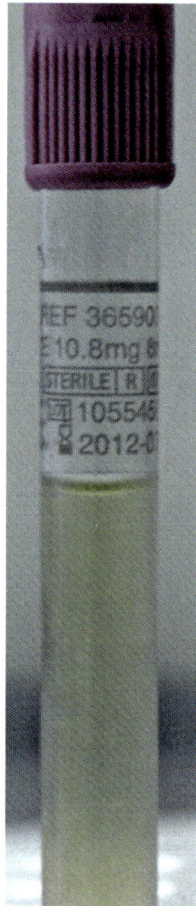

Fig. 15.1 Purulent synovial fluid aspirate

tissue, visible synovial fluid purulence at the time of aspiration or during surgery (Fig. 15.1), acute inflammation on histopathologic examination of periprosthetic tissue sections, or presence of a sinus tract communicating with the prosthesis.

Considering the aforementioned criteria as the strongest standard for diagnosing PJI, they found that the optimal synovial fluid WBC count and %PMN cutoff values for identifying patients with PJI were $1.7 \times 10^3/\mu L$ or >65 %, respectively (Fig. 15.2). A WBC count had a sensitivity of 94 % and specificity of 88 % for diagnosing PJI, whereas a %PMN had sensitivity of 97 % and specificity of 98 % [5]. By applying cutoff values, used for diagnosing septic arthritis in native joints (WBC count of more than 50,000 cells/μL and %PMN more than 90 %) [10], the sensitivity for diagnosing PJI was only 21 % for WBC and 59 % for %PMN [5]. Later, several other authors were trying to determine synovial fluid leukocyte count and %PMN cutoff values for infected total knee and hip joints as well. Mason et al. [16] found

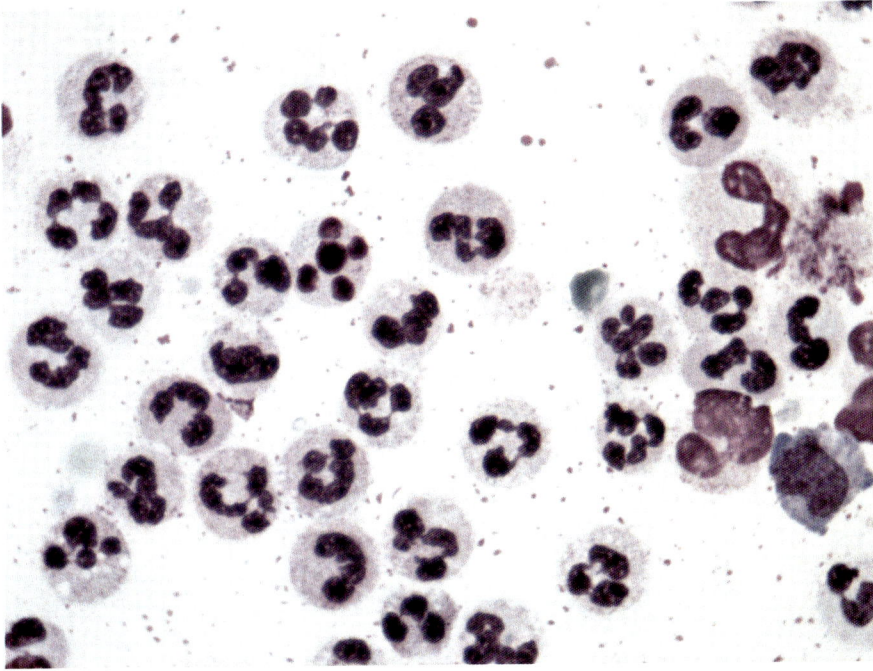

Fig. 15.2 Photomicrograph demonstration of purulent synovial fluid aspirate with predominant appearance of PMN (PMN differential of 92 %)

that WBC count of more than 2,500 cells/μL and %PMN greater than 60 % were highly suggestive of infection. Parvizi et al. [4] determined the optimal cutoff values for WBC count and %PMN as more than 1,760 cells/μL and more than 73 %, respectively. Those results for WBC count and %PMN had a positive predictive value of 99 and 96 %, respectively. Della Valle et al. [17] demonstrated that WBC count greater than 3,000 cells/μL yielded the sensitivity of 100 % and the specificity of 98 %. Ghanem et al. [18] reviewed 429 knees revised for multiple reasons, including infection. They observed that optimal cutoff values for WBC count and %PMN were more than 1,100 cells/μL and more than 64 %, respectively. Schinsky et al. [19] reviewed 201 painful total hip arthroplasties. The optimal cutoff values for WBC count and %PMN were more than 4,200 cells/μL and more than 80 %, respectively. A cutoff for WBC count %PMN had a positive predictive value of 81 and 65 %, respectively. Their results are shown in Table 15.1.

The authors of papers reviewed in Table 15.1 analyzed synovial fluid in patients where the reason for primary arthroplasty was primary osteoarthritis. The data from Table 15.1 suggests the optimal cutoff value for diagnosing PJI by calculating the %PMN to be around 65 % and the optimal cutoff value for WBC count around 1,700 cells/μL, independently on the joint involved. Studies reviewed in Table 15.1 showed strikingly comparable results with excellent sensitivity and specificity. Excellent accuracy makes synovial cytology an essential diagnostic tool in the evaluation of

Table 15.1 Results of different studies evaluating synovial fluid leukocyte count and %PMN cutoff values

Study	N	WBC	%PMN	S(WBC)%	Sp(WBC)%	S(PMN)%	Sp(PMN)%
Mason et al. [16]	86 K	2,500	60	69	98	76	89
Trampuz et al.[a] [5]	133 K	1,700	65	94	88	97	98
Parvizi et al. [4]	145 K 23 H	1,760	73	90	99	93	95
Della Valle et al. [17]	94 K	3,000	65	100	98	–	–
Ghanem et al. [18]	429 K	1,100	64	90.1	88.1	95.0	94.7
Schinsky et al. [19]	201 H	4,200	80	84	93	84	82

N number of cases, *WBC* leukocyte count (cells/μL), *PMN* polymorphonuclear leukocytes, *S* sensitivity, *Sp* specificity, *H* hip, *K* knee
[a]The first published prospective study

artificial joint disorders. The sensitivity and specificity of recommended cutoff values for diagnosing PJI are similar to other diagnostic procedures that serve related purposes like intraoperative tissue cultures and histopathology [5].

For reliable accuracy of the procedure, the samples should be acquired preoperatively and the aspiration performed through intact skin. Hip aspiration may require imaging guidance [3]. If samples could not be acquired preoperatively, they can still be obtained during surgery, just after the pseudocapsule is exposed. Care must be taken to avoid contamination with blood to avoid false-positive results. In case bloody aspirate is unavoidable, a correctional formula can help calculating the correct values of synovial fluid WBC and PMN percentage [20]. Correctional factor is defined as a ratio between RBC in peripheral blood and synovial fluid. Peripheral blood for correctional factor determination should be acquired within 48 h after the synovial aspiration.

$$\text{Correctional formula}: \text{WBC}_{adjusted} = \text{WBC}_{observed} - \left[\left(\text{WBC}_{blood} \times \text{RBC}_{fluid} / \text{RBC}_{blood} \right) \right]_{predicted}.$$

The PMN percentage can be determined in a similar fashion [20].

It is not yet known how long after an uncomplicated prosthetic replacement it takes for the synovial fluid cell counts to stabilize and become reliable for diagnostic cytology. In their study, Trampuz et al. [5] only used specimens obtained more than 6 months after the index surgery. We speculate that synovial cytology can probably be performed much earlier, even only a few weeks after index surgery, with similar accuracy, if correctional formula published by Ghanem et al. is used [20]. Trampuz et al. [5] found that antimicrobial treatment prior to the aspiration for synovial cytology did not decrease the sensitivity of WBC counts in diagnosing PJI.

Despite excellent accuracy, synovial cytology has its own inherent limitations influenced by several factors like the following: the PJI causative agents that fail to grow in vitro, the microbiological contaminations of samples, the contamination of synovial fluid samples with blood, and the presence of an underlying noninfectious inflammatory disease with influence on synovial fluid characteristics. For patients with inflammatory conditions, the PJI cutoff values for synovial WBC count and %PMN were not yet established. Cutoff values in these patients are probably higher and need to be established by further investigations.

15.4 Conclusion

Synovial fluid cytological analysis is a very efficient and economic method for evaluation of failed prosthetic joints. The recommended cutoff values for diagnosing PJI by WBC count are >1,700 cells/μL or >65 % of PMN. These cutoff criteria are useful only if the reason for the primary arthroplasty was primary osteoarthritis. In our opinion, synovial fluid cytological analysis is an essential diagnostic procedure in the evaluation of most artificial joint disorder.

References

1. Kurtz SM, Ong K, Lau E, Mowat F, Halpern M. Projections of primary and revision hip and knee arthroplasty in the United States from 2005 to 2030. J Bone Joint Surg Am. 2007;89:780–5.
2. Zimmerli W, Trampuz A, Ochsner PE. Prosthetic-joint infections. N Engl J Med. 2004; 351:1645–54.
3. del Pozo JL, Patel R. Clinical practice. Infection associated with prosthetic joints. N Engl J Med. 2009;361:787–94.
4. Parvizi J, Ghanem E, Menashe S, Barrack RL, Bauer TW. Periprosthetic infection: what are the diagnostic challenges? J Bone Joint Surg Am. 2006;88 Suppl 4:138–47.
5. Trampuz A, Hanssen AD, Osmon DR, Mandrekar J, Steckelberg JM, Patel R. Synovial fluid leukocyte count and differential for the diagnosis of prosthetic knee infection. Am J Med. 2004;117:556–62.
6. Terčič D, Božič B. The basis of the synovial fluid analysis. Clin Chem Lab Med. 2001; 39:1221–6.
7. Clohisy JC, Lindskog D, Abu-Amer Y. Bone and joint biology. In: Lieberman JR, editor. AAOS comprehensive orthopaedic review. Rosemont: American Academy of Orthopaedic Surgeons; 2009.
8. Brinker MR, O'Connor DP. Basic sciences. In: Miller MD, editor. Review of orthopaedics. Philadelphia: Saunders Elsevier; 2008.
9. Baker DG, Schumacher Jr HR. Acute monoarthritis. N Engl J Med. 1993;329:1013–20.
10. Guidelines for the initial evaluation of the adult patient with acute musculoskeletal symptoms. American College of Rheumatology Ad hoc Committee on Clinical Guidelines. Arthritis Rheum. 1996;39:1–8.
11. An YH, Friedman RJ. Concise review of mechanisms of bacterial adhesion to biomaterial surfaces. J Biomed Mater Res. 1998;43:338–48.
12. Zalavras CG, Costerton JW. Biofilm, biomaterials and bacterial adherence. In: Cierny G, McLaren AC, Wongworawat MD, editors. Orthopaedic knowledge update: musculoskeletal infection. Rosemont: American Academy of Orthopaedic Surgeons; 2009.

13. Ceri H, Olson ME, Stremick C, Read RR, Morck D, Buret A. The Calgary biofilm device: new technology for rapid determination of antibiotic susceptibilities of bacterial biofilms. J Clin Microbiol. 1999;37:1771–6.
14. Berbari EF, Hanssen AD, Duffy MC, Steckelberg JM, Ilstrup DM, Harmsen WS, Osmon DR. Risk factors for prosthetic joint infection: case control study. Clin Infect Dis. 1998; 27:1247–54.
15. Trampuz A, Piper KE, Jacobson MJ, Hanssen AD, Unni KK, Osmon DR, Mandrekar JR, Cockerill FR, Steckelberg JM, Greenleaf JM, Patel R. Sonication of removed hip and knee prostheses for diagnosis of infection. N Engl J Med. 2007;357:654–63.
16. Mason JB, Fehring TK, Odum SM, Griffin WL, Nussman DS. The value of white blood cell counts before revision total knee arthroplasty. J Arthroplasty. 2003;18:1038–43.
17. Della Valle CJ, Sporer SM, Jacobs JJ, Berger RA, Rosenberg AG, Paprosky WG. Preoperative testing for sepsis before revision total knee arthroplasty. J Arthroplasty. 2007;22 Suppl 2:90–3.
18. Ghanem E, Parvizi J, Burnett RS, Sharkey PF, Keshavarzi N, Agarwal A, Barrack RL. Cell count and differential of aspirated fluid in the diagnosis of infection at the site of total knee arthroplasty. J Bone Joint Surg Am. 2008;90:1637–43.
19. Schinsky MF, Della Valle CJ, Sporer SM, Paprosky WG. Perioperative testing for joint infection in patients undergoing revision total hip arthroplasty. J Bone Joint Surg Am. 2008;90:1869–75.
20. Ghanem E, Houssock C, Pulido L, Han S, Jaberi FM, Parvizi J. Determining "true" leukocytosis in bloody joint aspirate. J Arthroplasty. 2008;23:182–7.

Chapter 16
Histological Analysis of Periprosthetic Tissue for Detecting Prosthetic Joint Infection

Andrej Cör

Abstract The possibility of differentiating an aseptic loosening from prosthetic joint infection (PJI) is rather difficult when clinical findings are poor or even absent but is very important since the treatments are different. Unfortunately, to date, there is no preoperative or intraoperative test that is 100 % sensitive and specific for diagnosis of prosthetic infection. Several authors proposed analysis of either frozen or permanent histological sections of periprosthetic tissue as a reliable method for PJI detection. Histological analysis using various criteria for the determination of "positivity" has been touted as a rapid and inexpensive test that has a high specificity; however, its sensitivity has been widely inconsistent ranging from 18 to 100 % in various studies. Histological analysis of periprosthetic tissue at joint revision surgery could be helpful when preoperative tests are ambiguous, but careful attention to the application of criteria for a histological diagnosis must be made to preclude diagnostic errors.

Keywords Diagnosis • Histology • Frozen sections • Sampling

Since surgical treatment of joint prosthesis loosening (septic or aseptic) is different, it is very important to establish the correct diagnosis of prosthetic joint infection (PJI). Correct diagnosis of PJI is still a challenge in clinical practice. A misdiagnosis of prosthetic joint infection has crucial consequences for the patients. Different tests can be performed before surgery (C-reactive protein, erythrocyte sedimentation rate, white blood cell count, and different radiological techniques); however, those tests have low sensitivity and specificity. Microbiological cultures represent the gold standard for prosthesis joint infection diagnosis, but appropriateness of this method in determining surgical treatment is limited due to the time required for bacterial growth. Only two intraoperative tests, Gram stain and histology, give

A. Cör, M.D., Ph.D.
Faculty of Health Sciences, University of Primorska,
Polje 42, Izola, 6310 Slovenia
e-mail: andrej.coer@fvz.upr.si

R. Trebše (ed.), *Infected Total Joint Arthroplasty*,
DOI 10.1007/978-1-4471-2482-5_16, © Springer-Verlag London 2012

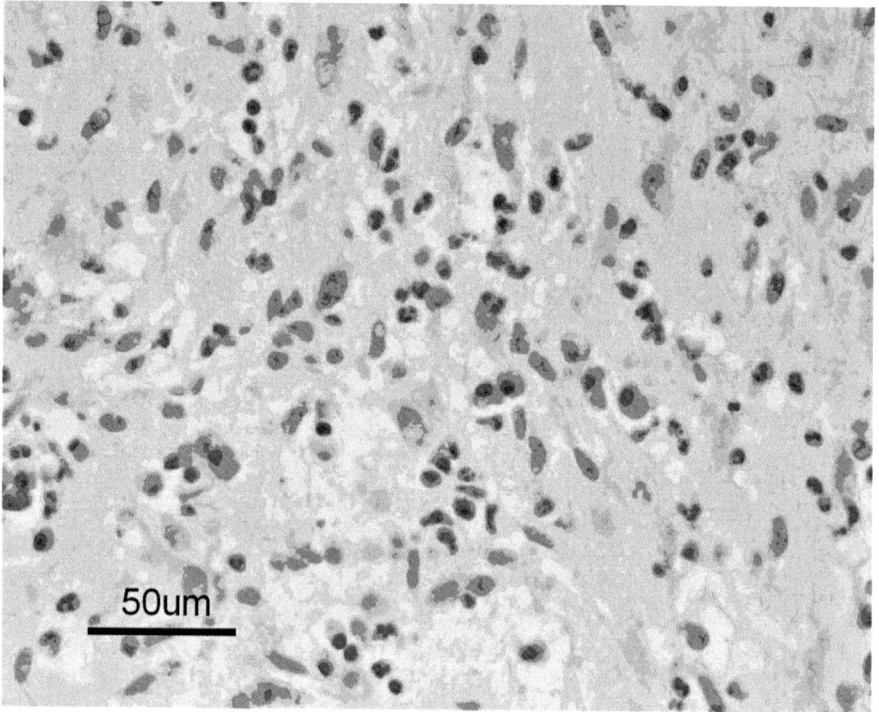

Fig. 16.1 Photomicrograph demonstration more than ten polymorphonuclear leukocytes per high-power field in a paraffin section from a patient with total hip prosthesis infection (hematoxylin and eosin, ×400)

immediate information about the etiology of the prosthesis loosening; however, Gram stain sensitivity is lower than 30 % [23]. Many authors suggested that frozen section analysis is the accurate and quick method to diagnose the PJI. [6, 25]

Between the bone and prosthesis, a fringe of connective tissue of varying width develops, named periprosthetic membrane, which has to be removed during revision surgery. This membrane is valuable specimen for histopathological analysis. Periprosthetic membranes show very heterogeneous morphological characteristics. In order to standardize histopathological diagnostic investigation, Morawietz et al. proposed a histological classification system that defines four different types of periprosthetic membranes based on the detection of foreign body particles, granulation tissue, and polymorphonuclear leukocytes (PMN) (type I is induced by wear particles, type II is infective type, type III is combined, and type IV is indeterminate). Infective and combined type reflects septic loosening [17]. The presence of significant number of neutrophils is the most important histological feature in establishing a diagnosis of PJI, since they are the most important cell population in the defense against bacterial infection (Fig. 16.1). The assessment of other cell types such as lymphocytes or plasma cells has not been proven to be suitable for diagnosing periprosthetic infections [5].

In 1973, Charosky et al. described a qualitative histological difference in the periprosthetic tissue response to infection as compared with particulate wear debris [9]. Those authors documented an infiltration of PMN cells that were characteristic for prosthetic joint infection. Later, in a series of 36 failed prostheses, Mirra et al. quantified the degree of inflammation in the presence of infection. They found more than five polymorphonuclear cells per high-power field (HPF) that were associated with infection. To minimize sampling error, Feldman et al. [12] described the criteria for histological diagnostic of PJI: (1) granulation tissue should be analyzed; (2) analysis should be performed at least on two samples of tissue from each patient; (3) the five most cellular fields per sample should be selected; (4) PMN cells have to be counted under high-power magnification; (5) only neutrophils with well-defined cytoplasmic borders should be included into counting [12].

There is an ongoing debate on the exact number of PMN leukocytes needed to diagnose PJI. Several cuts of criteria of the number of PMN cells have been published: e.g., Athanasou et al. require at least one PMN cell per HPF; Feldamn et al. use five PMN cells per HPF as cut of criterion; Pandey et al. described that >5 neutrophils should be diagnostic for PJI, but 1–5 neutrophils should be considered highly suggestive of infection; Bori et al. use five PMN cells as cut of criteria and described that the probability of infection is high when at least five PMN leukocytes per high-power field are found in the periprosthetic tissue; however, it is not possible to rule out infection when the number of neutrophils is less than five. Banit et al. [3] and Lonner et al. [14] propose that an infection should be diagnosed if at least ten neutrophils per HPF is found, and finally, Morawietz et al. [18] recommended a counting algorithm with threshold of ≥23 neutrophils in ten HPF.

Besides Feldman et al. [12] who reported 100 % sensitivity of PJI diagnosed by histological method, also Müller et al. [19] reported that among all preoperative and intraoperative tests, histopathology yielded the highest accuracy (94 %). The conclusions of these reports were questioned by Fehring and McAlister [11], who reported a sensitivity of only 18 %. Recently published articles that used the presence of microorganisms in periprosthetic tissue as a gold standard of PJI also reported lower value of sensitivity; however, even microbiological cultures are not 100 % reliable. Several authors reported worrisome prevalence of negative microbiological cultures of orthopedic specimens obtained intraoperatively [13, 16]. A discrepancy between microbiological and histological findings was found in 10.7 % of cases [17].

Upon close review of the literature, the sensitivity of histological diagnosis of PJI ranges between 18 and 100 %, but on the other side, it can be considered fairly specific, as reported in previous studies with range of 89.5–100 % (Table 16.1). Several authors concluded that analysis of histological sections of periprosthetic tissue is an important method to rule out the presence of infection, but not for detecting it [4, 10]. Nunez et al. [20] suggested that if there is no clinical suspicion of infection prior to operation and intraoperative frozen sections do not reveal five or more PMN leukocytes per HPF, reimplantation may be carried out at that moment, with 91 % chance of absence of infection. In suspected cases without positive preoperative diagnostic results but in a presence of more than five PMN cells in frozen

Table 16.1 Results of different studies evaluating histological method for prosthetic joint infection diagnosis

Study	N	PMN	S (%)	Sp (%)	PPV (%)	NPV (%)
Mira et al. [15]	34	>5	100	98	–	–
Fehring and McAlister [11]						
Feldman et al. [12]	33	>5	100	96	–	–
Lonner et al. [14]	175	>5	84	96	70	98
Athanasou et al. [2]	106	>5	90	96	88	98
Spangehl et al. (1998) [23]	202	>5	80	94	74	96
Abdul-Karim et al. [1]	64	>5	43	97	–	–
Pons et al. [22]	83	>5	100	98	94	100
Pandey et al. [21]	602	>5	100	97	92	100
Borrego et al. [8]	146	>10	91	87	81	94
Müller et al. [19]	50	>5	95	92	97	86
Morawietz et al. [18]	147	>23	73	95	91	91
Tothz et al. (2010) [24]	64	>5	86	100	100	95

N number of cases analyzed, *PMN* polymorphonuclear leukocytes, *S* sensitivity, *SP* specificity, *PPV* positive predictive value, *NPV* negative predictive value

section, the surgeon must proceed with caution and it could be convenient in such cases to defer reimplantation.

The reasons for the fact that the specificity and sensitivity of histology for diagnosis of PJI in several studies have never reached 100 % are different. False-positive results of histology could be due to one of several causes: a fastidious microorganism that fails to grow in vitro, the fact that samples for culture or histology are not taken from same area, or the presence of a loculated infection [14]. It has to be emphasized that a negative result of microbiological culture does not exclude the presence of infection.

False-negative results of histological analysis could be attributed to:

1. Bacteriological contamination of the specimen obtained for microbiology culture
2. The cut of criteria (number of PMN leukocytes per microscopic field) to establish the diagnosis of prosthetic joint infection
3. Low-virulent microorganisms like *Staphylococcus epidermidis* or *Propionibacterium* spp. that do not stimulate PMN cell infiltration
4. Type of specimen submitted to the laboratory for histological analysis [7]

There is a lot of variability in the specimens submitted for histological evaluation. The majority of orthopedic surgeons obtain specimens from pseudocapsule, synovial surface, periprosthetic membrane, or any tissue suspected for infection. Periprosthetic membrane is located at the interface between prosthesis component and bone or between bone cement and tissue and is not to be mistaken with pseudocapsule that forms around joint space. Several authors described that histological appearance of interface membrane and pseudocapsule is very similar in the same patient [17, 21]. However, Bori et al. found out that periprosthetic interface membrane is the best specimen for the histological diagnosis of prosthetic joint infection [7] and that interface membrane has a higher sensitivity and predictive values than pseudocapsule. Samples of the interface membrane should be sent to histological laboratory as soon as possible, and multiple small samples may be more effective in detecting focal areas of inflammation.

Several studies reported very good correlation between the results of the analysis of frozen sections and those of the analysis of the permanent sections. The agreement reported ranged between 78 and 100 %. The paraffin embedding used in the preparation of permanent histological sections makes sectioning easier and leaves less tissue artifacts; however, by frozen sections, we can get the information about possible PJI much faster.

Conclusions: Due to its high specificity, negative histological analysis of periprosthetic tissue indicates absence of infection; on the other hand, a positive histology not necessarily confirms infection because of its low sensitivity. To improve the results of PJI histopathological diagnosis, the pathologist must be well versed in the technique of preparation and the interpretation of frozen and permanent sections. Additionally, the orthopedic surgeon and the pathologist must have a close working relationship and a free exchange of information. The pathologist should be provided with clinical data such as type of prosthesis and type of fixation, lifetime of prosthesis, and previous microbiological findings by the orthopedic surgeon.

References

1. Abdul-Karim FM, McGinis MG, Kraay M, et al. Frozen section biopsy assessment for the presence of polymorphonuclear leukocytes in patients undergoing revision of arthroplasties. Mod Pathol. 1998;11:427–31.
2. Athanasou NA, Pandey R, de Steiger R, et al. The role of intraoperative frozen sections in revision total joint arthroplasty. J Bone Joint Surg Am. 1997;79:1433–4.
3. Banit DM, Kaufer H, Harford JM. Intraoperative frozen section analysis in revision total joint arthroplasty. Clin Orthop Relat Res. 2002;400:230–8.
4. Bori G, Soriano A, Garcia S, et al. Low sensitivity of histology to predict the presence of microorganisms in suspected aseptic loosening of a joint prosthesis. Mod Pathol. 2006;19:874–7. doi:10.1038/modpathol.3800606.
5. Bori G, Soriano A, Garcia S, Mallofre C, Riba J, Mensa J. Usefulness of histological analysis for predicting the presence of microorganisms at the time of reimplantation after hip resection arthroplasty for the treatment of infection. J Bone Joint Surg Am. 2007;89:1232–7. doi:10.2106/JBJS.F.00741.
6. Bori G, Soriano A, Garcia S, Gallart X, Mallofre C, Mensa J. Neutrophils in frozen sections and type of microorganism isolated at the time of resection arthroplasty for the treatment of infection. Arch Orthop Trauma Surg. 2009;129:591–5. doi:10.1007/s00402-008-0679-6.
7. Bori G, Monuz-Mahamud E, Garcia S, et al. Interface membrane is the best sample for histological study to diagnose prosthetic joint infection. Mod Pathol. 2011;24:579–84. doi:10.1038/modpathol.2010.219.
8. Borrego AF, Martinez FM, Parra JLC, Graneda DS, Crespo RG, Stern LLD. Diagnosis of infection in hip and knee revision surgery: intraoperative frozen section analysis. Int Orthop. 2007;31:33–7. doi:10.1007/s00264-005-0069-4.

9. Charosky CB, Bullough PG, Wilson PD. Total hip replacement failures. A histological evaluation. J Bone Joint Surg Am. 1973;55:49–58.

10. Della Valle CJ, Bogner E, Desai P, et al. Analysis of frozen sections of intraoperative specimens obtained at the time of reoperation after hip or knee resection arthroplasty for the treatment of infection. J Bone Joint Surg Am. 1999;81:684–9.

11. Fehring TK, McAlister Jr JA. Frozen histological section as a guide to sepsis in revision joint arthroplasty. Clin Orthop. 1994;304:229–37.

12. Feldman DS, Lonner JS, Desal P, Zuckerman JD. The role of intraoperative frozen sections in revision total joint arthroplasty. J Bone Joint Surg Am. 1995;77:1807–13.

13. Ince A, Rupp J, Fromelt L, Katzer A, Gille J, Lohr JF. Is "aseptic" loosening of the prosthetic cup after total hip replacement due to nonculturable bacterial pathogens in patients with low-grade infection? Clin Infect Dis. 2004;39:1599–603.

14. Lonner JH, Desai P, Dicesare PE, Steiner G, Zuckerman JD. The reliability of analysis of intraoperative frozen sections for identifying acute infection during revision hip or knee arthroplasty. J Bone Joint Surg Am. 1996;78:1553–8.

15. Mira JM, Amstutz HC, Matos M, et al. The pathology of the joint tissue and its clinical relevance in prosthesis failure. Clin Orthop. 1976;117:221–40.

16. Moran E, Byren I, Atkins L. Diagnosis and management of prosthetic joint infections. J Antimicrob Chemother. 2010;65 Suppl 3:45–54. doi:10.1093/jac/dkq305.

17. Morawietz L, Classen RA, Schroder JH, et al. Proposal of histopathological consensus classification of the periprosthetic interface membrane. J Clin Pathol. 2006;59:591–7. doi:10.1136/jcp.2005.027485.

18. Morawietz L, Tiddens O, Mueller M, et al. Twenty-three neutrophil granulocytes in 10 high-power fields is the best histopathological threshold to differentiate between aseptic and septic endopros-thesis loosening. Histopathology. 2009;847–853. doi:10.1111/j.1365-2559.2009.03313.x.

19. Müller M, Morawietz L, Hasart O, Strube P, Perka C, Tohtz S. Diagnosis of periprosthetic infection following total hip arthroplasty-evaluation of the diagnostic values of pre- and intra-operative parameters and the associated strategy to preoperatively select patients with a high probability of joint infection. J Orthop Surg Res. 2008;3:31. doi:10.1186/1749-799X-3-31.

20. Nunez LV, Buttaro MA, Morandi A, Pusso R, Piccaluga F. Frozen sections of samples taken intraoperatively for diagnosis of infection in revision hip surgery. Acta Orthop. 2007;78:226–30. doi:10.1080/17453670710013726.

21. Pandey R, Drakoulakis E, Athanasou NA. An assessment of the histological criteria used to diagnose infection in hip revision arthroplasty tissues. J Clin Pathol. 1999;52:118–23.

22. Pons M, Angels F, Sanchez C, et al. Infected total hip arthroplasty-the value of intraoperative histology. Int Orthop. 1999;23:34–6.

23. Spangehl MJ, Masri BA, O'Connel JX, et al. Prospective analysis of preoperative and intraoperative investigational for the diagnosis of infection at the sites of two hundred and two revision total hip arthroplasties. J Bone Joint Surg Am. 1999;81:672–83.

24. Tohtz SW, Muller M, Morawietz L, Winkler T, Parka C. Validity of frozen sections for analysis of periprosthetic loosening membranes. Clin Orthop Relat Res. 2010;468:762–8. doi:10.107/s!1999-009-1102-5.

25. Wong YC, Lee QJ, Wai YL, Ng WF. Intraoperative frozen section for detecting active infection in failed hip and knee arthroplasties. J Arthroplasty. 2005;20:1015–20. doi:10.1016/j.arth.2004.08.003.

Chapter 17
Microbiological Diagnosis of Prosthetic Joint Infection

Jaime Esteban, Concepción Pérez-Jorge, Ramón Pérez-Tanoira, and Enrique Gómez-Barrena

Abstract Diagnosis of Prosthetic Joint Infection is still a complex matter in clinical practice. Syndromic diagnosis includes the presence of several symptoms and signs together with the use of a combination of different techniques, including image analysis, biochemical markers and intraoperatory histopatology. Microbiological diagnosis is an essential part of this process, because it allows selection of the best possible antibiotic therapy, and even orients the surgical management and the potential outcome of the patient in some cases. Cultures of synovial fluids, periprosthetic tissues and implant sonication are the commonly recommended techniques, and a combination of these techniques allows reaching an etiologic diagnosis in most cases. However, rapid diagnosis is still a problem, because the lack of sensitivity and specificity of Gram stain of surgical products.

Keywords Cultures • Imaging • Aspiration • Sonication

17.1 Introduction

The use of joint prosthesis is one of the most important advances in orthopedics. It allows millions of people to improve their quality of life with the recovery from a chronic impairment not possible with any other solution but prosthetic joint reconstruction. The use of prosthetic joints is currently increasing, and it is expected that more than three million prosthesis per year will be implanted in 2050 [1]. Despite

J. Esteban, M.D., Ph.D. • C. Pérez-Jorge • R. Pérez-Tanoira
Bone and Joint Infection Unit, Department of Clinical Microbiology,
IIS-Fundación Jiménez Díaz,
Av. Reyes Católicos 2, Madrid 28040, Spain
e-mail: jestebanmoreno@gmail.com; cperemarch@fjd.es; rptanoira@fjd.es

E. Gómez-Barrena, M.D., Ph.D. (✉)
Department of Orthopaedic Surgery and Traumatology, Hospital "La Paz",
Paseo de la Castellana 261, Madrid 28046, Spain
e-mail: enrique.gomezbarrena@uam.es

R. Trebše (ed.), *Infected Total Joint Arthroplasty*,
DOI 10.1007/978-1-4471-2482-5_17, © Springer-Verlag London 2012

all these advantages, the use of implants is not without complications. Among these, one of the most devastating problems is the development of infection, which appears in 1–3 % of all the cases [2], and raises patient morbidity and mortality. Due to the increasing number of implant surgeries, it is expected that the number of infected patients will grow parallel to the number of implanted prostheses, so the problem will be even greater in the next future [3].

One of the key issues in the management of these patients is diagnosis. Clinical diagnosis has been considered the gold standard for decades and still is extremely important. Clinical suspicion is the first step that triggers all other tests leading to a final diagnosis of prosthetic joint infection (PJI) [2, 4–6]. However, there are cases of PJI in which clinical data are scanty or appear to mimic aseptic loosening, but even these cases can be diagnosed correctly if proper diagnostic tools are applied [7]. Moreover, despite general confirmation of PJI diagnosis is important, etiologic diagnosis is essential for proper management of these patients [2, 4–6], because an adequate selection of antibiotics is the key for a proper patient management [2, 8]. This is due to the high number of organisms that can be the cause of these infections, even if 60–70 % of all the cases are caused by the members of the genus *Staphylococcus* [4]. Identification and susceptibility testing is an extremely important issue, and the techniques used for this purpose will be revised in this chapter.

17.2   Rapid Conventional Diagnosis

Rapid diagnosis of PJI can lead to establish a different management of the patient even during the surgery. These techniques are based on the use of different stains, most of them available elsewhere.

17.2.1   Histopathology

Although this technique cannot provide an etiologic diagnosis, several authors have shown a high correlation between the presence of acute and chronic inflammatory cells on frozen sections of periprosthetic tissues and the existence of PJI (Table 17.1). Mirra et al. [9] found the presence of an infiltrate of acute inflammatory cells on frozen-section histology in 15 cases with evidence of infection and reported the absence of such infiltrate in 21 noninfected cases. This study allowed designing the criterion of the presence of several polymorphonuclear leukocytes/high-power field (HPF) as a diagnostic feature of PJI. Different studies have used various cutoff points, but usually, 5–10 polymorphonuclear leukocytes per HPF typically indicate acute inflammation and are considered the breakpoint to confirm the diagnosis of PJI [1, 4–6, 10–14]. However, although this test is quite specific to diagnose PJI, it is not highly sensitive. Some other issues must be taken into account: the number of areas to be scanned in frozen sections is not standardized [15]. Because the degree of infiltration with inflammatory cells may vary considerably between tissue sections,

Table 17.1 Frozen section/histopathology in diagnosis of PJI

Reference	No. and type of arthroplasty	Cutoff	S (%)	Sp (%)	PPV (%)	NPV (%)
Fehring et al. [59]	107	No cutoff	18.2	89.5		
Athanasou et al. [60]	106 (hip-knee)	1	90	96	88	98
Lonner et al. [12]	175 (hip-knee)	5	84	96	70	98
		10	84	99	89	98
Pandey et al. [61]	602 (hip)	1	98	97	92	100
Banit et al. [62]	121 (hip-knee)	10	67	93	67	93
Bori et al. [13]	21 (hip)	5	28.5	100	100	74
		1	71.4	64.2	50	81.8

S sensitivity, *Sp* specificity, *PPV* positive predictive value, *NPV* negative predictive value

at least ten HPFs should be examined to obtain an average count. Another major limitation of histopathological examination is that it does not identify the causative organism. In addition, interpretation of tissue histopathology from patients with underlying inflammatory joint disorders may be difficult [10].

Frozen-section analysis of biopsy specimens must be taken from several different sites in order to increase the sensitivity. It is also important that the tissue adequately represents the fibrous membrane and does not contain only superficial fibrin.

17.2.2   Gram Stain

Gram stain is one of the most useful techniques to perform a rapid diagnosis in the clinical microbiology laboratory. It is a technique with extremely long experience which allows to detect bacteria and to perform an initial classification of these organisms according to their shape and staining characteristics [16]. Its use in synovial fluid has been claimed to be highly specific, although sensitivity is only 40–45 % [5]. However, its use in periprosthetic tissues for PJI diagnosis (Table 17.2) has many other disadvantages. In fact, although a positive result of a Gram stain can predict infection, the sensitivity is so poor that multiple samples from a large number of infected patients must be examined for each positive result [17]. Moreover, Ghanem et al. [18] have reported that such sensitivity did not show major improvement with increasing number of samples. In other study, Chimento et al. [19] conclude that the absence of organisms on intraoperative Gram staining during revision arthroplasty does not confirm the absence of infection and even the presence and number of polymorphonuclear cells did not correlate with the presence or absence of infection. Because of these limitations, rapid diagnosis of PJI by using Gram stain can be abandoned as a diagnostic tool at elective revision arthroplasty [17, 20].

Table 17.2 Gram stain in diagnosis of PJI

Reference	Number cases analyzed	Type sample	Positive result if presence of[a]:	S % (hip-knee)	Sp % (hip-knee)	PPV % (hip-knee)	NPV % (hip-knee)
Atkins et al.[17]	297	Pre-intra	Organism	12[b]	98.8[b]	–	–
				6[c]	99.7[c]	–	–
Chimento et al. [19]	169	Intra	Organism	0	–	–	–
			>10PMN	18.8	95.6	50	83
Feldman et al. [63]	33	Intra	Organism	22.2	–	–	–
Pandey et al. [61]	602 (hip)		Organism	21.5	–	–	–
Della Valle et al. [64]	413	Intra		14.7			
Spangehl et al. [65]	202 (hip)	Intra	Organism	19	98	63	89
Ghanem et al. [18]	321 infected and 683 uninfected	Intra	Organism	31–30	100	100–98	79–70
			>5PMN	31–53	99	89–96	79–78
			Both[d]	18–21	100	100	77–68
			Both[e]	43–64	99	93–97	82
Parvizi et al. [66]	453(knee)	Intra	Organism	30	98	89	70
			>5PMN	50	100	100	79
			Both	43-64	100	100	82

Pre preoperative, *Intra* intraoperative, *S* sensitivity, *Sp* specificity, *PPV* positive predictive value, *NPV* negative predictive value

[a]The result was considered positive for infection if there were organisms, more than five or ten PMN per high-power field (×40) in at least five separate microscopic fields or both

[b]Sensitivity and specificity was measured against positive histology (presence of at least five neutrophils per high-power field)

[c]Sensitivity and specificity was measured against positive culture (isolation of an indistinguishable microorganism from three or more independent specimens)

[d]Series combination testing requires both tests to be positive (and not just either one) to reach a diagnosis of PPI

[e]Parallel combination testing requires any one or both of the tests to be positive to diagnose infection

17.2.3 *Immunofluorescence*

Another technique that can be used for a rapid diagnosis is immunofluorescence microscopy (IFM). In this technique, monoclonal antibodies labeled with fluorescent markers are used to detect the microorganisms with a fluorescence microscopy. There are different studies in the literature about the use of direct visualization of bacteria from sonication fluid with pathogen-targeted antibodies as a nonculture method for the microbiological diagnosis of PJI. Tunney et al. [21] used polyclonal antibodies against *Staphylococcus* sp. from fluid obtained after sonication of retrieved implants in patients with PJI and controls. The IFM results indicated that 63 % of retrieved hip prostheses were colonized with bacteria, although the species could not be identified. Piper et al. also evaluated the use of IFM for the diagnosis of PJI in shoulder prosthesis processed by sonication of the retrieved implants, using monoclonal antibodies directed against *Propionibacterium acnes* and *Staphylococcus* sp., and compared it with the use of molecular biology. The sensitivity of IFM and PCR with sonicate fluid for the detection of definite prosthetic shoulder infection (from any cause) was 39.4 % (13/33) and 57.6 % (19/33), respectively; the specificity was 98.0 % (99/101) and 99.0 % (100/101), respectively [22].

Yet, the value of this technique for the microbiological diagnosis of PJI outside from a research study is unclear. According to the authors, the IFM did not improve the culture sensitivity from the sonicate fluid due to the fact that all IFM positive specimens had positive cultures [22]. According to some authors [21, 23], the characteristics in the visualization from large aggregates to single bacteria could help distinguish between contaminating and pathogen bacteria. However, the main limitation of the technique is its specificity regarding identification of the pathogen at the species level. If a specific monoclonal antibody is used [22], a high number of stains must be used in order to identify all potential pathogens, and those which are not sought cannot be identified. If an unspecific antibody is used [21], identification of the detected bacteria cannot be performed. Because of these limitations, IFM is not currently used for diagnosis of PJI in a clinical setting by most laboratories.

17.2.4   Other Image Studies

Stoodley et al. [24] described the case of a patient who had chronic recurring symptoms of infection that persisted for years. Confocal microscopy was performed using Molecular Probes Live/Dead BacLight kit on fluid, tissue, and cement at the final surgical revision and demonstrated the presence of biofilms with living coccoid bacterial cells in an infected elbow case that yielded negative cultures over a period of 5 years. Therefore, confocal laser scanning microscopy permits the observation of biofilm-embedded bacteria on the surfaces of the explanted prostheses, although its use still remains experimental [25, 26].

A periprosthetic biopsy under fluoroscopy is an alternative and may increase the chances of sampling the area with the highest density of organisms in chronic infections (the bone/cement or bone/prosthesis interface) [27].

17.3   Preoperative Conventional Microbiological Diagnosis

The microbiological study can help to preoperatively (before the arthroplasty revision surgery) diagnose a PJI when used together with other specific analytics parameters, clinical history, physical examination, and imaging, especially because all these data are separately associated with a high level of false positives and negatives [28]. The microbiological diagnosis allows the identification of the causative organism, facilitating the management of the patient through the choice of the antimicrobial therapy and the adequate evaluation of a surgical treatment. Moreover, it could help to differentiate between PJI and aseptic loosening in some patients [28, 29].

17.3.1   Synovial Fluid Culture

Synovial fluid culture is one of the main microbiological techniques used to perform the PJI diagnosis in patients with underlying inflammation. Usually, the synovial fluid analysis includes the evaluation of inflammatory markers and synovial fluid cell counts [4]. In many cases, there are no reliable results with the use of these techniques, and in these cases, the synovial fluid culture may be useful in diagnosing the PJI [29]. The main advantage of the synovial culture is that it allows the identification and susceptibility testing of microorganisms independently of the presence of underlying inflammatory diseases, which can affect the results of other tests [1, 4].

The value of the synovial fluid culture has been studied in depth [1, 4]. However, there are a lot of factors that are still under study. One of the most recent issues is the inoculation of blood culture bottles compared to the use of conventional solid media cultures. There are different theories that tried to explain the low sensitivity of conventional cultures [30–33]. First, the amount of microorganisms present in the sample is often quite low, and the inoculation of the sample in blood culture bottles could improve this lack and increase the sensitivity through the use of a higher amount of sample (approximately 5 mL/flask) than that used in solid media cultures. Secondly, the presence of inhibitors in the sample, such as antibiotics, may inhibit the growth of microorganisms. Nowadays, blood culture bottles include different methods to overcome this problem. Third, it must be taken into account the fact that the microorganisms may be phagocytozed by white blood cells in synovial fluid and therefore may not be recovered by culture. Most of the blood culture systems contain lytic agents (such as saponin), which release phagocytized organisms, allowing them to grow freely in the liquid medium. Finally, there is a possible contamination of the plates of culture media when the sample is inoculated, while in blood cultures the sample manipulation is reduced, and therefore the risk of contamination could decrease. The different factors aforementioned suggest that inoculation of synovial fluid in blood culture bottles may improve the sensitivity of the technique. There are several studies in the literature comparing the inoculation of synovial fluid in blood culture bottles using different systems, such as BACTEC PEDS PLUS/F Medium bottle (BD, USA) [30, 31], BACTEC 460 aerobic blood culture bottles (BD, USA) [33] or BACTEC 9240 bottles [32], against the use of conventional solid media culture (Table 17.3). These studies showed a statistically significant greater amount of isolated pathogens than with conventional cultures, using different protocols.

However, there could be discordance between synovial fluid and intraoperative cultures. Most studies remark that synovial biopsy studies are superior to joint aspiration in the diagnosis of PJI. Fink et al. [31] evaluated synovial biopsy culture in comparison with joint aspiration and C- reactive protein in total knee replacements. Synovial fluid was collected in BD BACTEC PEDS PLUS/F Medium, and after 14 days, they reported a positive result if the same organism was identified in at least two samples. The results showed that the combination of the bacteriological and the histological study of the synovial biopsy had the highest diagnostic value to identify a late periprosthetic infection. These results could be due to the fact that, in the infected prosthesis, organisms are

Table 17.3 Comparison of cultures of fluid samples injected into standard blood culture vials (SBC), periprosthetic tissue and swab samples cultured in standard media

Reference	No. of patients	Type of samples	S %	Sp %
Font-Vizcarra et al. [32]	63	SBC	86	100
		Periprosthetic tissue	69	81
		Swab	61	99
Levine et al. [67]	24	SBC	92	100
		Periprosthetic tissue	46	100
		Swab	64	100

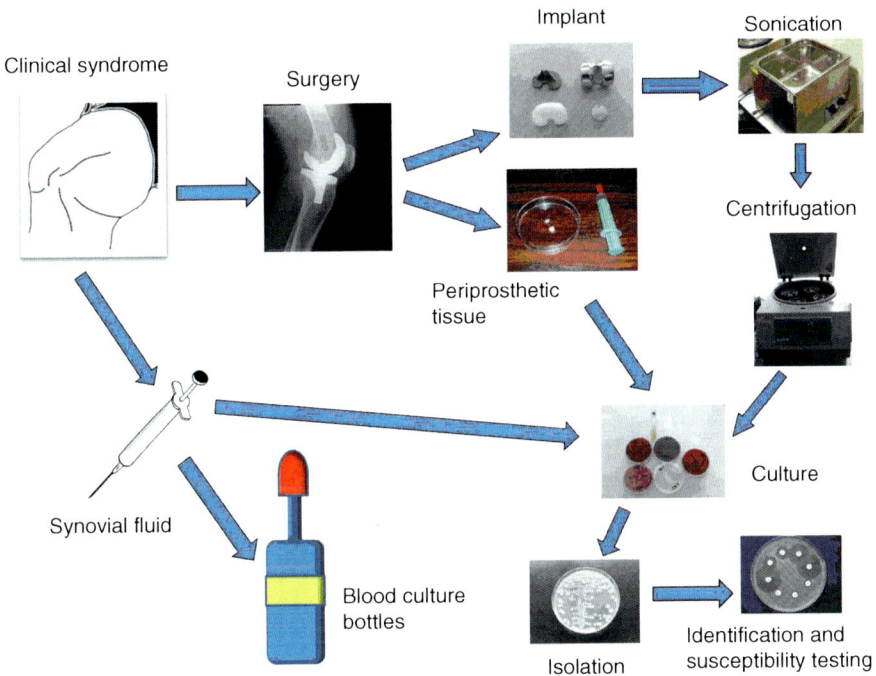

Fig. 17.1 Proposed scheme for microbiological diagnosis of PJI

embedded in biofilms firmly attached to the implant surface, and only a low percentage appeared as planktonic bacteria [32, 34]. In acute infections, synovial fluid is abundant, the number of planktonic bacteria is high, and the characteristic symptoms and signs of infection are present, while in chronic infections, the volume of synovial fluid is low and most of the bacteria are in a sessile state, attached to the implant surface.

In conclusion, as can be stated by the results obtained from the literature, the synovial fluid culture in automatic systems increase the sensitivity and specificity to diagnose PJI compared to conventional tests and should be introduced in a general practice (Fig. 17.1).

17.3.2 Sinus Tract Cultures

Sinus tract specimens are reported as a poor sample for the diagnosis of PJI [5], although, because these are easy to obtain, they are commonly sent to clinical microbiology laboratories in many areas. In a study of chronic osteomyelitis, cultures obtained from sinus tracts detected the infecting pathogen only in 44 % of cases, as compared to cultures of intraoperative tissue specimens, and only isolation of *Staphylococcus aureus* from sinus tracts is predictive of the causative pathogen [15]. A bacteriologic diagnosis of chronic osteomyelitis based on isolation of common pathogens other than *S. aureus* from sinus tracts must be verified by an appropriate operative culture [27, 35]. Moreover, because the most frequently isolated pathogen in PJI is the group of coagulase-negative staphylococci, cultures of sinus tract exudates should be avoided; these are often positive because of microbial skin colonization and poorly correlate with cultures of surgical specimens [4]. Another study by Cune et al. [36] in patients with acute PJI analyzed the concordance defined as the isolation of one microorganism in the superficial samples that was also found in the deep samples. They concluded that superficial samples could help surgeons to identify resistant microorganism early and to start specific antibiotic treatment. However, the efficacy of superficial swabbing was greater when the isolated microorganism was *S. aureus* or aerobic gram-negative bacilli, and not for other organisms [36]. Moreover, other studies showed lower rate of correlation between sinus tract cultures and biopsy cultures than that of Cune et al. [5, 37].

Despite this result, swab cultures have been reported to sustain a high rate of false-positive results due to contamination with coagulase-negative *Staphylococcus* and/or *Propionibacterium* sp., so these cannot be recommended for the diagnosis of chronic PJI, although they could have some usefulness in some cases of acute PJI [1, 4, 5, 32].

17.4 Intraoperative Conventional Microbiological Diagnosis

When diagnosis of PJI is performed, surgical therapy is an essential part of the management of the patient [2, 8]. During surgery, it is essential to obtain or confirm the etiologic diagnosis by sending different samples to the microbiology laboratory. These samples include from synovial fluid to the implant itself.

17.4.1 Synovial Fluid Aspiration

Spangehl et al. [38] prospectively analyzed the value of preoperative and intraoperative synovial fluid culture for the diagnosis of infection in 178 patients who had a total of 202 revision hip replacements. The results of preoperative aspiration of the joint were 86 % sensitivity, 94 % specificity, 67 % positive predictive value, and 98 % negative predictive value, while the results of intraoperative cultures were 94 % sensitivity, 97 % specificity, 77 % positive predictive value, and 99 % negative predictive value. Its use together with tissue samples also increases its value for diagnosis of PJI [39].

17.4.2 Periprosthetic Tissue Cultures

Periprosthetic tissue cultures provide the most accurate specimens for detecting the infecting microorganism, and the results of culture of tissue and/or fluid obtained during revision arthroplasty are usually considered the gold standard for determining the presence or absence of periprosthetic infection [20].

Sensitivity of periprosthetic tissue culture may be low (between 37 and 61 %) [25, 40], and probably this may be related to the state of the surrounding tissue. To increase the sensitivity of these cultures, it has been recommended the use of a minimum of three different samples [10, 15], although the number can be increased to at least five of them [4, 17, 20]. Kamme and Lindberg [41] described that the growth in one or two of five biopsy samples was a strong indicator of contamination, while growth in five of five biopsy samples of one or two bacterial species strongly indicated an infection. According to other authors, the growth of the same organism in at least three samples differentiates contaminants from true pathogens [20]. Atkins et al. proposed the use of a cutoff of ≥2 positive tissue cultures [17]. A combination of different samples could also increase the sensitivity. In the study of Meermans and Haddad [39], the combination of tissue biopsy and aspiration provided improved sensitivity and accuracy. Nevertheless, a strong recommendation regarding the use of strictly sterile procedures to obtain and manipulate the samples must be done in all cases.

In the microbiology laboratory, processing of the samples is usually performed by inoculation of culture media after grinding the samples. A recent report [42] suggests that sensitivity could be increased by using bead mill sample processing, which releases the infected organisms in a higher proportion than classical processing. Another controversial issue in the laboratory concerns the incubation time. Some organisms causing PJI may be slow growing due to either their phenotypic state (sessile forms inside the biofilm) or inherent characteristics (like *P. acnes* or other slow-growing organisms). According to Schafer et al. [43], an extended incubation period of 15 days improves the sensitivity of cultures from periprosthetic samples, with only 73.6 % of the samples being positive before day 7 of incubation.

Whenever possible, antibiotics should be removed before all diagnostic microbiological tests have been completed. It is not clear how long a patient should be off antibiotics prior to the diagnostic procedures being performed, but a 14-day antibiotic-free period has been recommended [4, 10, 27]. Moreover, it has been reported that administration of antimicrobials within 3 months of arthroplasty revision is associated with negative cultures [1, 44, 45].

17.4.3   Retrieved Implants

One of the most important issues related to the pathogenesis of PJI is the fact that microorganisms form a biofilm on the prosthesis [34, 46–48]. This phenomenon also has extremely important implications for the diagnosis of the patient, because bacteria could be firmly attached to the implant, and so cultures from other samples could give negative results. If the implanted material is removed, it can be send to the microbiology laboratory to be processed, looking for sessile organisms. The obvious advantage of this approach is that the sample to be tested is the actual site of infection [46]. However, the risk of contamination during processing is high. Several approaches have been used for implant processing, including scrapping or swabbing the implant surface or culturing all the implant in liquid media. However, these approaches usually lack of sensitivity and/or specificity and are not used in current clinical microbiology routine [5, 10, 11, 25]. Recently, the use of low-intensity ultrasounds (sonication) became a useful system to perform implant processing and is currently used in many laboratories as part of their diagnostic routine.

17.4.3.1   Sonication

According to the "race for the surface" theory by Gristina [48], biomaterial-related infections started when bacteria adhere to these devices and develop an extracellular matrix with specific characteristics which starts biofilm formation. The biofilm protects the bacteria from the activity of antimicrobials and from the host defense mechanisms [34, 46, 49]. One of the main consequences of this phenomenon is the difficulty to manage biomaterial-related infections, which usually need to remove the devices in order to obtain a good patient outcome [8, 10, 46, 50]. The periprosthetic tissue cultures are the gold standard method for microbiological diagnosis, but sessile organisms are sometimes impossible to detect by common culture techniques because they are attached to the implant, and not in the surrounding samples [8, 21, 46].

The use of ultrasounds to release bacteria attached to different surfaces has been used several years ago. However, this technique has been used only for experimental purposes, and not to obtain a diagnosis in the clinical setting. Sonication protocols have been developed to obtain the highest amount of viable bacteria from the surface. Monsen et al. [51] analyzed this problem and suggested a protocol for sonication in which different effects were taken into account to improve the sensitivity of sonication. The effects of the temperature, duration, composition of sonication buffer, and material in the sonication tube during bacteria sonication were variables evaluated by these authors. They concluded that sterilized buffer should be used for sonication of removed implants and transportation to the laboratory should be as quick as possible. Once in the laboratory, the implant could be transferred for sonication, preferably to a glass tube. The conditions of the sonication proposed by these authors are as follow: 7 min at room temperature (22 °C), with further concentration of the sonicate solution by centrifugation to obtain a final volume of 400 μL. The suspended pellet is divided into four portions of 100 μL for culture in different agar medium. The duration of the sonication is important in order to isolate gram-negative bacilli, which can be eradicated after 15 min of exposure, while there are some authors that used protocols sonicating the sample during longer time periods [52].

At the end of the 1990s, Tunney et al. [21] developed a sonication protocol for hip-infected prostheses which showed a high specificity and sensitivity. The study showed the need of anaerobic cultures to improve the detection of anaerobic bacteria isolates. However, this study showed also a high number of positive results in patients without clinical symptoms or signs of infection, so this method was not incorporated into clinical routine [21]. A later study by Trampuz et al. [6] about the use of bags in a sonication suggests that the use of solid containers could avoid the contamination of cultures by waterborne microorganism when there is a bag leakage, a phenomenon associated with false-positive results [53]. Using a protocol designed to avoid this problem, the same authors evaluated sonication in a high number of patients with PJI, with extremely good results that improved the sensitivity of periprosthetic tissue culture without diminution of specificity [40]. In this later study, samples were processed in rigid plastic containers and vortexed prior to sonication in a high volume of buffer. Several months later, other studies were published that confirmed the usefulness of sonication, even with different protocols [54, 55]. In the study performed by Esteban et al. [54], the risk of bag contamination was overcome by performing changes of the water in the sonicator before each procedure and by a careful inspection of the bags, looking for leakages [54]. In this study, a concentration step using centrifugation of the sonicate and the use of a broad spectrum of culture media (designed to isolate uncommon organisms) was suggested to improve the sensitivity of the technique. Further studies used a combined approach with rigid plastic containers and centrifugation with good result, not only for joint prosthesis but also for other orthopedic implants [22, 56, 57].

The implications of one significant problem of the periprosthetic tissue culture, such as the previous therapy with antibiotics, were studied by Trampuz et al. [40]. Sonication showed a greater sensitivity than tissue culture in patients who received antimicrobial therapy within the previous 14 days [40]. In this study, the authors also suggested a quantification of the number of microorganisms isolated from a sonicate fluid that may help to distinguish infected from contaminated prostheses [40]. However, other results did not confirmed this issue [54], and no breakpoint for diagnosis of infection has been established yet. Differentiating sonication of the implant pieces has also been suggested as an aid to determine if the isolate was a true pathogen or a contamination [54]. Nevertheless, even with all these differences, the studies showed that sonication was, at least, as sensitive as periprosthetic tissue culture and most studies, in fact, showed a better performance of sonication for the diagnosis of PJI [21, 22, 40, 54–58]. Therefore, its use must be recommended as an aid to other microbiological procedures in order to isolate the causative organisms of PJI (Fig. 17.1).

All the previously cited protocols are similar: after the implant retrieval, it is introduced in a sterile container and sent to the laboratory with a maximum delay of

24 h (samples could be stored at 4 °C). In the laboratory, samples are introduced in sterile containers, and a specific quantity of buffer is added. Samples are then vortexed and sonicated during 5 min or a similar time period, and the sonicate is then concentrated by centrifugation. The sediment is resuspended and inoculated in different media using a quantitative approach. Fungal cultures, mycobacterial cultures, or both may be considered because samples are not easy to obtain and a maximum effort must be done to reach the most specific diagnosis.

17.5   Conclusions

Etiologic diagnosis is one of the cornerstones in the management of the patient with PJI. Without such diagnosis, treatment of the patient must be empirical, and the risks of a bad outcome increase. Such diagnosis still is performed using classical methods such as stains and cultures in different media, but new technologies have increased the sensitivity and specificity of the different techniques, so the number of undiagnosed patients has markedly decreased. However, despite these advances, there is still a number of patients which have negative results with these techniques, so further studies are necessary to improve the currently used techniques. The use of molecular biology or similar approaches could be extremely important in the next years, and a better management of these patients is expected to be developed in the near future.

References

1. Gomez E, Patel R. Laboratory diagnosis of prosthetic joint infection, part I. Clin Microbiol Newslett. 2011;33(8):55–60. doi:10.1016/j.clinmicnews.2011.03.004.
2. Darouiche RO. Treatment of infections associated with surgical implants. N Engl J Med. 2004;350:1422–9.
3. Kurtz SM, Lau E, Schmier J, Ong KL, Zhao K, Parvizi J. Infection burden for hip and knee arthroplasty in the United States. J Arthroplasty. 2008;23(7):984–91.
4. Del Pozo JL, Patel R. Clinical practice. Infection associated with prosthetic joints. N Engl J Med. 2009;361(8):787–94.
5. Zimmerli W, Trampuz A, Ochsner PE. Prosthetic-joint infections. N Engl J Med. 2004; 351(16):1645–54.
6. Trampuz A, Widmer AF. Infections associated with orthopedic implants. Curr Opin Infect Dis. 2006;19:349–56.
7. Nelson CL, McLaren AC, McLaren SG, Johnson JW, Smeltzer MS. Is aseptic loosening truly aseptic? Clin Orthop Relat Res. 2005;437:25–30.
8. Esteban J, Cordero-Ampuero J. Treatment of prosthetic osteoarticular infections. Expert Opin Pharmacother. 2011;12(6):899–912.
9. Mirra JM, Amstutz HC, Matos M, Gold R. The pathology of the joint tissues and its clinical relevance in prosthesis failure. Clin Orthop Relat Res. 1976;117:221–40.
10. Trampuz A, Zimmerli W. Prosthetic joint infections: update in diagnosis and treatment. Swiss Med Wkly. 2005;135(17–18):243–51.

11. Zimmerli W. Prosthetic-joint-associated infections. Best Pract Res Clin Rheumatol. 1996;20(6):1045–63.

12. Lonner JH, Desai P, Dicesare PE, Steiner G, Zuckerman JD. The reliability of analysis of intraoperative frozen sections for identifying active infection during revision hip or knee arthroplasty. J Bone Joint Surg Am. 1996;78(10):1553–8.

13. Bori G, Soriano A, Garcia S, Mallofre C, Riba J, Mensa J. Usefulness of histological analysis for predicting the presence of microorganisms at the time of reimplantation after hip resection arthroplasty for the treatment of infection. J Bone Joint Surg Am. 2007;89(6):1232–7.

14. Della Valle CJ, Bogner E, Desai P, Lonner JH, Adler E, Zuckerman JD, et al. Analysis of frozen sections of intraoperative specimens obtained at the time of reoperation after hip or knee resection arthroplasty for the treatment of infection. J Bone Joint Surg Am. 1999;81:684–9.

15. Widmer AF. New developments in diagnosis and treatment of infection in orthopedic implants. Clin Infect Dis. 2001;33 Suppl 2:S94–106.

16. Atlas RM, Snyder JW. Reagents, stains and media: bacteriology. In: Versalovic J, Carroll KC, Funke G, Jorgensen JH, Landry ML, Warnock DW, editors. Manual of clinical microbiology. 10th ed. Washington, DC: ASM Press; 2011. p. 272–303.

17. Atkins BL, Athanasou N, Deeks JJ, Crook DW, Simpson H, Peto TE, et al. Prospective evaluation of criteria for microbiological diagnosis of prosthetic-joint infection at revision arthroplasty. The OSIRIS Collaborative Study Group. J Clin Microbiol. 1998;36(10):2932–9.

18. Ghanem E, Ketonis C, Restrepo C, Joshi A, Barrack R, Parvizi J. Periprosthetic infection: where do we stand with regard to Gram stain? Acta Orthop. 2009;80(1):37–40.

19. Chimento GF, Finger S, Barrack RL. Gram stain detection of infection during revision arthroplasty. J Bone Joint Surg Br. 1996;78(5):838–9.

20. Bauer TW, Parvizi J, Kobayashi N, Krebs V. Diagnosis of periprosthetic infection. J Bone Joint Surg Am. 2006;88(4):869–82.

21. Tunney MM, Patrick S, Curran MD, Ramage G, Hanna D, Nixon JR, et al. Detection of prosthetic hip infection at revision arthroplasty by immunofluorescence microscopy and PCR amplification of the bacterial 16S rRNA gene. J Clin Microbiol. 1999;37(10):3281–90.

22. Piper KE, Jacobson MJ, Cofield RH, Sperling JW, Sanchez-Sotelo J, Osmon DR, et al. Microbiologic diagnosis of prosthetic shoulder infection by use of implant sonication. J Clin Microbiol. 2009;47(6):1878–84.

23. McDowell A, Patrick S. Evaluation of nonculture methods for the detection of prosthetic hip biofilms. Clin Orthop Relat Res. 2005;437:74–82.

24. Stoodley P, Nistico L, Johnson S, Lasko LA, Baratz M, Gahlot V, et al. Direct demonstration of viable *Staphylococcus aureus* biofilms in an infected total joint arthroplasty. A case report. J Bone Joint Surg Am. 2008;90(8):1751–8.

25. Neut D, van Horn JR, van Kooten TG, van der Mei HC, Busscher HJ. Detection of biomaterial-associated infections in orthopaedic joint implants. Clin Orthop Relat Res. 2003;413:261–8.

26. Stoodley P, Kathju S, Hu FZ, Erdos G, Levenson JE, Mehta N, et al. Molecular and imaging techniques for bacterial biofilms in joint arthroplasty infections. Clin Orthop Relat Res. 2005; 437:31–40.

27. Moran E, Byren I, Atkins BL. The diagnosis and management of prosthetic joint infections. J Antimicrob Chemother. 2010;65 Suppl 3:iii45–54.

28. Virolainen P, Lahteenmaki H, Hiltunen A, Sipola E, Meurman O, Nelimarkka O. The reliability of diagnosis of infection during revision arthroplasties. Scand J Surg. 2002;91(2):178–81.

29. Patel R, Osmon DR, Hanssen AD. The diagnosis of prosthetic joint infection: current techniques and emerging technologies. Clin Orthop Relat Res. 2005;437:55–8.

30. Hughes JG, Vetter EA, Patel R, Schleck CD, Harmsen S, Turgeant LT, et al. Culture with BACTEC Peds Plus/F bottle compared with conventional methods for detection of bacteria in synovial fluid. J Clin Microbiol. 2001;39(12):4468–71.

31. Fink B, Makowiak C, Fuerst M, Berger I, Schafer P, Frommelt L. The value of synovial biopsy, joint aspiration and C-reactive protein in the diagnosis of late peri-prosthetic infection of total knee replacements. J Bone Joint Surg Br. 2008;90(7):874–8.

32. Font-Vizcarra L, Garcia S, Martinez-Pastor JC, Sierra JM, Soriano A. Blood culture flasks for culturing synovial fluid in prosthetic joint infections. Clin Orthop Relat Res. 2010;468(8): 2238–43.

33. Yagupsky P, Dagan R, Howard CW, Einhorn M, Kassis I, Simu A. High prevalence of *Kingella kingae* in joint fluid from children with septic arthritis revealed by the BACTEC blood culture system. J Clin Microbiol. 1992;30(5):1278–81.

34. Costerton JW, Montanaro L, Arciola CR. Biofilm in implant infections: its production and regulation. Int J Artif Organs. 2005;28:1062–8.

35. Mackowiak PA, Jones SR, Smith JW. Diagnostic value of sinus-tract cultures in chronic osteomyelitis. JAMA. 1978;239(26):2772–5.

36. Cune J, Soriano A, Martinez JC, Garcia S, Mensa J. A superficial swab culture is useful for microbiologic diagnosis in acute prosthetic joint infections. Clin Orthop Relat Res. 2009; 467(2):531–5.

37. Sadiq S, Wootton JR, Morris CA, Northmore-Ball MD. Application of core biopsy in revision arthroplasty for deep infection. J Arthroplasty. 2005;20(2):196–201.

38. Spangehl MJ, Masri BA, O'Connell JX, Duncan CP. Prospective analysis of preoperative and intraoperative investigations for the diagnosis of infection at the sites of two hundred and two revision total hip arthroplasties. J Bone Joint Surg Am. 1999;81(5):672–83.

39. Meermans G, Haddad FS. Is there a role for tissue biopsy in the diagnosis of periprosthetic infection? Clin Orthop Relat Res. 2010;468(5):1410–7.

40. Trampuz A, Piper KE, Jacobson MJ, Hanssen AD, Unni KK, Osmon DR, et al. Sonication of removed hip and knee prostheses for diagnosis of infection. N Engl J Med. 2007; 357(7):654–63.

41. Kamme C, Lindberg L. Aerobic and anaerobic bacteria in deep infections after total hip arthroplasty: differential diagnosis between infectious and non-infectious loosening. Clin Orthop Relat Res. 1981;154:201–7.

42. Roux AL, Sivadon-Tardy V, Bauer T, Lortat-Jacob A, Herrmann JL, Gaillard JL, et al. Diagnosis of prosthetic joint infection by beadmill processing of a periprosthetic specimen. Clin Microbiol Infect. 2011;17(3):447–50.

43. Schafer P, Fink B, Sandow D, Margull A, Berger I, Frommelt L. Prolonged bacterial culture to identify late periprosthetic joint infection: a promising strategy. Clin Infect Dis. 2008;47(11): 1403–9.

44. Berbari EF, Marculescu C, Sia I, Lahr BD, Hanssen AD, Steckelberg JM, et al. Culture-negative prosthetic joint infection. Clin Infect Dis. 2007;45(9):1113–9.

45. Malekzadeh D, Osmon DR, Lahr BD, Hanssen AD, Berbari EF. Prior use of antimicrobial therapy is a risk factor for culture-negative prosthetic joint infection. Clin Orthop Relat Res. 2010;468(8):2039–45.

46. Costerton JW. Biofilm theory can guide the treatment of device-related orthopaedic infections. Clin Orthop Relat Res. 2005;437:7–11.

47. Costerton JW, Post JC, Ehrlich GD, Hu FZ, Kreft R, Nistico L, et al. New methods for the detection of orthopedic and other biofilm infections. FEMS Immunol Med Microbiol. 2011; 61(2):133–40.

48. Gristina AG. Biomaterial-centered infection: microbial adhesion versus tissue integration. Science. 1987;237:1588–95.

49. Donlan RM, Costerton JW. Biofilms: survival mechanisms of clinically relevant microorganisms. Clin Microbiol Rev. 2002;15(2):167–93.

50. Trampuz A, Osmon DR, Hanssen AD, Steckelberg JM, Patel R. Molecular and antibiofilm approaches to prosthetic joint infection. Clin Orthop Relat Res. 2003;414:69–88.

51. Monsen T, Lovgren E, Widerstrom M, Wallinder L. In vitro effect of ultrasound on bacteria and suggested protocol for sonication and diagnosis of prosthetic infections. J Clin Microbiol. 2009;47(8):2496–501.

52. Nguyen LL, Nelson CL, Saccente M, Smeltzer MS, Wassell DL, McLaren SG. Detecting bacterial colonization of implanted orthopaedic devices by ultrasonication. Clin Orthop Relat Res. 2002;403:29–37.

53. Trampuz A, Piper KE, Hanssen AD, Osmon DR, Cockerill FR, Steckelberg JM, et al. Sonication of explanted prosthetic components in bags for diagnosis of prosthetic joint infection is associated with risk of contamination. J Clin Microbiol. 2006;44(2):628–31.
54. Esteban J, Gomez-Barrena E, Cordero J, Martin-de-Hijas NZ, Kinnari TJ, Fernandez-Roblas R. Evaluation of quantitative analysis of cultures from sonicated retrieved orthopedic implants in diagnosis of orthopedic infection. J Clin Microbiol. 2008;46(2):488–92.
55. Dora C, Altwegg M, Gerber C, Bottger EC, Zbinden R. Evaluation of conventional microbiological procedures and molecular genetic techniques for diagnosis of infections in patients with implanted orthopedic devices. J Clin Microbiol. 2008;46(2):824–5.
56. Sampedro MF, Huddleston PM, Piper KE, Karau MJ, Dekutoski MB, Yaszemski MJ, et al. A biofilm approach to detect bacteria on removed spinal implants. Spine (Phila Pa 1976). 2010; 12:1218–24.
57. Holinka J, Bauer L, Hirschl AM, Graninger W, Windhager R, Presterl E. Sonication cultures of explanted components as an add-on test to routinely conducted microbiological diagnostics improve pathogen detection. J Orthop Res. 2011;29(4):617–22.
58. Achermann Y, Vogt M, Leunig M, Wust J, Trampuz A. Improved diagnosis of periprosthetic joint infection by multiplex PCR of sonication fluid from removed implants. J Clin Microbiol. 2010;48(4):1208–14.
59. Fehring TK, McAlister JA, Jr. Frozen histologic section as a guide to sepsis in revision joint arthroplasty. Clin Orthop Relat Res. 1994;(304):229–37
60. Athanasou NA, Pandey R, de Steiger R, Crook D, Smith PM. Diagnosis of infection by frozen section during revision arthroplasty. J Bone Joint Surg Br. 1995;77(1):28–33.
61. Pandey R, Berendt AR, Athanasou NA. Histological and microbiological findings in non-infected and infected revision arthroplasty tissues. The OSIRIS Collaborative Study Group. Oxford Skeletal Infection Research and Intervention Service. Arch Orthop Trauma Surg. 2000;120(10):570–4.
62. Banit DM, Kaufer H, Hartford JM. Intraoperative frozen section analysis in revision total joint arthroplasty. Clin Orthop Relat Res. 2002;(401):230–8.
63. Feldman DS, Lonner JH, Desai P, Zuckerman JD. The role of intraoperative frozen sections in revision total joint arthroplasty. J Bone Joint Surg Am. 1995;77(12):1807–13.
64. Della Valle CJ, Scher DM, Kim YH, Oxley CM, Desai P, Zuckerman JD, et al. The role of intraoperative Gram stain in revision total joint arthroplasty. J Arthroplasty. 1999;14(4):500–4.
65. Spangehl MJ, Masri BA, O'Connell JX, Duncan CP. Prospective analysis of preoperative and intraoperative investigations for the diagnosis of infection at the sites of two hundred and two revision total hip arthroplasties. J Bone Joint Surg Am. 1999;81(5):672–83.
66. Parvizi J, Ghanem E, Sharkey P, Aggarwal A, Burnett RS, Barrack RL. Diagnosis of infected total knee: findings of a multicenter database. Clin Orthop Relat Res. 2008;466(11):2628–33.
67. Levine BR, Evans BG. Use of blood culture vial specimens in intraoperative detection of infection. Clin Orthop Relat Res. 2001;(382):222–31.

Chapter 18
Microbiological Processing of Samples in the Investigation of Suspected Prosthetic Joint Infection

David G. Partridge and Rob Towsend

Abstract Microbiological diagnosis is the most important issue in the evaluation of a PJI. It guides further treatment. The outcomes of PJI treatment reflect the quality if the initial microbiological assessment. Aspiration and tissue cultures are still the most important samples for microbiological evaluation of PJI. The chapter presents the appropriate workout for the specimens and the potential pitfalls in the sampling and handling of specimens obteined for microbiological analysis.

Keywords Sampling • Bacterial cultures • Identification • Susceptibility

18.1 Introduction

The results of aspirate and tissue cultures are key to the diagnosis of prosthetic joint infection (PJI) and to its subsequent management. The production of these results is a multistep process with surgeons, hospital transport systems, laboratory scientists and technicians, and clinical microbiologists or infection specialists all playing pivotal roles. Breakdown at any stage of the collection, transport, processing, or interpretation of the samples has the potential to give rise to misleading results and inappropriate management (Fig. 18.1).

The basic materials used for the culture of microbiological samples have changed little over the past century, but methods of organism identification are rapidly evolving with molecular techniques now accessible to an increasing number of laboratories and likely to play an ever greater role over the next decade and beyond.

The principal difficulty in interpretation of PJI tissue culture results lies in the discrimination of true etiological pathogens from contaminating organisms. Prolonged broth culture is a very sensitive tool for the detection of the bacteria, and

D.G. Partridge • R. Towsend (✉)
Infectious Diseases and Microbiology, Sheffield Teaching Hospitals NHS Trust,
Herries Road, Sheffield, South Yorkshire S5 7AU, UK
e-mail: c.david.partridge@sth.nhs.uk; rob@ukoms.co.uk

R. Trebše (ed.), *Infected Total Joint Arthroplasty*,
DOI 10.1007/978-1-4471-2482-5_18, © Springer-Verlag London 2012

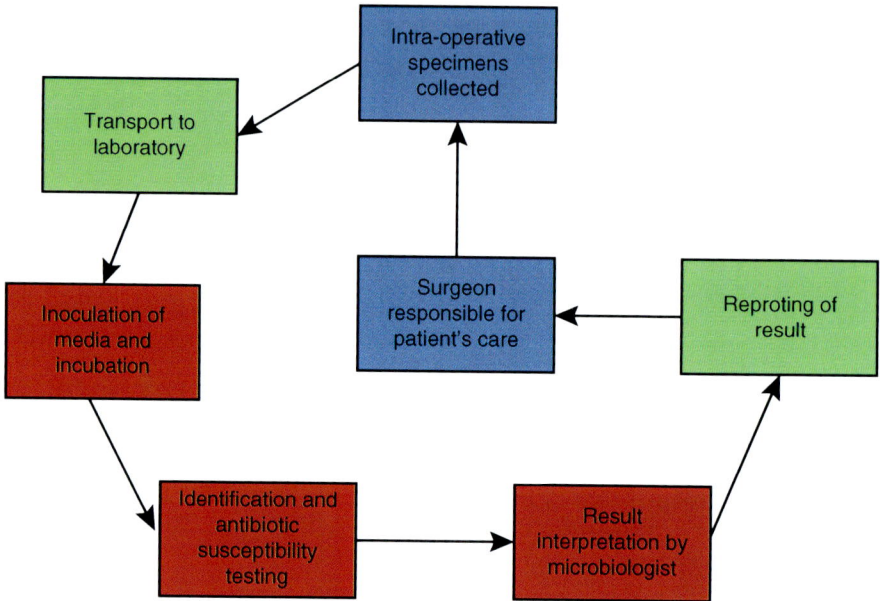

Fig. 18.1 Steps involved in the processing of prosthetic joint tissue culture from surgeon to surgeon

even minor degrees of contamination may therefore hinder diagnostic accuracy as the most common infecting organisms, such as coagulase negative staphylococci, are also those most likely to be found as contaminants [1].

Collection and microbiological processing of samples from suspected PJI therefore has the dual focus of optimizing detection of significant pathogens while minimizing contamination and ensuring that true pathogens are not mislabeled as contaminants or vice versa. The remainder of this chapter will examine each of the stages illustrated in the flow chart in Fig. 18.1 to outline how this can best be achieved.

18.2 Specimen Collection

18.2.1 Timing of Sample Collection

Samples taken at the time of initial debridement form the mainstay of PJI diagnosis, but initial radiologically guided aspiration or biopsy of the affected joint enables more rapid confirmation of the presence of infection and can guide selection of local or systemic antibiotic therapy around the time of surgery [2]. Early confirmation of the etiological pathogen and its antimicrobial susceptibility is becoming increasingly important in the management of PJI, given the rising rates of resistance seen in both gram-positive and gram-negative organisms over recent years [2]. Culture of joint aspirate also has a role in the distinction of PJI from aseptic loosening and has a sensitivity of 56–75 %

and specificity of 95–100 % when used for this purpose [3]. If more than one biopsy is performed, this also permits histological examination of the tissue to aid diagnosis.

Antibiotic therapy can adversely affect yield from periprosthetic tissue culture for days to weeks after cessation of the antimicrobial [4]. Although antibiotics must be initiated early in the acutely septic patient, in the context of the more usual indolent presentation of PJI, sensitivity of preoperative sampling will be improved by allowing an antibiotic-free period of at least 2 weeks before sampling [4–6].

18.2.2 Type of Specimen to Collect

Appropriate operative samples for microbiological processing may be biopsies of the inflammatory tissues around the infected joint or fluid from within the joint space. Little evidence has been published on the relative sensitivity of different specimen types, but in studies examining the diagnostic accuracy of orthopedic tissue culture, surgeons are typically requested to sample the most inflamed or abnormal tissues in the region of the joint including any periprosthetic membranes [5, 7]. Each specimen should be taken using different sterile instruments into separate sterile specimen pots so as to minimize the risk of contamination and, in particular, to ensure that contaminants are not transferred from specimen to specimen, making correct interpretation of culture results impossible. Specially assembled kits should be available with at least five sets of sterile, leakproof containers and instruments for specimen collection to facilitate the process. Specimens should be collected in a manner that minimizes contact with the operative field or with gloves in an effort to reduce contamination, and perioperative prophylactic antibiotics are usually administered after sample collection in order to optimize culture yield. In laboratories where Ballotini beads are utilized to disrupt specimens, sterile containers containing the beads in saline or Ringer's solution may be provided to the operating theater to minimize subsequent specimen handling [7].

There is now increasing interest in the use of sonication of entire removed implants to improve sensitivity of tissue culture by disruption of the biofilm on the prosthetic surface. A study by Trampuz et al. demonstrated an increase in sensitivity where sonication was performed as compared with standard tissue cultures in 331 patients, of whom 79 were defined as having PJI by macroscopic or histopathological examination [4]. Sensitivity of sonicated implant culture for the diagnosis of PJI was 78.5 % as compared with 60.8 % for standard tissue culture ($p < 0.001$) with specificity exceeding 98 % in both arms. There appeared to be a particular benefit in patients who had received antibiotics within 2 weeks prior to sampling with sensitivity increasing from 45 to 75 % ($p < 0.001$). Unfortunately, conventional microbiological processing was somewhat suboptimal in the study with no terminal subculture of non-cloudy broths and varying numbers of samples submitted for conventional culture. The latter flaw seems of particular relevance as when analysis was restricted to those patients who had at least four periprosthetic tissue samples sent, sensitivity of conventional culture increased to 72.7 %, emphasizing the need for adequate numbers of specimens. The authors of this study also suggested that sonication of a removed implant could obviate the need for standard tissue cultures with the result that only a single specimen needed processing but such an approach would make correct interpretation of contaminating flora impossible. However, it is possible that there may be a role for sonication as an adjunct to conventional tissue culture [8].

As mentioned above, preoperative biopsies or fluid aspirates may also be cultured. Sensitivity and specificity of joint aspirate culture are maximized by immediate inoculation directly into blood culture bottles. Direct inoculation into broth preserves the viability of organisms that may not survive transport to the laboratory and also involves less manual handling with the potential for introduction of contaminants.

Whichever samples are taken, it is of the utmost importance that specimens sent to the laboratory are correctly labeled with patient details and specimen type. A large hospital microbiology laboratory may receive over 1,000 specimens on any given day, which require different methods of processing depending on type of specimen and the pathogens which are most likely to be isolated. Specimens which may present a hazard to the laboratory workers should be clearly labeled as such. It is also important that the clinical team consider the possibility of infection with pathogens which would require specialist media such as *Mycobacterium tuberculosis*, which is an uncommon but well reported cause of PJI [9].

18.2.3 Number of Specimens to Collect

The optimal number of periprosthetic tissue samples required for diagnosis of PJI remains a subject of some debate. Sufficient samples are required to ensure that sensitivity of culture is adequate while at the same time ensuring that contaminating organisms can be confidently excluded from treatment decisions. In a prospective study of nearly 300 patients who underwent revision of a prosthetic joint at a single, large center, Atkins et al. determined the diagnostic sensitivity and specificity of positive results from varying numbers of periprosthetic tissue cultures against a histological gold standard. Mathematical modeling based upon their results determined that five or six samples provided optimal diagnostic accuracy when indistinguishable isolates from two or three different samples was used as the cutoff to define infection [10].

18.3 Transport to the Laboratory

It should be ensured that efficient methods for transport of collected specimens to the laboratory exist. Delay in transport and processing of specimens may adversely affect the accuracy of results provided as small numbers of contaminating organisms may outgrow significant pathogens or more fastidious pathogens may die prior to processing. The latter is a particular problem encountered in the detection of anaerobic organisms, many of which tolerate aerobic conditions for only a short time [11].

18.4 Specimen Handling in the Laboratory

18.4.1 Sample Preparation

Following arrival in the laboratory, specimens should be inoculated into appropriate media as soon as is practicable, but extreme care is required to prevent contamination at this stage. Gram stain is of very poor sensitivity in the context of prosthetic joint infection, with as few as 6 % of confirmed infections found to have positive results on Gram stain [10], and is therefore not routinely performed except in the context of the acutely septic joint. Even in this context, gram film results should be interpreted with caution, especially if negative. Each specimen should be handled separately using different instruments, and ideally all manipulation should be performed within a class 2 laminar flow safety cabinet (see Figure 18.2), which provides a constant flow of filtered air from the hood and resists the ingress contaminating organisms from the technician handling the sample.

Samples may be divided before inoculation into different media by means of a sterile scalpel, but sample homogenization by means of Ballotini beads has become popular. Homogenization in this manner is performed by placing the sample in a sterile container with around ten glass beads and 5 mL of saline or Ringer's solution.

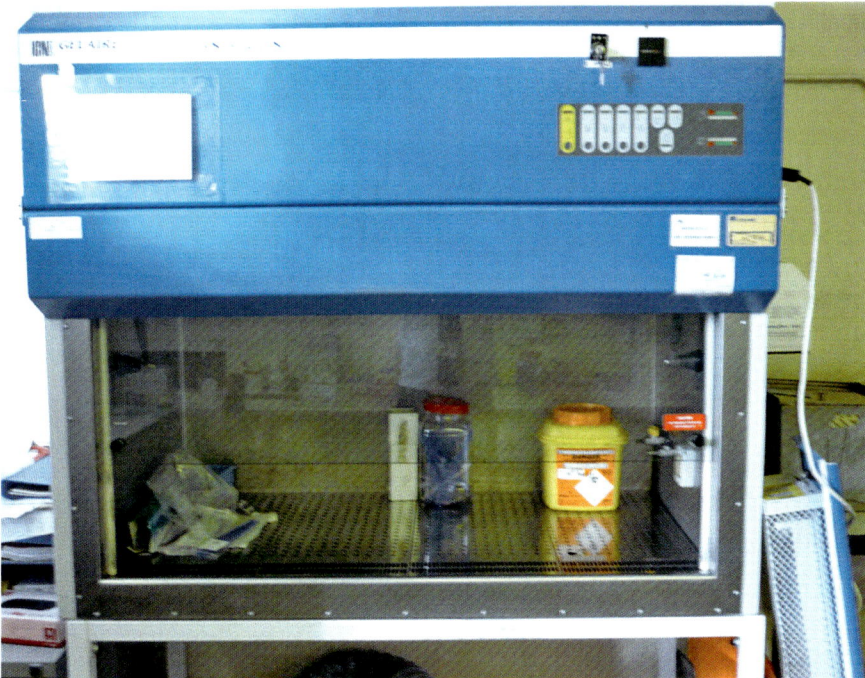

Fig. 18.2 Class 2 laminar flow safety cabinet

The sample is then either shaken at 250 rpm for 10 min or is vortexed for 15 s [7]. As stated above, in order to reduce specimen handling and consequent risk of contamination, specimen pots containing Ballotini beads may be provided directly to the operating theater. If polymerase chain reaction is to be employed as a diagnostic technique (see below), then use of sterile water may be more appropriate than saline or Ringer's.

The increasing interest in the use of sonication of entire prostheses to disrupt biofilm before microbiological processing is discussed above but is not without its drawbacks. Use of beads or sonication also allows inoculation of automated blood culture system broths, which has proved to be of high sensitivity [12] and reduces hands-on processing time.

18.4.2   Culture Conditions

Sensitivity of culture is influenced by the type of media used, temperature and atmosphere of incubation, and its duration. Broth culture has been demonstrated to be of superior sensitivity to use of solid media [12], which is likely to be due to improved isolation of organisms lying dormant in biofilms. In the context of vascular prosthetic devices, *Staphylococcus epidermidis* was significantly more likely to be cultured from experimentally infected grafts when broth culture was performed compared with solid agar media [13]. However, broth culture has the disadvantage that mixed infections may be detected less easily.

We would therefore recommend that both methods are used simultaneously on each specimen. A variety of broth types may be used, but in a recent study, the sensitivity of Robertson's cooked meat broth and of commercial blood culture broth both appeared to be superior to that of fastidious anaerobic broth [12]. Broths should be observed daily for development of turbidity consistent with organism growth and should be subcultured if this is suspected. Duration of broth culture should be at least 5 days, and the likelihood of detecting fastidious organisms will be increased if culture time is prolonged further, with one recent study confirming that an incubation time of 13 days is required to optimally detect slow-growing species such as propionibacteria [14]. At the end of the incubation period, all broths should undergo terminal subculture, even if there is no obvious evidence of turbidity to further enhance the detection of fastidious organisms.

Although solid media have inferior sensitivity compared to broth, their use may improve the detection of mixed cultures as rapidly growing organisms are less likely to prevent the detection of others. With regard to media and incubation conditions, the recommendations of the United Kingdom National Standard Method seem reasonable with blood and chocolate agar in 5–10 % CO_2 for 2 days at 37° C and fastidious anaerobic agar incubated for 5 days at 37° C [7, 15]. Concurrently inoculated broths which have become cloudy or have completed their incubation period should be subcultured onto similar media and, in addition, onto Sabouraud's agar, which should be incubated at 30° C for 14 days to detect fungi.

18.4.3   Organism Identification

All organisms growing from prosthetic joint samples should ideally be identified to species level. For the past century, biochemical tests of carbohydrate and amino acid utilization and assimilation have formed the cornerstone of such identification in the routine laboratory. Gradually such techniques are being replaced by molecular identification, which is becoming increasingly accessible to routine laboratories.

Matrix-assisted laser desorption-ionization time-of-flight mass spectrometry (MALDI-TOF MS) is already widely available and provides rapid and accurate speciation of an organism from pure subculture [16]. This technique relies upon the acceleration of high abundance proteins within the pathogen into gas phase by a laser. These ions pass down a tube across a charge and their time-of-flight is proportional to their mass/charge ratio. The produced profile can be compared to a database of profiles for different species and in most cases provides robust and rapid speciation. Discrimination between different strains of the same organism may also be possible, if their MALDI-TOF MS profile is sufficiently distinct.

Nucleic acid sequencing is reducing in both cost and time requirement, and, although it is not yet available to routine clinical microbiology laboratories for routine specimens, there is the potential for low-cost high-throughput sequencing techniques to revolutionize clinical microbiology over the coming decades.

18.4.4   Antimicrobial Susceptibility Testing

Following the identification of an infecting organism, the next important task for the laboratory is to provide accurate antimicrobial susceptibility results to guide decisions over systemic and local therapy and confirm the susceptibility of pathogens to the constituents of antibiotic laden cement or spacers incorporated at revision arthroplasty. Unlike organism identification, molecular methods for determination of antimicrobial susceptibility have only a limited role in the routine clinical laboratory at present. Instead, susceptibility testing is performed by attempting to grow the subcultured organism in the presence of a defined concentration of antibiotic which correlates with the likelihood of clinical success, termed the breakpoint. If the organism can grow in the presence of the breakpoint concentration of antimicrobial, it is deemed to be resistant to that agent, whereas if all growth is inhibited, the organism is deemed susceptible. Confirmation of susceptibility can be achieved by inoculating agar containing the breakpoint concentration of antimicrobial and inspecting for growth or by allowing the antibiotic to diffuse into the medium in a predictable manner from antibiotic impregnated discs or strips. Although the same principles hold, there has been a trend toward increasing automation of susceptibility testing over recent years with several automated platforms now available. When interpreting susceptibility results to any given antimicrobial, it is important to appreciate that this is only an in vitro test and that clinical outcome cannot be directly inferred from it if antibiotic concentrations at the infected site are low because of poor drug penetration or are very high as is the case with locally implanted cement-based antimicrobials. Similarly, organisms residing in biofilm are less metabolically active and have a higher degree of resistance to some antimicrobials than might be predicted from in vitro data.

18.4.5   Strain Typing

The growth of indistinguishable isolates from multiple tissue samples is pivotal in the differentiation of contaminating from pathogenic organisms as is discussed above. However, the depth of investigation performed before two isolates are deemed indistinguishable may vary. Speciation of the organisms and comparison of antimicrobial susceptibilities are likely to be sufficient in most cases, but the advent of molecular techniques such as nucleic acid sequencing and mass spectrometry and their increasing accessibility to the diagnostic laboratory promises routine discrimination of organisms to a higher degree in future.

18.4.6   Molecular Methods

The basic methods and techniques of pathogen isolation have changed relatively little in the past century, with the culture of organisms on solid or in liquid agar still at the foundations of the diagnostic process, to the extent that Louis Pasteur would probably feel fairly comfortable in a modern routine diagnostic bacteriology laboratory. The genomic revolution, which has occurred over the past 25 years, promises to change this somewhat. The polymerase chain reaction (PCR) amplifies microbial nucleic acids and is already a valuable addition to the microbiologist's toolkit. PCR relies upon the separation of DNA strands by heat and subsequent binding of a selected "primer," a short chain of nucleic acids, to each of the resulting single strands on cooling. A thermally stable DNA polymerase is then used to replicate each strand from the point of primer binding with the resultant potential to double the amount of the DNA target. This cycle is then repeated multiple times until detectable levels of nucleic acid are present. An individual PCR assay can detect a broad or narrow range of species depending upon the primers selected. Use of genus or species-specific primers enables confident identification of the organism at the time of amplification without the need for further processing but will obviously miss any organisms present from other genera or species. Broad-range PCRs target areas of the genome common to a large number of pathogens, such as the 16S ribosomal RNA gene. Following the initial amplification of the 16S gene, sequencing may be performed to identify the bacterium to species level.

The potential sensitivity of PCR is very good, and, as it detects bacterial nucleic acid regardless of whether the organism is replicating, the technique may be particularly useful in the context of antibiotic treatment or where organisms are metabolically inactive in biofilm. Unfortunately, thus far, PCR has not lived up to its potential. A number of studies have been performed comparing broad-range PCR to culture in the context of PJI. As yet, the sensitivity benefit of the molecular test is relatively marginal [17, 18], and the technique is also prone to detection of contaminants [19]. At present, PCR does not yield any information about antimicrobial sensitivity other than that which can be inferred from knowledge of the infecting bacterial species. One study has demonstrated that PCR may improve the sensitivity of preoperative joint fluid aspirate [20].

18.5 Interpretation of Results

Data generated by the laboratory may be misleading to the clinician if reported in its raw format, especially when all tests have not yet been completed. Antibiotic susceptibility results are particularly subject to change based upon the results of further testing and the application of expert rules for their interpretation. Similarly, clinical details about the case may impact upon the significance of laboratory findings. For these reasons, it is important to have a strong 2-way interface between the microbiology and surgical teams.

18.6 Provision of Results

The quality of service provided by a microbiology department to an orthopedic surgeon is only as strong as its weakest link. Careful specimen collection, transport, and microbiological processing are of limited value if the clinician responsible for making decisions regarding therapy does not have access to the results in a suitable format which is easy to interpret. Computerized result reporting systems allow rapid retrieval of reports, but the content has to be of high quality and should always be supported by availability of specialist microbiology advice when required.

18.7 Conclusion

Accurate microbiological results from prosthetic tissue samples and their correct interpretation are a cornerstone in the appropriate management of prosthetic joint infection. The production of these results is a multistep process which is only as robust as its weakest link and requires every effort to be made to perfect existing methods and embrace any new technologies demonstrated to confer a diagnostic advantage.

References

1. Stefansdottir A, Johansson D, Knutson K, Lidgren L, Robertsson O. Microbiology of the infected knee arthroplasty: report from the Swedish Knee Arthroplasty Register on 426 surgically revised cases. Scand J Infect Dis. 2009;41(11–12):831–40. doi:10.3109/00365540903186207.
2. Fink B, Makowiak C, Fuerst M, Berger I, Schafer P, Frommelt L. The value of synovial biopsy, joint aspiration and C-reactive protein in the diagnosis of late peri-prosthetic infection of total knee replacements. J Bone Joint Surg Br. 2008;90(7):874–8. doi:10.1302/0301-620X.90B7.20417. PII:90-B/7/874.
3. Del Pozo JL, Patel R. Clinical practice. Infection associated with prosthetic joints. N Engl J Med. 2009;361(8):787–94. doi:10.1056/NEJMcp0905029. PII:361/8/787.
4. Trampuz A, Piper KE, Jacobson MJ, Hanssen AD, Unni KK, Osmon DR, Mandrekar JN, Cockerill FR, Steckelberg JM, Greenleaf JF, Patel R. Sonication of removed hip and knee prostheses for diagnosis of infection. N Engl J Med. 2007;357(7):654–63. doi:10.1056/NEJMoa061588. PII:357/7/654.
5. Della Valle C, Parvizi J, Bauer TW, DiCesare PE, Evans RP, Segreti J, Spangehl M, Watters 3rd WC, Keith M, Turkelson CM, Wies JL, Sluka P, Hitchcock K. American Academy of Orthopaedic Surgeons clinical practice guideline on: the diagnosis of periprosthetic joint infections of the hip and knee. J Bone Joint Surg Am. 2011;93(14):1355–7.
6. Moran E, Byren I, Atkins BL. The diagnosis and management of prosthetic joint infections. J Antimicrob Chemother. 2010;65 Suppl 3:iii45–54. doi:10.1093/jac/dkq305. PII:dkq305.
7. Health Protection Agency. Investigation of prosthetic joint infection samples. National Standard Method BSOP 44 Issue 1.1. 2009.
8. Holinka J, Bauer L, Hirschl AM, Graninger W, Windhager R, Presterl E. Sonication cultures of explanted components as an add-on test to routinely conducted microbiological diagnostics improve pathogen detection. J Orthop Res. 2011;29(4):617–22.
9. Khater FJ, Samnani IQ, Mehta JB, Moorman JP, Myers JW. Prosthetic joint infection by Mycobacterium tuberculosis: an unusual case report with literature review. South Med J. 2007; 100(1):66–9.
10. Atkins BL, Athanasou N, Deeks JJ, Crook DW, Simpson H, Peto TE, McLardy-Smith P, Berendt AR. Prospective evaluation of criteria for microbiological diagnosis of prosthetic-joint infection at revision arthroplasty. The OSIRIS Collaborative Study Group. J Clin Microbiol. 1998;36(10):2932–9.
11. Brook I. Comparison of two transport systems for recovery of aerobic and anaerobic bacteria from abscesses. J Clin Microbiol. 1987;25(10):2020–2.
12. Hughes HC, Newnham R, Athanasou N, Atkins BL, Bejon P, Bowler IC. Microbiological diagnosis of prosthetic joint infections: a prospective evaluation of four bacterial culture media in the routine laboratory. Clin Microbiol Infect. 2011;17(10):1528–30.
13. Bergamini TM, Bandyk DF, Govostis D, Vetsch R, Towne JB. Identification of Staphylococcus epidermidis vascular graft infections: a comparison of culture techniques. J Vasc Surg. 1989;9(5):665–70. PII:S0741-5214(89)70037-9.
14. Butler-Wu SM, Burns EM, Pottinger PS, Magaret AS, Rakeman JL, Matsen 3rd FA, Cookson BT. Optimization of periprosthetic culture for diagnosis of Propionibacterium acnes prosthetic joint infection. J Clin Microbiol. 2011;49(7):2490–5. doi:10.1128/JCM.00450-11. PII:JCM.00450-11.
15. Bailey C, Duckett S, Davies S, Townsend R, Stockley I. Haemophilus parainfluenzae prosthetic joint infection. The importance of accurate microbiological diagnosis and options for management. J Infect. 2011;63(6):474–6. doi:10.1016/j.jinf.2011.08.009. PII:S0163-4453(11)00461-0.
16. Harris LG, El-Bouri K, Johnston S, Rees E, Frommelt L, Siemssen N, Christner M, Davies AP, Rohde H, Mack D. Rapid identification of staphylococci from prosthetic joint infections using MALDI-TOF mass-spectrometry. Int J Artif Organs. 2010;33(9):568–74. PII:2213A231-7A27-44BF-A569-CAC6A2777982.
17. Fenollar F, Roux V, Stein A, Drancourt M, Raoult D. Analysis of 525 samples to determine the usefulness of PCR amplification and sequencing of the 16S rRNA gene for diagnosis of

bone and joint infections. J Clin Microbiol. 2006;44(3):1018–28. doi:10.1128/JCM.44.3.1018-1028.2006. PII:44/3/1018.

18. Fihman V, Hannouche D, Bousson V, Bardin T, Liote F, Raskine L, Riahi J, Sanson-Le Pors MJ, Bercot B. Improved diagnosis specificity in bone and joint infections using molecular techniques. J Infect. 2007;55(6):510–7. doi:10.1016/j.jinf.2007.09.001. PII:S0163-4453(07)00755-4.

19. Panousis K, Grigoris P, Butcher I, Rana B, Reilly JH, Hamblen DL. Poor predictive value of broad-range PCR for the detection of arthroplasty infection in 92 cases. Acta Orthop. 2005;76(3):341–6.

20. Gallo J, Kolar M, Dendis M, Loveckova Y, Sauer P, Zapletalova J, Koukalova D. Culture and PCR analysis of joint fluid in the diagnosis of prosthetic joint infection. New Microbiol. 2008;31(1):97–104.

Chapter 19
Molecular Diagnosis of Prosthetic Joint Infection

**Jaime Esteban, Diana Molina-Manso, Gema del-Prado,
and Enrique Gómez-Barrena**

Abstract Diagnosis of Prosthetic Joint Infection remains as a challenge in modern medicine. Conventional techniques lead to the diagnosis of many patients with a classical infectious syndrome, but differential diagnosis with other entities (particularly aseptic failure) is still a problem. Several molecular markers have been studied in the diagnosis of infection (like cytokines, procalcitonin, specific IgG, sICAM-1, VEGF or alpha2-Macroglobulin), and even for microbiological diagnosis (lipid S, PIA, icaADBC operon), with variable success. PCR-based genetic amplification procedures have also been studied for the detection of microbial genes in different clinical samples, and will be probably included in the next future as part of the diagnostic schemes for this kind of infections.

Keywords Diagnosis • Markers • Antigens • Genes • Polymerase • Chain reaction

19.1 Diagnosis of Prosthetic Join Infections: An Overview

Total joint arthroplasty is considered one of the most successful surgical procedures currently available, but it has been estimated that just under 10 % of patients develop complications during their lifetime. Although implant failure is mostly due to biomechanical aseptic loosening, prosthetic joint infection (PJI) is the second leading cause of implant retrieval, with incidence rates between 0.5 and 5 % for a primary

J. Esteban, M.D., Ph.D. • D. Molina-Manso • G. del-Prado
Bone and Joint Infection Unit, Department of Clinical Microbiology,
IIS-Fundación Jiménez Díaz, Av. Reyes Católicos 2,
Madrid 28040, Spain
e-mail: jestebanmoreno@gmail.com; Dmolina@fjd.es; Gprado@fjd.es

E. Gómez-Barrena, M.D., Ph.D. (✉)
Department of Orthopaedic Surgery and Traumatology, Hospital "La Paz",
Paseo de la Castellana 261, Madrid 28046, Spain
e-mail: enrique.gomezbarrena@uam.es

R. Trebše (ed.), *Infected Total Joint Arthroplasty*,
DOI 10.1007/978-1-4471-2482-5_19, © Springer-Verlag London 2012

arthroplasty [1–4], but higher after revision [5]. Therefore, PJI is a serious complication that not only causes great morbidity but also increases socioeconomic concern [6, 7].

Diagnosis of PJI prior to revision would be desirable to establish an appropriate treatment [8]. Discriminating between septic and aseptic failures is critical in order to avoid extended hospital stays, exposure to surgical risks, and unnecessary antimicrobial therapies. On the other hand, failure in the detection of PJI may result in persistent infection [9–12]. To date, conventional diagnostic methods exhibit lacks and limitations in detecting and defining PJI. Although it is well known that *Staphylococcus aureus* and *Staphylococcus epidermidis* are the two bacterial species being the major cause of PJI [13, 14], the etiology can include a wide range of microorganisms, a fact that increases the diagnostic difficulties. Moreover, polymicrobial infections are also common [13–15]. The implementation of microbiological methods of diagnosis not only has increased the probability of detecting a PJI but also allows the characterization of causative microorganisms. Conventional techniques are focused in microorganism retrieval from infected sources after sample inoculation on different culture media [3, 5, 8, 14, 16, 17], and, despite being the gold standard for diagnosis, several problems can affect the final result. Among these, we find sampling errors, inappropriate sample transport and manipulation, presence of contaminants, inadequate quantities of vital microbes retrieved, presence of biofilms, and some fastidious microorganisms that do not grow in media culture resulting in as many as 20 % false negatives [17], even if new biofilm-based methods are applied [15, 18–21].

These problems could be overcome by the use of culture-independent molecular detection methods for the diagnosis of PJI [21–26]. Molecular diagnosis is based on the detection and sometimes the quantification of macromolecules, like DNA, RNA, or proteins unique to the infecting pathogens; optimally, the target molecule should be present in the target and absent in the host cells [27]. Detection of new inflammation-related molecules is also another approach for molecular diagnosis of PJI. Molecular techniques are being used increasingly in clinical microbiology laboratories to establish the cause of infectious diseases, and several molecular diagnostic assays have been developed with good results, so they could be of interest in the diagnosis of PJI [2, 21, 28].

19.2　Clinical Diagnostics by Molecular Markers

19.2.1　Blood and Serum Markers

Blood tests are noninvasive procedures essentially based on the detection of inflammation markers, since complete white blood cell count (WBC) has shown a poor sensitivity for the diagnosis of PJI despite being increased in patients with infection compared to aseptic loosening [1, 29]. To date, the erythrocyte sedimentation rate (ESR) and the C-reactive protein (CRP) are commonly used in the preoperative assessment of PJI [8, 14, 30]. Another new molecular approaches recently proposed as serum biomarkers are interleukin 6 (IL-6), interleukin 1β

(IL-1β), tumor necrosis factor alpha (TNF-α), procalcitonin (PTC), immuno-globulin G (IgG), and soluble intercellular adhesion molecule-1 (sICAM-1).

19.2.1.1   Cytokines: IL-6, IL-1β, and TNF-α

IL-6, IL-1β, and TNF-α belong to an important family of mediators involved in the regulation of the acute-phase response to injury and infection [31], and their increased levels are intimately related to elevations of acute-phase proteins like CRP [32, 33]. IL-1β and TNF-α are exclusively pro-inflammatory cytokines, but IL-6 has a dual activity, both pro-inflammatory and anti-inflammatory [33]. Such pro-inflammatory activity induces osteoclast activation which leads to bone resorption, osteolysis, and finally prosthetic loosening [34]. Then, it is a critical issue to identify significant differences in serum or synovial fluid levels of these cytokines when infection is present [35]. On the other hand, the serum levels of IL-6, IL-1β, and TNF-α can be increased in the presence of certain bacterial components such as the S-peptide, a short-glycerophosphate-chain-length form of lipoteichoic acid (sce-LTA) from *S. epidermidis* cell wall [36]. This finding strongly justifies their testing as PJI indicators.

Although high IL-6 levels can be observed in patients with chronic inflammatory diseases both in serum and synovial fluid of affected joints [33], a recent study by Worthington et al. has shown that serum levels of IL-6 were significantly more raised in patients with septic loosening than in other patients [29]. However, IL-6 tests have not yet been adopted for routine use in the evaluation of arthroplasty dysfunction, although the high rates of sensitivity and specificity found for 58 patients undergoing knee and hip arthroplasty (100 and 95 %, respectively, for a cutoff established at ≥10 pg/mL) (Table 19.1) [37] suggest that IL-6 could be the most accurate inflammatory marker, together with CRP (minimal validated cutoff of >10 mg/mL) [32]. On the contrary to IL-6, TNF-α serum test has showed a low sensitivity (43 %) in spite of being quite specific (94 %), so it is not a really useful PJI indicator presently [38].

19.2.1.2   Procalcitonin (PTC)

PCT is a peptidic precursor of the calcitonin hormone. Under normal conditions, PCT is synthesized in small amounts by the C neuroendocrine cells of thyroid and lung. However, when a bacterial infection develops, it can be released by adipose tissue and other organs such as spleen, liver, testes, or brain to activate the immune system and thus increasing their blood levels [39]. PCT serum levels have been successfully used to differentiate viral from bacterial infection, predict prognosis in severe sepsis, and guide antimicrobial therapy [39, 40]. Nevertheless, PCT does not show any advantage in the diagnosis of PJI compared to classic markers such as CRP. In previous studies, the sensitivity and specificity in the PCT test were estimated as 76 and 70 %, respectively [41]. According to Bottner et al., while specificity rates were similar (98 % for PTC, 96 % for CRP), the PCT test was significantly less sensitive than the CRP test (33 % vs. 95 %) (Table 19.1) [38]. Such limitations in sensitivity have been later corroborated by the work of Worthington et al. [29], where PCT was not found of value in differentiating septic and

Table 19.1 Evaluation of different molecules for the diagnosis of PJI

| Molecules | Source | Percentage of (%)[a] | | | | | References |
		Sensitivity	Specificity	Positive predictive value (PPV)	Negative predictive value (NPV)	Accuracy	
Inflammatory markers							
Interleukin 6	Serum	81–100	77–95	65–89	50–100	78–97	[29, 37]
	Synovial fluid	87.1–100	100	100	91.5–100	94.6–100	[47, 48]
Interleukin 1-β	Synovial fluid	59–100	83–100	56–100	85–100	100	[35, 47]
Interleukin 8	Synovial fluid	90.3	97.7	96.6	93.5	94.7	[48]
Tumor necrosis factor alpha (TNF-α)	Serum	43	94	75	85	83	[38]
	Synovial fluid	76	72	50	89	NA	[35]
Procalcitonin (PCT)	Serum	33–76	70–98	87	80	81	[38, 41]
Soluble intercellular adhesion molecule-1 (sICAM-1)	Serum	94	74	65	65	80	[29]
Vascular endothelial growth factor (VEGF)	Synovial fluid	77.4	91.5	85.7	86	85.9	[48]
α₂-Macroglobulin (α2M)	Synovial fluid	80.6	95.6	92.6	87.8	89.5	[48]
Serological markers							
Immunoglobulin G (IgG)	Serum	93.3	96.9	NA	97	75	[43]

NA not available

[a] Rates from several studies are cutoff value dependent

aseptic implant loosening. Despite its low sensitivity, PCT could be used as an additional high specific test in identifying patients with true positive CRP and/or IL-6 levels [38].

19.2.1.3 IgG

Detecting antibodies against microorganisms associated with PJI lacks specificity due to the presence of basal antibody levels against organisms which can be part of the normal human flora, like coagulase-negative staphylococci (CNS) [42]. However, serum IgG directed against the bacterial antigen sce-LTA has been previously reported as a good indicator of PJI (Table 19.1), with sensitivity and specificity rates of 93 and 97 %, respectively [43]. Recently, the potential usefulness of IgG has been confirmed, being elevated in 75 % of patients with infection due to CNS [29].

19.2.1.4 sICAM-1

sICAM-1 is an endothelium-derived inflammatory marker from ICAM, an immuno-globulin-like cell adhesion molecule expressed by different cell types, whose expression is enhanced by pro-inflammatory cytokines [44]. Moreover, sICAM-1 has also signaling properties and invokes a broad range of pro-inflammatory responses. The circulating form sICAM-1 has been measured in several body fluids and found elevated in patients with a broad range of diseases [45, 46]. Recently, serum sICAM-1 has been found significantly raised in patients with septic loosening, which suggests a possible use as PJI indicator (Table 19.1) [29].

19.2.2 Synovial Fluid Markers

The screening of increased inflammatory proteins in synovial fluid from patients who are undergoing revision arthroplasty for septic or aseptic failures can be especially useful in the identification of novel PJI biomarkers [47, 48]. In the present moment, analysis of cytokines such as IL-6 and IL-1β has been suggested as a new approach in the intraoperative diagnosis of PJI [8, 49, 50] and also can be extended to interleukin 8 (IL-8), vascular endothelial growth factor (VEGF), and α2-macroglobulin (α2M) [48].

19.2.2.1 Cytokines: IL-6, IL-1β, IL-8, and TNF-α

IL-6, IL-1β, and TNF-α levels have been found significantly higher in the synovial fluid than in the serum from patients with septic loosening (Table 19.1) [35, 47]. In a posterior study, the rates of specificity and positive predictive value for IL-6 were maintained, but the sensitivity was reduced to 87.1 %, negative predictive value to

91.5 %, and accuracy to 94.6 %, probably due to methodological differences [48]. IL-8 can also be an interesting candidate for PJI detection, because high rates of sensitivity, (90.3 %) specificity (97.7 %), and accuracy (94.7 %) have been reported [48].

19.2.2.2   Vascular Endothelial Growth Factor (VEGF)

VEGF is a signaling protein released in rheumatoid arthritis in response to TNF-α, which increases the permeability and endothelial swelling, and stimulates angiogenesis [51]. Elevated concentrations of VEGF have been found in synovial fluid from patients with septic loosening. The test was less sensitive than specific (Table 19.1). Because the estimated accuracy was of 85.9 %, VEGF has been considered one promising molecular method for PJI diagnosis [48].

19.2.2.3   α2-Macroglobulin (α2M)

α2M is a large plasma protein of hepatic origin that can be increased in nephropathy, in diabetes mellitus, and also in infectious diseases and joint rheumatism. Similarly to VEGF, α2M test was less sensitive than specific, but the positive and negative predictive values and also the test accuracy were high (Table 19.1) [48].

19.3   Microbiological Diagnosis

19.3.1   Bacterial Antigens

19.3.1.1   Lipid S (sce-LTA)

sce-LTA is an exocellular compound released from *S. epidermidis* biofilms into the medium during bacterial growth. After being characterized using cell cultures, sce-LTA has been pointed as the prime mediator of the host inflammatory response to device-related infection by *S. epidermidis*. In this sense, its functionality has been equated to lipopolysaccharide (LPS) in Gram-negative sepsis, although it has been resulted to be quite less active than LPS from *Escherichia coli* [36]. The ability of these components to stimulate the production of IL-6, IL-1β, and TNF-α and also to induce immunity responses mediated by IgG has remade their role as diagnostics tools, providing promising serological tests for PJI diagnosis [29, 43].

19.3.1.2   Polysaccharide Intercellular Adhesin (PIA)

PIA is a molecule of relevant importance in the first attachment phase of biofilm development [52], and its role in PJIs caused by *S. aureus* and *S. epidermidis*, along with other protein factors, has been investigated. While in *S. aureus* PIA contributes to biofilm formation regardless of the infection site, such protein resulted differently in the pathogenesis of *S. epidermidis* [53]. This dependence on the causative microorganism is a serious inconvenient for its use as infection marker, although it could be useful to identify PJIs caused by *S. aureus*.

19.3.1.3 *ica*ADBC Operon

The *ica*ADBC operon, which not only has been well characterized in *S. epidermidis* and *S. aureus* but also has been identified in several other CNS, encodes the biosynthetic products responsible for the generation of PIA [54]. Although it has been previously reported that the *ica*ADBC may be used to discriminate pathogenic strains from normal human flora isolates [55, 56], there are two major drawbacks that lack *ica*ADBC reliability as PJI indicator. First, a study by Frank et al. did not found significant difference in the frequency of detection of *icaA* between CNS PJI isolates and arthroplasty-associated non-PJI CNS isolates [54]. Second, the presence of *ica*ADBC operon could not be a prerequisite for establishing infection with CNS. Related to Frank's findings, a later study suggests the phenotypic and/or genotypic heterogeneity of CNS isolated from PJI, with only one-third of the infections caused by *S. epidermidis* being *ica*ADBC positive [57]. Other studies have confirmed this finding in orthopedic infection-related strains of *Staphylococcus* [58].

19.3.2 Gene Detection

Polymerase chain reaction (PCR) is the most widely used molecular tool and has been applied to many different infection agents from a variety of sources [25, 27, 59, 60]. Several studies have addressed the usefulness of PCR in the diagnosis of PJI. This technique is based in the amplification of a selected fragment of DNA using a thermostable DNA polymerase enzyme and forward and reverse oligodeoxynucleotide primers designed to match the selected sequences of target DNA, resulting in a large number of copies (Fig. 19.1) [2, 16, 61–66]. PCR assays allow for a rapid and high sensitive amplification of the genetic material of a pathogen directly from a clinical specimen, without relying on microbial proliferation, and could be an aid for the diagnosis in the early stages of infection [2, 25]. This method needs to be followed by detection and identification of the PCR product in order to characterize their lengths and sequences (such as electrophoresis or hybridization with specific probes) [2]. In the PCR technique, the search is directed and limited to a well-known sequence in the DNA, but it is not possible to detect the presence of other sequences. Thus, the search could be incomplete. Then, it is necessary to know very well the most frequent pathogens in each infection in order to know what organisms are necessary to detect [67].

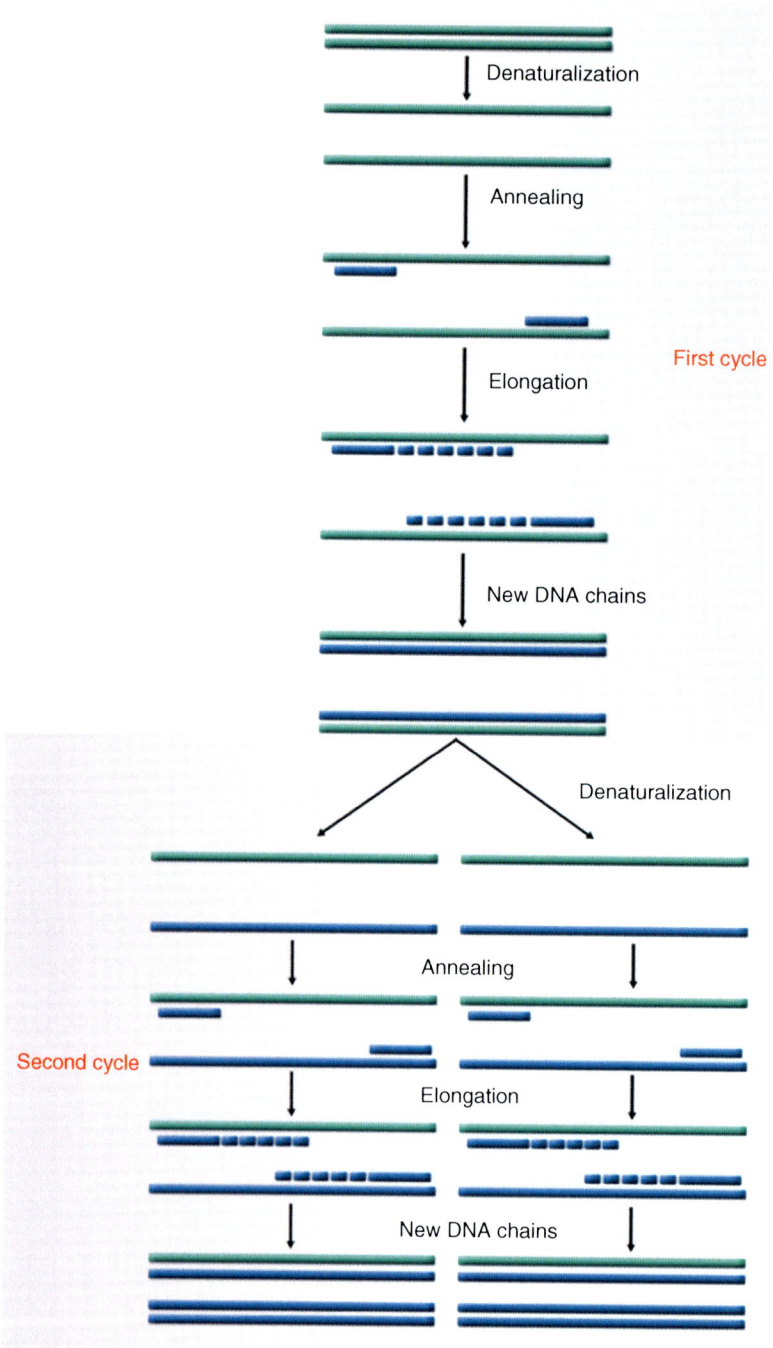

Fig. 19.1 Scheme of the Polymerase Chain Reaction (PCR)

Since its introduction, several improvements have been developed in the technique due to problems that appeared with its use, such as the risk of contamination, and, consequently, the false-positive results that can appear due to the post-amplification manipulation [2, 49, 68].

19.3.2.1 Broad-Range PCR

Conventional PCR is usually used when there is evidence or suspicion of a particular agent or group of pathogen agents, so that a specific PCR could be designed. However, when the goal is the detection of any bacterial pathogen in a clinical sample and the identity of the organism is not known (as in almost all cases of PJI), broad-range PCR amplification, also called "universal," must be used [25]. In this technique, universal primers are used to anneal with conserved regions of the DNA which appear in the genomes of most bacterial species. The targets most commonly employed are ribosomal genes, especially 16S rRNA gene [2, 25, 27, 59, 69–74], which is highly conserved in nearly all species of bacteria and is used as a phylogenetic "fingerprint" [16, 27, 62, 65, 67, 72, 75–78]. This gene is present in multiple copies in the bacterial genome, a fact that facilitates its amplification, and contains alternating regions of nucleotide conservation and heterogeneity. The conserved region makes it possible to amplify the target from all or almost all bacterial species, including human pathogens [2, 25, 63, 79, 80], and practically all of the orthopedically relevant bacterial pathogens can be rapidly identified with universal primers [63]. It has been used successfully for the identification of bacteria associated with PJI in several reports [21, 25, 26, 64].

In addition, other ribosomal targets have been previously tested for broad-range PCR, such as 23 S rDNA, RNase P, housekeeping genes (such as *groEL*) [72], citrate synthetase gene, and heat shock protein genes. Nevertheless, 16S rRNA is the target which has shown the best results, probably because of the high sequence conservation [2].

However, bacterial 16S rRNA amplification alone only detects the presence of bacteria, but it does not identify the infecting organisms [2, 21, 65]. After the amplification process, the variability between genomes allows the microbial identification by means of different techniques that have been developed over the years, such as oligonucleotide array, restriction digestion, sequencing, or hybridization using different sets of specific probes [2, 21, 59, 64, 68, 79, 81–87].

Despite these promising results, the high sensitivity of the technique and the fact that each bacterial species is a target for this PCR make it highly susceptible to contamination [65], leading to potentially false-positive results [2, 18, 21, 27, 59, 62–64, 70, 81, 88, 89]. It must be taken in account that the etiological agents of PJI are mainly opportunistic pathogens and members of the human microbiota; thus, the potential contamination of samples must be addressed [21, 70, 87, 90].

Another problem associated with broad-range PCR assays may be caused by the reagents, specifically the Taq polymerase, in which traces of *E. coli* DNA could be detected because this enzyme is obtained from a recombinant *E. coli* source

[27, 62, 70, 91, 92]. The primers cannot differentiate this *E. coli* DNA from that present in pathogenic bacteria. This problem could be overcome by using specific primers targeting the major causative agents of orthopedic infections [27, 62, 93] or with the elimination of residual bacterial DNA by pretreatment of the mixture of reagents, including primers with restriction enzymes [65].

However, some authors defend that PCR is not appropriate for the identification of each pathogen in case of mixed infection [2, 3, 18, 26, 94], although if a mixture of bacterial species is present in a clinical specimen, interpretation of multiple PCR products generated using broad-range PCR may only be resolved by a subjecting amplified DNA to cloning, high-performance liquid chromatography (HPLC), or denaturing or temperature gradient gel electrophoresis to obtain a pure template for sequencing of individual 16S rDNA [2]. However, a recent research showed that some cases of mixed infections can be detected using broad-range PCR amplification followed by solid-phase hybridization with specific probes against several pathogens, with good results [87].

Broad-range PCR has been a great step for the diagnosis of infectious diseases, but the main limitations are the problems related to specificity, sensitivity, and provision of antimicrobial susceptibility [2, 64, 94]. Quantitative real-time PCR in a closed system, in which amplification and detection are coupled, could avoid these problems, and so it could be useful for the diagnosis of PJI infections [64].

19.3.2.2   Quantitative Real-Time PCR (Q-PCR)

Q-PCR had been developed over the past decade as a sophisticated technique and is recognized as a rapid and reliable alternative assay in many settings [28, 95, 96]. This assay allows to detect at real time the amplification of the DNA molecules and quantify the fluorescently labeled PCR product using reference controls [2, 59, 95, 97], being faster, more objective, and consistent than traditional molecular methods [59, 95, 98, 99].

In this type of assay, amplification and detection are realized in the same vessel, and therefore the probability of contamination is reduced [2]. This technique presents several advantages over conventional PCR, like speed, simplicity, reproducibility, quantitative capacity, and low risk of contamination. In addition, pathogen-specific PCR is useful also when contamination is suspected [64]. It must be noted that, as for conventional PCR, it is impossible to confirm the viability of the bacteria identified by Q-PCR [95], but it is possible to perform a modification of the technique through an mRNA-based RT-qPCR reverse transcription where mRNA is converted to cDNA by reverse transcriptase before PCR amplification. This technique permits to demonstrate the viability of the organisms [63, 67, 95, 100], so bacterial mRNA rather than DNA could be a better option to identify transcriptionally active bacteria that are thought to be involved in PJI [26]. However, the sensitivity of this method is limited by the low number of mRNA transcripts in bacteria from a clinical sample and the high rate of degradation of mRNA after cell death [49, 63, 101]. In this sense, some studies have also tried to identify transcriptionally active bacteria within the biofilms on the surface of failed prostheses through detecting bacterial mRNA amplifying bacterial 16S rRNA genes and generating cDNA acting as a template and followed by cloning, RFLP, and DNA sequencing [26].

19.3.2.3   PCR Modifications

Several variations of the original PCR have been developed to improve both the detection and the identification of PJI, such as PCR which distinguishes between *S. aureus* and CNS [62, 70, 87, 102]. This assay is desirable in cases of orthopedic infection, given the high frequency of the *Staphylococcus* species as a causative agent of infection [14, 70].

Another adaptation are the PCR and sequencing which detect Gram-positive and Gram-negative bacteria [62, 103]; the 16S rRNA PCR combined with reverse line blot hybridization with use of oligonucleotide probes to detect and identify bacterial species followed by sequencing analysis [65, 87, 104]; the PCR combined with pyrosequencing technology that can identify bacterial subgroups [105]; the multiplex PCR technique, which amplifies separate regions of DNA instead of the whole molecule, reducing the risk of false negatives [68, 106]; or the nested PCR technique, which uses a second pair of primers, producing a second PCR product that will be shorter and discernable from the first one [68, 107]. Multiplex-real-time PCR, in which multiple specific PCR assays are run simultaneously to test for multiple different DNA templates for species verification, combined with sonication of removed implants has been also tested as a diagnostic method [18, 25]. This approach may be hampered by the interference between primers within the same reaction, but well-designed assays targeted at the bacteria most frequently implicated in PJI may be useful in this molecular diagnosis [2, 18, 87].

Finally, the genetic fingerprinting techniques, the denaturing gradient gel electrophoresis (DGGE), and the temperature gradient gel electrophoresis (TGGE) allow the identification of a variety of microorganism for comparison of the diversity of microbial communities and for monitoring population dynamics [68, 108], but these techniques have not been tested in PJI.

19.3.2.4   Microarrays and Proteomics

Other new molecular techniques that may have a role in diagnosing PJI include the use of microarrays and proteomics technologies [47, 62]. The microarrays are analytical devices containing hundreds or thousands of probes attached to a solid support [75, 82, 109]. PCR-microarray analysis based on specific oligonucleotide probes offers several advantages in patients requiring a prompt diagnosis when used to complement culture results [75]. Proteomics-based techniques allow simultaneous isolation and evaluation of numerous proteins [62].

The premise of these techniques is to identify organism-specific genes or proteins, and the most important advantage of these techniques is that they allow detection of the causative organism even when the conventional culture results are negative.

However, as with all other techniques, false-positive and false-negative results can also be obtained [75, 110].

19.3.2.5 IBIS Technology

Recently, IBIS technology has been developed as a novel molecular strategy in which multiple pairs of primers, 16S rRNA and 23S rRNA, as well as sequences that are phylum or class specific and others, are used to amplify certain regions of the genome of the microorganism of interest [67]. The amplicons obtained by PCR would be weighted by mass spectrometry (ESI-MS), and the results of the nucleotide composition obtained used to calculate the base composition which allows the identification of the bacteria present in the sample by comparison with a database [67, 72].

Theoretically, this system enables the identification and quantification of bacteria, fungi, and viruses that cause disease in humans [62], even to recognize new species [67].

Primer sets have to be designed to focus on the most typical pathogens of a specific disease, such as orthopedic infection, so that sensitivity and accuracy can be enhanced [67]. Until the moment, this technique has not yet been used for detection of PJI, but it has to be taken into account in the near future.

19.4 Use and Limitations of PJI Molecular Diagnosis

Several authors have evaluated the role of PCR-based methods in the diagnosis of PJI [18, 21, 23, 24, 63, 111, 112], mainly investigating synovial fluid or periprosthetic tissue, whereas sonication fluid was evaluated only recently [15, 18, 87]. The detection of bacterial DNA in culture-negative clinical samples by PCR amplification by several researchers shows the potential of this kind of techniques in PJI diagnosis [21, 75, 87, 94]. These molecular approaches based on amplification and sequencing have shown high sensitivity in identifying microorganisms in samples where traditional culture have failed or nongrowing or slow-growing bacterial agents could be implicated [2, 21, 88, 89, 93]. Broad-range PCR and more advanced molecular methods have shown a high specificity (96–100 %) [27, 64, 65, 81, 87, 88, 94], but often a reduced sensitivity (≤50 %) in diagnosing PJI [27, 81, 88, 94].

Most of these studies have been performed using homemade protocols. One common problem from homemade techniques is the lack of standardization, which made problematic the use of the technique in a routine setting. Commercial techniques have been standardized, and they are currently used in most laboratories for the diagnosis of many infectious diseases [113]. The study performed by Achermann et al. [18] was based on modifying the standard protocol of a commercial multiplex PCR assay originally designed to identify microorganisms from blood cultures. The study combined this technique with a sonication protocol for retrieved implants and showed an important increase in the number of positive results. Another study used a similar approach with a commercial PCR-hybridization technique also designed for its use with blood culture bottles [87], with an increase of positive diagnosis of 10 % of patients with clinical diagnosis of infection. Both studies had the same problem: the commercial techniques were designed to detect common blood culture isolates, and some PJI pathogens cannot be detected by these kits (especially *Propionibacterium acnes*, *Corynebacterium* sp., or anaerobic bacteria).

On the other hand, some authors have criticized these techniques due to the potentially high false-positive results because of its sensitivity [16, 89, 94, 112], so both DNAs present in dead bacteria and in the recombinant prepared reagents would be amplified and detected [63]. Moreover, there are patients without clinical diagnosis of infection which gave positive results with molecular techniques [21, 87], the actual significance of these results being problematic because it is difficult to determine if these are subclinical infections or contaminations.

One important problem common to these techniques is related to the knowledge of the antimicrobial susceptibilities of the microorganisms, because none of the non-culture methods allows for it [21, 49]. However, it is possible to detect several known resistance genes by PCR, such as the methicillin-resistance gene *mecA* or quinolone- and rifampin-resistance gene [16, 18, 49, 67, 87, 114]. However, not all the mechanisms of antibiotic resistances are known, so in the present moment it is impossible to predict the antibiotic susceptibility only by using molecular methods [16].

Nowadays, molecular methods are a support in the detection of PJI, rather than the replacement of conventional techniques, especially in complicated cases such as culture-negative cases when aseptic loosening and subclinical infections are difficult to differentiate [75, 87]. Further research is needed before routinely apply molecular methods in PJI diagnosis. Moreover, to date, no single clinical or laboratory test has shown to achieve ideal sensitivity and specificity for the PJI diagnosis [2], and molecular techniques are not yet routinely employed in orthopedic practice [25, 65], although the integration of these techniques in the PJI diagnostic may be expected.

Today, the appropriate combination of traditional culture-based diagnosis, histopathology, and molecular techniques, together with other approaches and clinical assessment, may contribute to improve the PJI diagnosis [2, 8, 26, 49, 63]. New diagnostic methods and improvement of those that already exist are still needed for the diagnosis of PJI [49].

References

1. Virolainen P, Lahteenmaki H, Hiltunen A, Sipola E, Meurman O, Nelimarkka O. The reliability of diagnosis of infection during revision arthroplasties. Scand J Surg. 2002;91(2): 178–81.
2. Trampuz A, Osmon DR, Hanssen AD, Steckelberg JM, Patel R. Molecular and antibiofilm approaches to prosthetic joint infection. Clin Orthop Relat Res. 2003;414(414):69–88.
3. Zimmerli W, Trampuz A, Ochsner PE. Prosthetic-joint infections. N Engl J Med. 2004;351(16):1645–54.

4. Roberts VI, Esler CN, Harper WM. A 15-year follow-up study of 4606 primary total knee replacements. J Bone Joint Surg Br. 2007;89(11):1452–6.

5. Cataldo MA, Petrosillo N, Cipriani M, Cauda R, Tacconelli E. Prosthetic joint infection: recent developments in diagnosis and management. J Infect. 2010;61(6):443–8.

6. Azanza JR. What is the cost of a prosthesis infection? Enferm Infecc Microbiol Clin. 2001;19(1):44–5.

7. Poultsides LA, Liaropoulos LL, Malizos KN. The socioeconomic impact of musculoskeletal infections. J Bone Joint Surg Am. 2010;92(11):e13.

8. Gomez E, Patel R. Laboratory diagnosis of prosthetic joint infection, part I. Clin Microbiol Newslett. 2011;33(8):55–60. doi:10.1016/j.clinmicnews.2011.03.004.

9. Burger RR, Basch T, Hopson CN. Implant salvage in infected total knee arthroplasty. Clin Orthop Relat Res. 1991;273(273):105–12.

10. Gallo J, Smizansky M, Radova L, Potomkova J. Comparison of therapeutic strategies for hip and knee prosthetic joint infection. Acta Chir Orthop Traumatol Cech. 2009;76(4):302–9.

11. Moyad TF, Thornhill T, Estok D. Evaluation and management of the infected total hip and knee. Orthopedics. 2008;31(6):581–8.

12. Tattevin P, Cremieux AC, Pottier P, Huten D, Carbon C. Prosthetic joint infection: when can prosthesis salvage be considered? Clin Infect Dis. 1999;29(2):292–5.

13. Berbari EF, Hanssen AD, Duffy MC, Steckelberg JM, Osmon DR. Prosthetic joint infection due to Mycobacterium tuberculosis: a case series and review of the literature. Am J Orthop (Belle Mead NJ). 1998;27(3):219–27.

14. Del Pozo JL, Patel R. Clinical practice. Infection associated with prosthetic joints. N Engl J Med. 2009;361(8):787–94.

15. Piper KE, Jacobson MJ, Cofield RH, Sperling JW, Sanchez-Sotelo J, Osmon DR, et al. Microbiologic diagnosis of prosthetic shoulder infection by use of implant sonication. J Clin Microbiol. 2009;47(6):1878–84.

16. Gallo J, Raska M, Dendis M, Florschutz AV, Kolar M. Molecular diagnosis of prosthetic joint infection. A review of evidence. Biomed Pap Med Fac Univ Palacky Olomouc Czech Repub. 2004;148(2):123–9.

17. Trampuz A, Widmer AF. Infections associated with orthopedic implants. Curr Opin Infect Dis. 2006;19:349–56.

18. Achermann Y, Vogt M, Leunig M, Wust J, Trampuz A. Improved diagnosis of periprosthetic joint infection by multiplex PCR of sonication fluid from removed implants. J Clin Microbiol. 2010;48(4):1208–14.

19. Esteban J, Gomez-Barrena E, Cordero J, Martin-de-Hijas NZ, Kinnari TJ, Fernandez-Roblas R. Evaluation of quantitative analysis of cultures from sonicated retrieved orthopedic implants in diagnosis of orthopedic infection. J Clin Microbiol. 2008;46(2):488–92.

20. Trampuz A, Piper KE, Jacobson MJ, Hanssen AD, Unni KK, Osmon DR, et al. Sonication of removed hip and knee prostheses for diagnosis of infection. N Engl J Med. 2007;357(7): 654–63.

21. Tunney MM, Patrick S, Curran MD, Ramage G, Hanna D, Nixon JR, et al. Detection of prosthetic hip infection at revision arthroplasty by immunofluorescence microscopy and PCR amplification of the bacterial 16S rRNA gene. J Clin Microbiol. 1999;37(10):3281–90.

22. Clarke MT, Roberts CP, Lee PT, Gray J, Keene GS, Rushton N. Polymerase chain reaction can detect bacterial DNA in aseptically loose total hip arthroplasties. Clin Orthop Relat Res. 2004;427:132–7.

23. Dempsey KE, Riggio MP, Lennon A, Hannah VE, Ramage G, Allan D, et al. Identification of bacteria on the surface of clinically infected and non-infected prosthetic hip joints removed during revision arthroplasties by 16S rRNA gene sequencing and by microbiological culture. Arthritis Res Ther. 2007;9(3):R46.

24. Levine MJ, Mariani BA, Tuan RS, Booth Jr RE. Molecular genetic diagnosis of infected total joint arthroplasty. J Arthroplasty. 1995;10(1):93–4.

25. Mariani BD, Tuan RS. Advances in the diagnosis of infection in prosthetic joint implants. Mol Med Today. 1998;4(5):207–13.

26. Riggio MP, Dempsey KE, Lennon A, Allan D, Ramage G, Bagg J. Molecular detection of transcriptionally active bacteria from failed prosthetic hip joints removed during revision arthroplasty. Eur J Clin Microbiol Infect Dis. 2010;29(7):823–34.
27. Hoeffel DP, Hinrichs SH, Garvin KL. Molecular diagnostics for the detection of musculoskeletal infection. Clin Orthop Relat Res. 1999;360:37–46.
28. Kobayashi H, Oethinger M, Tuohy MJ, Procop GW, Hall GS, Bauer TW. Limiting false-positive polymerase chain reaction results: detection of DNA and mRNA to differentiate viable from dead bacteria. Diagn Microbiol Infect Dis. 2009;64(4):445–7.
29. Worthington T, Dunlop D, Casey A, Lambert R, Luscombe J, Elliott T. Serum procalcitonin, interleukin-6, soluble intercellular adhesin molecule-1 and IgG to short-chain exocellular lipoteichoic acid as predictors of infection in total joint prosthesis revision. Br J Biomed Sci. 2010;67(2):71–6.
30. Zimmerli W. Prosthetic-joint-associated infections. Best Pract Res Clin Rheumatol. 1996;20(6):1045–63.
31. Heinrich PC, Behrmann I, Haan S, Hermanns HM, Muller-Newen G, Schaper F. Principles of interleukin (IL)-6-type cytokine signalling and its regulation. Biochem J. 2003;374(Pt 1):1–20.
32. Berbari E, Mabry T, Tsaras G, Spangehl M, Erwin PJ, Murad MH, et al. Inflammatory blood laboratory levels as markers of prosthetic joint infection: a systematic review and meta-analysis. J Bone Joint Surg Am. 2010;92(11):2102–9.
33. Cronstein BN. Interleukin-6 – a key mediator of systemic and local symptoms in rheumatoid arthritis. Bull NYU Hosp Jt Dis. 2007;65 Suppl 1:S11–5.
34. Andersson MK, Lundberg P, Ohlin A, Perry MJ, Lie A, Stark A, et al. Effects on osteoclast and osteoblast activities in cultured mouse calvarial bones by synovial fluids from patients with a loose joint prosthesis and from osteoarthritis patients. Arthritis Res Ther. 2007;9(1):R18.
35. Nilsdotter-Augustinsson A, Briheim G, Herder A, Ljunghusen O, Wahlstrom O, Ohman L. Inflammatory response in 85 patients with loosened hip prostheses: a prospective study comparing inflammatory markers in patients with aseptic and septic prosthetic loosening. Acta Orthop. 2007;78(5):629–39.
36. Jones KJ, Perris AD, Vernallis AB, Worthington T, Lambert PA, Elliott TS. Induction of inflammatory cytokines and nitric oxide in J774.2 cells and murine macrophages by lipoteichoic acid and related cell wall antigens from Staphylococcus epidermidis. J Med Microbiol. 2005;54(Pt 4):315–21.
37. Di Cesare PE, Chang E, Preston CF, Liu CJ. Serum interleukin-6 as a marker of periprosthetic infection following total hip and knee arthroplasty. J Bone Joint Surg Am. 2005;87(9):1921–7.
38. Bottner F, Wegner A, Winkelmann W, Becker K, Erren M, Gotze C. Interleukin-6, procalcitonin and TNF-alpha: markers of peri-prosthetic infection following total joint replacement. J Bone Joint Surg Br. 2007;89(1):94–9.
39. Gilbert DN. Use of plasma procalcitonin levels as an adjunct to clinical microbiology. J Clin Microbiol. 2010;48(7):2325–9.
40. Gendrel D, Raymond J, Coste J, Moulin F, Lorrot M, Guerin S, et al. Comparison of procalcitonin with C-reactive protein, interleukin 6 and interferon-alpha for differentiation of bacterial vs. viral infections. Pediatr Infect Dis J. 1999;18(10):875–81.
41. Jones AE, Fiechtl JF, Brown MD, Ballew JJ, Kline JA. Procalcitonin test in the diagnosis of bacteremia: a meta-analysis. Ann Emerg Med. 2007;50(1):34–41.
42. Kamme C, Lindberg L. Aerobic and anaerobic bacteria in deep infections after total hip arthroplasty: differential diagnosis between infectious and non-infectious loosening. Clin Orthop Relat Res. 1981;154(154):201–7.
43. Rafiq M, Worthington T, Tebbs SE, Treacy RB, Dias R, Lambert PA, et al. Serological detection of Gram-positive bacterial infection around prostheses. J Bone Joint Surg Br. 2000;82(8):1156–61.
44. van de Stolpe A, van der Saag PT. Intercellular adhesion molecule-1. J Mol Med (Berl). 1996;74(1):13–33.

45. Lawson C, Wolf S. ICAM-1 signaling in endothelial cells. Pharmacol Rep. 2009;61(1):22–32.
46. Pare G, Ridker PM, Rose L, Barbalic M, Dupuis J, Dehghan A, et al. Genome-wide association analysis of soluble ICAM-1 concentration reveals novel associations at the NFKBIK, PNPLA3, RELA, and SH2B3 loci. PLoS Genet. 2011;7(4):e1001374.
47. Deirmengian C, Hallab N, Tarabishy A, Della Valle C, Jacobs JJ, Lonner J, et al. Synovial fluid biomarkers for periprosthetic infection. Clin Orthop Relat Res. 2010;468(8):2017–23.
48. Jacovides CL, Parvizi J, Adeli B, Jung KA. Molecular markers for diagnosis of periprosthetic joint infection. J Arthroplasty. 2011;12:12.
49. Gomez E, Patel R. Laboratory Diagnosis of Prosthetic Joint Infection, Part II. Clin Microbiol Newslett. 2011;33(9):63–70. doi:10.1016/j.clinmicnews.2011.04.001.
50. Mertens MT, Singh JA. Biomarkers in arthroplasty: a systematic review. Open Orthop J. 2011;5:92–105.
51. Holmes K, Roberts OL, Thomas AM, Cross MJ. Vascular endothelial growth factor receptor-2: structure, function, intracellular signalling and therapeutic inhibition. Cell Signal. 2007;19(10):2003–12.
52. O'Gara JP. ica and beyond: biofilm mechanisms and regulation in Staphylococcus epidermidis and Staphylococcus aureus. FEMS Microbiol Lett. 2007;270(2):179–88.
53. Rohde H, Burandt EC, Siemssen N, Frommelt L, Burdelski C, Wurster S, et al. Polysaccharide intercellular adhesin or protein factors in biofilm accumulation of Staphylococcus epidermidis and Staphylococcus aureus isolated from prosthetic hip and knee joint infections. Biomaterials. 2007;28(9):1711–20.
54. Frank KL, Hanssen AD, Patel R. icaA is not a useful diagnostic marker for prosthetic joint infection. J Clin Microbiol. 2004;42(10):4846–9.
55. Arciola CR, Campoccia D, Gamberini S, Rizzi S, Donati ME, Baldassarri L, et al. Search for the insertion element IS256 within the ica locus of Staphylococcus epidermidis clinical isolates collected from biomaterial-associated infections. Biomaterials. 2004;25(18):4117–25.
56. Galdbart JO, Allignet J, Tung HS, Ryden C, El Solh N. Screening for Staphylococcus epidermidis markers discriminating between skin-flora strains and those responsible for infections of joint prostheses. J Infect Dis. 2000;182(1):351–5.
57. Nilsdotter-Augustinsson A, Koskela A, Ohman L, Soderquist B. Characterization of coagulase-negative staphylococci isolated from patients with infected hip prostheses: use of phenotypic and genotypic analyses, including tests for the presence of the ica operon. Eur J Clin Microbiol Infect Dis. 2007;26(4):255–65.
58. Esteban J, Molina-Manso D, Spiliopoulou I, Cordero-Ampuero J, Fernandez-Roblas R, Foka A, et al. Biofilm development by clinical isolates of Staphylococcus spp. from retrieved orthopedic prostheses. Acta Orthop. 2010;81(6):674–9.
59. Yang S, Lin S, Kelen GD, Quinn TC, Dick JD, Gaydos CA, et al. Quantitative multiprobe PCR assay for simultaneous detection and identification to species level of bacterial pathogens. J Clin Microbiol. 2002;40(9):3449–54.
60. Tompkins LS. The use of molecular methods in infectious diseases. N Engl J Med. 1992;327(18):1290–7.
61. Mullis KB, Faloona FA. Specific synthesis of DNA in vitro via a polymerase-catalyzed chain reaction. Methods Enzymol. 1987;155:335–50.
62. Bauer TW, Parvizi J, Kobayashi N, Krebs V. Diagnosis of periprosthetic infection. J Bone Joint Surg Am. 2006;88(4):869–82.
63. Bergin PF, Doppelt JD, Hamilton WG, Mirick GE, Jones AE, Sritulanondha S, et al. Detection of periprosthetic infections with use of ribosomal RNA-based polymerase chain reaction. J Bone Joint Surg Am. 2010;92(3):654–63.
64. Fenollar F, Roux V, Stein A, Drancourt M, Raoult D. Analysis of 525 samples to determine the usefulness of PCR amplification and sequencing of the 16S rRNA gene for diagnosis of bone and joint infections. J Clin Microbiol. 2006;44(3):1018–28.

65. Moojen DJ, Spijkers SN, Schot CS, Nijhof MW, Vogely HC, Fleer A, et al. Identification of orthopaedic infections using broad-range polymerase chain reaction and reverse line blot hybridization. J Bone Joint Surg Am. 2007;89(6):1298–305.

66. Tarkin IS, Henry TJ, Fey PI, Iwen PC, Hinrichs SH, Garvin KL. PCR rapidly detects methicillin-resistant staphylococci periprosthetic infection. Clin Orthop Relat Res. 2003;414: 89–94.

67. Costerton JW, Post JC, Ehrlich GD, Hu FZ, Kreft R, Nistico L, et al. New methods for the detection of orthopedic and other biofilm infections. FEMS Immunol Med Microbiol. 2011;61(2):133–40.

68. Hogdall D, Hvolris JJ, Christensen L. Improved detection methods for infected hip joint prostheses. APMIS. 2010;118(11):815–23.

69. Kolbert CP, Persing DH. Ribosomal DNA sequencing as a tool for identification of bacterial pathogens. Curr Opin Microbiol. 1999;2(3):299–305.

70. Kobayashi N, Procop GW, Krebs V, Kobayashi H, Bauer TW. Molecular identification of bacteria from aseptically loose implants. Clin Orthop Relat Res. 2008;466(7):1716–25.

71. Wilson KH, Blitchington RB, Greene RC. Amplification of bacterial 16S ribosomal DNA with polymerase chain reaction. J Clin Microbiol. 1990;28(9):1942–6.

72. Ecker DJ, Sampath R, Massire C, Blyn LB, Hall TA, Eshoo MW, et al. Ibis T5000: a universal biosensor approach for microbiology. Nat Rev Microbiol. 2008;6(7):553–8.

73. Nikkari S, Lopez FA, Lepp PW, Cieslak PR, Ladd-Wilson S, Passaro D, et al. Broad-range bacterial detection and the analysis of unexplained death and critical illness. Emerg Infect Dis. 2002;8(2):188–94.

74. Kroes I, Lepp PW, Relman DA. Bacterial diversity within the human subgingival crevice. Proc Natl Acad Sci USA. 1999;96(25):14547–52.

75. Uchida K, Yayama T, Kokubo Y, Miyazaki T, Nakajima H, Negoro K, et al. Direct detection of pathogens in osteoarticular infections by polymerase chain reaction amplification and microarray hybridization. J Orthop Sci. 2009;14(5):471–83.

76. Patel JB. 16S rRNA gene sequencing for bacterial pathogen identification in the clinical laboratory. Mol Diagn. 2001;6(4):313–21.

77. Yang S, Rothman RE. PCR-based diagnostics for infectious diseases: uses, limitations, and future applications in acute-care settings. Lancet Infect Dis. 2004;4(6):337–48.

78. Janda JM, Abbott SL. 16S rRNA gene sequencing for bacterial identification in the diagnostic laboratory: pluses, perils, and pitfalls. J Clin Microbiol. 2007;45(9):2761–4.

79. McCabe KM, Zhang YH, Huang BL, Wagar EA, McCabe ER. Bacterial species identification after DNA amplification with a universal primer pair. Mol Genet Metab. 1999;66(3):205–11.

80. Chakravorty S, Helb D, Burday M, Connell N, Alland D. A detailed analysis of 16S ribosomal RNA gene segments for the diagnosis of pathogenic bacteria. J Microbiol Methods. 2007; 69(2):330–9.

81. Fihman V, Hannouche D, Bousson V, Bardin T, Liote F, Raskine L, et al. Improved diagnosis specificity in bone and joint infections using molecular techniques. J Infect. 2007;55(6):510–7.

82. Anthony RM, Brown TJ, French GL. DNA array technology and diagnostic microbiology. Expert Rev Mol Diagn. 2001;1(1):30–8.

83. Lu JJ, Perng CL, Lee SY, Wan CC. Use of PCR with universal primers and restriction endonuclease digestions for detection and identification of common bacterial pathogens in cerebrospinal fluid. J Clin Microbiol. 2000;38(6):2076–80.

84. Rantakokko-Jalava K, Nikkari S, Jalava J, Eerola E, Skurnik M, Meurman O, et al. Direct amplification of rRNA genes in diagnosis of bacterial infections. J Clin Microbiol. 2000; 38(1):32–9.

85. McDowell A, Patrick S. Evaluation of nonculture methods for the detection of prosthetic hip biofilms. Clin Orthop Relat Res. 2005;437:74–82.

86. Goldenberger D, Kunzli A, Vogt P, Zbinden R, Altwegg M. Molecular diagnosis of bacterial endocarditis by broad-range PCR amplification and direct sequencing. J Clin Microbiol. 1997;35(11):2733–9.

87. Esteban J, Alonso-Rodriguez N, Sandoval E, Del Prado G, Ortiz-Perez A, Molina-Manso D, et al. Improved diagnosis of orthopaedic implant-related infection by PCR-hybridization after sonication. Acta Orthopaedica. 2012;83(3):299–304.

88. Mariani BD, Martin DS, Levine MJ, Booth Jr RE, Tuan RS. The Coventry Award. Polymerase chain reaction detection of bacterial infection in total knee arthroplasty. Clin Orthop Relat Res. 1996;331:11–22.

89. Stoodley P, Kathju S, Hu FZ, Erdos G, Levenson JE, Mehta N, et al. Molecular and imaging techniques for bacterial biofilms in joint arthroplasty infections. Clin Orthop Relat Res. 2005;437:31–40.

90. Borst A, Box AT, Fluit AC. False-positive results and contamination in nucleic acid amplification assays: suggestions for a prevent and destroy strategy. Eur J Clin Microbiol Infect Dis. 2004;23(4):289–99.

91. Grahn N, Olofsson M, Ellnebo-Svedlund K, Monstein HJ, Jonasson J. Identification of mixed bacterial DNA contamination in broad-range PCR amplification of 16S rDNA V1 and V3 variable regions by pyrosequencing of cloned amplicons. FEMS Microbiol Lett. 2003;219(1):87–91.

92. Corless CE, Guiver M, Borrow R, Edwards-Jones V, Kaczmarski EB, Fox AJ. Contamination and sensitivity issues with a real-time universal 16S rRNA PCR. J Clin Microbiol. 2000;38(5): 1747–52.

93. Vandercam B, Jeumont S, Cornu O, Yombi JC, Lecouvet F, Lefevre P, et al. Amplification-based DNA analysis in the diagnosis of prosthetic joint infection. J Mol Diagn. 2008; 10(6):537–43.

94. De Man FHR, Graber P, Lüem M, Zimmerli W, Ochsner PE, Sendi P. Broad-range PCR in selected episodes of prosthetic joint infection. Infection. 2009;37(3):292–4.

95. Kobayashi N, Inaba Y, Choe H, Iwamoto N, Ishida T, Yukizawa Y, et al. Rapid and sensitive detection of methicillin-resistant Staphylococcus periprosthetic infections using real-time polymerase chain reaction. Diagn Microbiol Infect Dis. 2009;64(2):172–6.

96. Mackay IM. Real-time PCR in the microbiology laboratory. Clin Microbiol Infect. 2004;10(3):190–212.

97. Heid CA, Stevens J, Livak KJ, Williams PM. Real time quantitative PCR. Genome Res. 1996;6(10):986–94.

98. Gerard CJ, Olsson K, Ramanathan R, Reading C, Hanania EG. Improved quantitation of minimal residual disease in multiple myeloma using real-time polymerase chain reaction and plasmid-DNA complementarity determining region III standards. Cancer Res. 1998;58(17):3957–64.

99. Schmittgen TD, Zakrajsek BA, Mills AG, Gorn V, Singer MJ, Reed MW. Quantitative reverse transcription-polymerase chain reaction to study mRNA decay: comparison of endpoint and real-time methods. Anal Biochem. 2000;285(2):194–204.

100. Birmingham P, Helm JM, Manner PA, Tuan RS. Simulated joint infection assessment by rapid detection of live bacteria with real-time reverse transcription polymerase chain reaction. J Bone Joint Surg Am. 2008;90(3):602–8.

101. Sheridan GE, Masters CI, Shallcross JA, MacKey BM. Detection of mRNA by reverse transcription-PCR as an indicator of viability in *Escherichia coli* cells. Appl Environ Microbiol. 1998;64(4):1313–8.

102. Sakai H, Procop GW, Kobayashi N, Togawa D, Wilson DA, Borden L, et al. Simultaneous detection of Staphylococcus aureus and coagulase-negative staphylococci in positive blood cultures by real-time PCR with two fluorescence resonance energy transfer probe sets. J Clin Microbiol. 2004;42(12):5739–44.

103. Kobayashi N, Bauer TW, Togawa D, Lieberman IH, Sakai H, Fujishiro T, et al. A molecular gram stain using broad range PCR and pyrosequencing technology: a potentially useful tool for diagnosing orthopaedic infections. Diagn Mol Pathol. 2005;14(2):83–9.

104. Kaufhold A, Podbielski A, Baumgarten G, Blokpoel M, Top J, Schouls L. Rapid typing of group A streptococci by the use of DNA amplification and non-radioactive allele-specific oligonucleotide probes. FEMS Microbiol Lett. 1994;119(1–2):19–25.

105. Kobayashi N, Bauer TW, Tuohy MJ, Lieberman IH, Krebs V, Togawa D, et al. The comparison of pyrosequencing molecular Gram stain, culture, and conventional Gram stain for diagnosing orthopaedic infections. J Orthop Res. 2006;24(8):1641–9.
106. Edwards MC, Gibbs RA. Multiplex PCR: advantages, development, and applications. PCR Methods Appl. 1994;3(4):S65–75.
107. Siebert PD, Chenchik A, Kellogg DE, Lukyanov KA, Lukyanov SA. An improved PCR method for walking in uncloned genomic DNA. Nucleic Acids Res. 1995;23(6):1087–8.
108. Muyzer G. DGGE/TGGE a method for identifying genes from natural ecosystems. Curr Opin Microbiol. 1999;2(3):317–22.
109. Tillib SV, Mirzabekov AD. Advances in the analysis of DNA sequence variations using oligonucleotide microchip technology. Curr Opin Biotechnol. 2001;12(1):53–8.
110. Jordan JA, Durso MB. Comparison of 16S rRNA gene PCR and BACTEC 9240 for detection of neonatal bacteremia. J Clin Microbiol. 2000;38(7):2574–8.
111. Dora C, Altwegg M, Gerber C, Bottger EC, Zbinden R. Evaluation of conventional microbiological procedures and molecular genetic techniques for diagnosis of infections in patients with implanted orthopedic devices. J Clin Microbiol. 2008;46(2):824–5.
112. Panousis K, Grigoris P, Butcher I, Rana B, Reilly JH, Hamblen DL. Poor predictive value of broad-range PCR for the detection of arthroplasty infection in 92 cases. Acta Orthop. 2005;76(3):341–6.
113. Nolte FS, Caliendo AM. Molecular microbiology. In: Versalovic J, Carroll KC, Funke G, Jorgensen JH, Landry ML, Warnock DW, editors. Manual of clinical microbiology. 10th ed. Washington, DC: ASM Press; 2011. p. 27–59.
114. Huletsky A, Giroux R, Rossbach V, Gagnon M, Vaillancourt M, Bernier M, et al. New real-time PCR assay for rapid detection of methicillin-resistant *Staphylococcus aureus* directly from specimens containing a mixture of staphylococci. J Clin Microbiol. 2004;42(5):1875–84.

Part II

Chapter 20
Current Treatment Strategies in Prosthetic Joint Infections

Rihard Trebše and Aleš Berce

Abstract There are many ways to approach the problem of PJI. The most frequently used is the two-step approach in which the first step serves for prosthetic joint removal, while in the second step, the artificial joint is reimplanted. There are, however, other options like amputation, joint fusion, implant removal, two-stage replacement, one-stage replacement, debridement and retention of implant, and permanent antibiotic suppression. Every treatment type has its indications that overlap to some extent and its advantages and disadvantages. In this chapter, these are discussed in detail for the reader to get familiar with the contemporary treatment strategies for easier implementation in own clinical praxis.

Keywords Debridement and retention • One-stage replacement • Two-stage replacement • Antibiotic suppression

20.1 Introduction

Actual surgical treatment options for PJI include in decreasing order of invasiveness: amputation, joint fusion, implant removal, two-stage replacement, one-stage replacement, debridement and retention of implant, and permanent antibiotic suppression. Traditionally, the choice of the strategy depended on the knowledge and experience of the treating orthopedic surgeon, hospital tradition, patient inclination, duration of symptoms, type of infection, virulence of the pathogen and its antibiotic sensitivity, soft tissue conditions, and patient comorbidities. Choices did not change a lot recently despite the improvements in diagnostic evaluation and treatment.

R. Trebše, M.D., Ph.D. (✉) • A. Berce, M.D.
Department for Bone Infections and Adult reconstructions,
Orthopaedic Hospital Valdoltra,
Jadranska cesta 31, Ankaran SI-6286, Slovenia
e-mail: rihard.trebse@ob-valdoltra.si; ales.berce@ob-valdoltra.si

R. Trebše (ed.), *Infected Total Joint Arthroplasty*,
DOI 10.1007/978-1-4471-2482-5_20, © Springer-Verlag London 2012

20.2 Amputation

Amputation is the most radical treatment option for PJI and fortunately also very seldom adopted in medically developed world. It comes into consideration when life-threatening infections cannot be controlled by other modalities or when the extent of bone and/or soft tissue loss precludes any less invasive solution like fusion and other procedures seem inadequate.

It is most frequently performed for TKA infections, [1] but it is also carried out for other peripheral artificial joint infections, occasionally for infected THA as well. Reasons that most frequently induce the adoption of this surgical solution include repetitive revisions, bone loss, and excruciating pain [2].

When considering various treatment options for a particular TKA infection, it is prudent to consider fusion early in the treatment algorithm when it is still feasible and reasonable to avoid extreme bone and soft tissue loss that can leave the amputation as the only solution.

It is difficult to estimate the incidence of amputations after total joint arthroplasty infections. Probably, the rate ranges around 1–10/10,000 primary THA [3, 4]. The incidence is higher after TKR [5–7] and total ankle arthroplasty [8] reaching up to 6 %. Our rate of above the knee amputations due to consequences of TKA infection is 0.05 %.

Functional performance of old patients after above-the-knee amputation is very limited, and more than half of them are consequently wheelchair bound [9].

20.3 Joint Fusion: Arthrodesis

Joint fusion is a rarely adopted option for treatment of chronic uncontrollable device-related infections of certain artificial joints especially knees. Successfully performed procedure stabilizes the joint and eliminates pain. According to the same concepts as for septic total joint revisions, one can perform a one- or two-step fusion of a joint, depending on the patient characteristics, germ, and local joint status. When considering appropriate surgical treatment several issues like poor general health status, i.v. drug abuse, immunodeficiency, limited mobility, dementia, and some other favor a fusion against a revision.

Fusion after removal of an infected artificial joint – usually a TKA, is technically a demanding procedure due to limited amounts of poor quality bone stock. Nonunion rate is consequently high, and despite a successful fusion, the limb is usually shorter.

The indications for fusion vary depending on the joint involved. It is the primary and the most appropriate treatment for total ankle arthroplasty infection in cases when retention of the device is not considered a viable option (Figs. 20.1 and 20.2). The functionality of a fused ankle is surprisingly good (Fig. 20.3) and disfavors other potential treatment options like one- or two-stage revision.

Fusion is relatively frequently adopted for treatment of chronic TKA infection especially if the function of the extensor mechanism is impaired because it grants stability, eliminates pain, and provides good setting for healing of the infection.

Fig. 20.1 Loosened infected prosthetic ankle

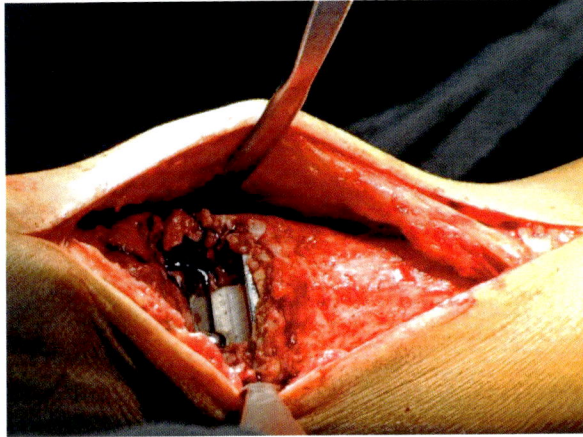

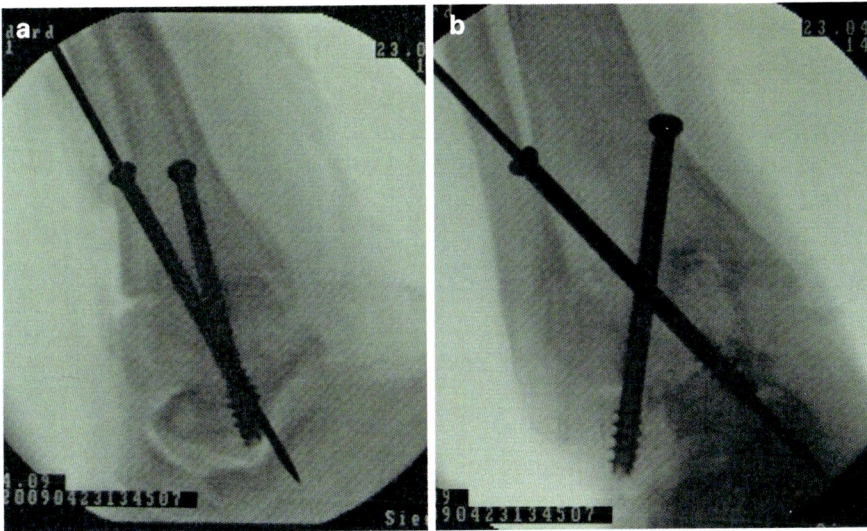

Fig. 20.2 Ankle fusion after loosened infected prosthetic ankle joint with bulk femoral head allograft (**a**) Lateral view (**b**) AP view

There are, however, many inconveniences with knee fusion. Walking is very difficult and awkward, but the most uncomfortable is sitting. Interestingly, despite these functional impairments, patients achieved similar Oxford University scores after fusion or two-stage revision of an infected TKA [10].

There are some patient circumstances in which fusion is particularly indicated. It probably is the best solution for a young active patient with single-joint disease and irreparable extensor mechanism insufficiency with or without skin and soft tissue deficiency, for an immunocompromised patient and when the infection is caused by a multi resistant or difficult to treat organism [11].

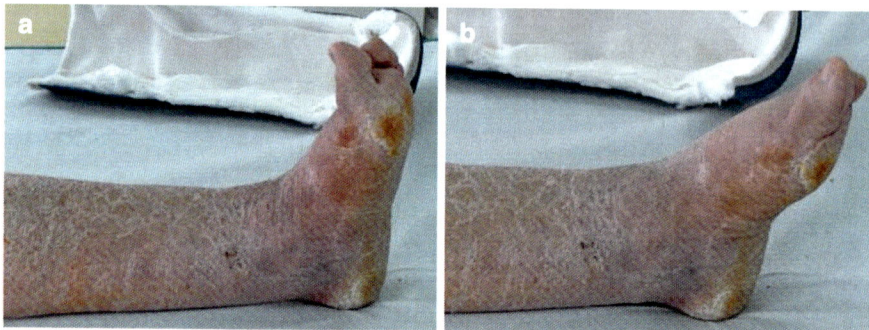

Fig. 20.3 Ankle fused after removed total ankle arthroplasty, ROM just after cast removal (**a**) dorsal flexion (**b**) plantar flexion

Fusion rate is lower than in primary cases and is limited mainly by persistent infection and bone stock deficiency. It is actually possible to achieve fusion despite persistent infection, but the rates are much lower in these circumstances [12].

There are several techniques for knee fusion after TKA infection. We can use an external fixator (Fig. 20.5), an intramedullary nail (Fig. 20.6), or plates with screws (Fig. 20.4).

The technique consists of meticulous necrectomy or debridement, removal of fibrous tissues, apposition of well-vascularized bony surfaces of distal femur and proximal tibia, and stabilization with one of the aforementioned devices. The advantage of the external fiksater is the avoidance of having any foreign material at the site of the infection. The disadvantage is that stability achieved by external fixator is inferior to stability obtained by plates or nails especially in cases with severe bone loss. In these cases, it is very difficult to realize sufficient long-term stability to consistently attain bony fusion. Application of the device in all three planes increases fusion rates [6, 11]. An additional concern related to external fiksater is the risk of acquiring pin tract infections that need further treatment. Nevertheless, the external fiksater is the most appropriate device in selected cases if a single stage fusion is considered.

Intramedullary rod gives the best fusion rates (from 80 to 100 %) for knee joint after removal of infected TKA [13]. The disadvantage is that it is possible to spread the infection along the intramedullary canals in the case of persistent unrecognized infection or if the rod is used for one-stage fusion in persistent active infections.

The third option is the use of two long plates placed in two planes at right angle. With the plates, it is readily possible to apply compression over the arthrodesis [14]. Plates allow for superior stability. The shortcoming with this technique is the need for increased bone exposure that negatively influences bone vitality and the biology of the healing. Soft tissue closure might be challenging with the use of plates.

Although theoretically possible, fusions are rarely attempted in hips and shoulders after a septic alloarthroplasty failure. The reasons comprise poor fusion rates and acceptable results with simple resection arthroplasty. There is no reliable information regarding fusion rates and results for fusion after removal of an infected total elbow arthroplasty [15].

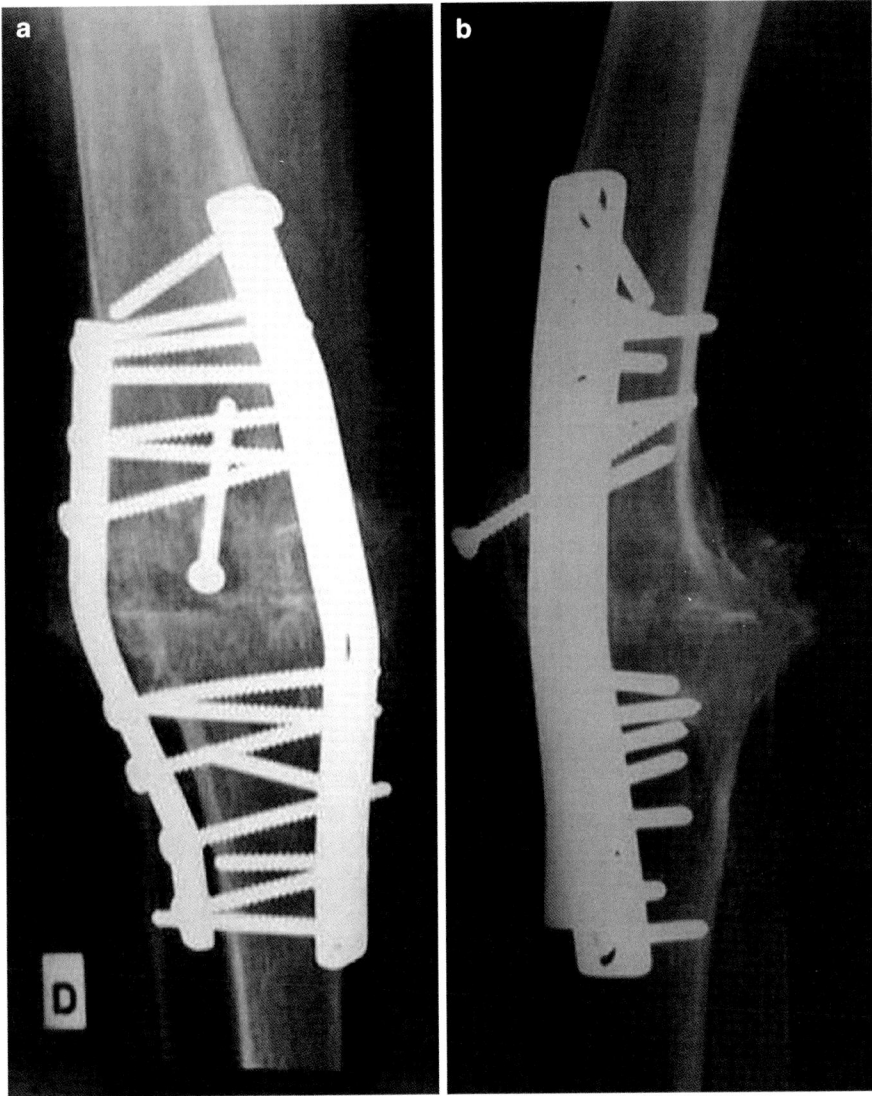

Fig. 20.4 Knee arthrodesis with plates and screws. (**a**) AP view (**b**) Lateral view

20.4   Resection Arthroplasty

Resection arthroplasty (Fig. 20.7) may be permanent in cases where no attempt of reimplantation of an artificial joint is intended, but it may also be temporary like between the two acts of a two-stage revision of a septic total joint arthroplasty (TJA). When it is used in the hip joint, it is known as a Girdlestone procedure after an English surgeon who introduced the method for treating various surgical conditions.

Fig. 20.5 Knee fusion with external fixator. (**a**) Oblique view (**b**) AP view

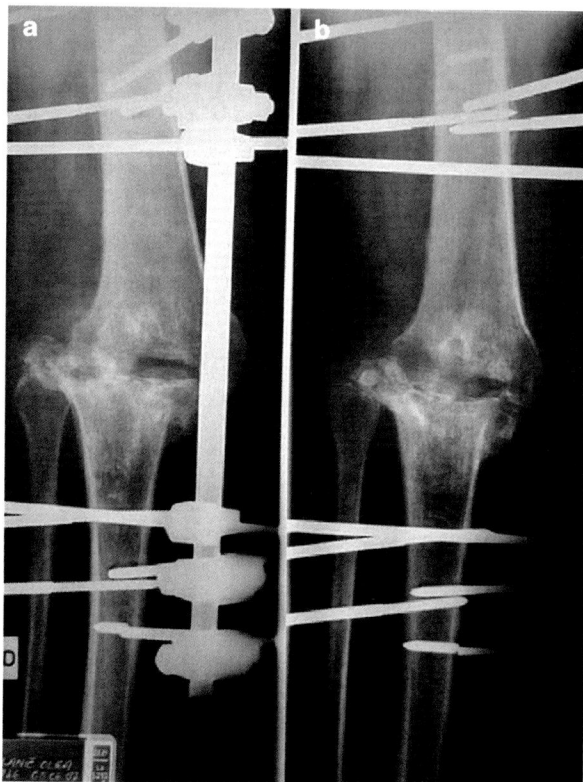

Permanent resection arthroplasty is indicated in patients with PJI caused by difficult to treat and multy resistant organisms, when there is deficient bone stock (Fig. 20.8) and soft tissue coverage, induced by septic process, and when general conditions of the patient do not allow repeat surgery.

Even though cure rates after resection arthroplasty are high, permanent infection due to infected joint cavity is a serious problem. Simple repeat revision does not provide a reliable solution. The best approach for this difficult situation is to implant a viable soft tissue flap into the cavity to close the dead space and to improve the blood flow within the infected region. Enhanced vascularity improves the efficacy of host defense mechanisms and allows for better local delivery of antibiotics.

Gluteus medius, rectus abdominis (Fig. 20.9), and vastus lateralis flaps (Fig. 20.10) are frequently employed for closing the cavity after a Girdlestone procedure in hip joint [16].

Since gluteus medius is the most important hip stabilizer, its sacrifice with the adoption of the gluteus medius flap precludes the prospective to have a functional hip joint after a potential reimplantation. Rectus abdominis flap is readily available, but it seriously weakens the abdominal wall, and the long-term consequences are unknown. The most reliable is probably the vastus lateralis flap because the function of the quadriceps is still acceptable after its transfer into the hip joint cavity. The flap

Fig. 20.6 Knee fusion with intramedullary nail. (**a**) AP view (**b**) Lateral view

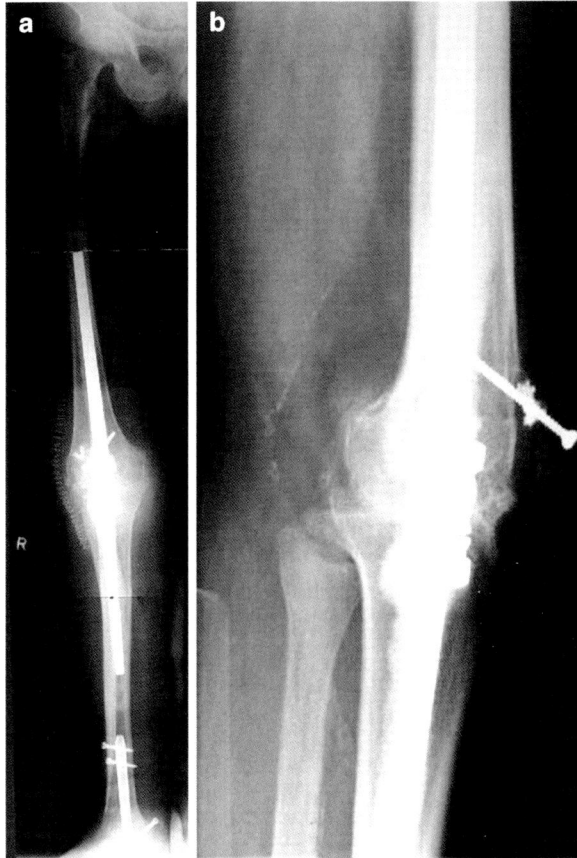

is easy to rise, and it is available in most situations as long as the proximal vascular pedicles are not destroyed by previous surgeries which seldom happen.

In a study of 120 chronic infections after failed hip resection arthroplasty, Suda and Hepperd [17] evaluated the potential of a vastus lateralis muscle flap in controlling infection. The infected cavity was the source of persistent infection in all patients. They fixed the muscular flap to acetabular rim with bone anchors. With this procedure, they were able to control the infection in all patients.

Permanent resection arthroplasty is an acceptable solution only in rare cases because the functionality of the patient after this procedure is poor [18, 19]. It is most frequently acceptable in hips but rarely in shoulders and elbows (Fig. 20.11). An 86–96 % infection cure rates in hips were reported with a poor function in all cases frequently poorer than before the resection arthroplasty [20]. Pain was, however, consistently alleviated with the procedure [18, 19].

Knee resection arthroplasty (Figs. 20.12 and 20.13) is mainly indicated in bedridden patients with multiple joint disease [6] and rarely in other patients because it is very difficult to achieve a functional stability of the joint with this procedure.

Fig. 20.7 Girdlestone hip –
resection arthroplasty

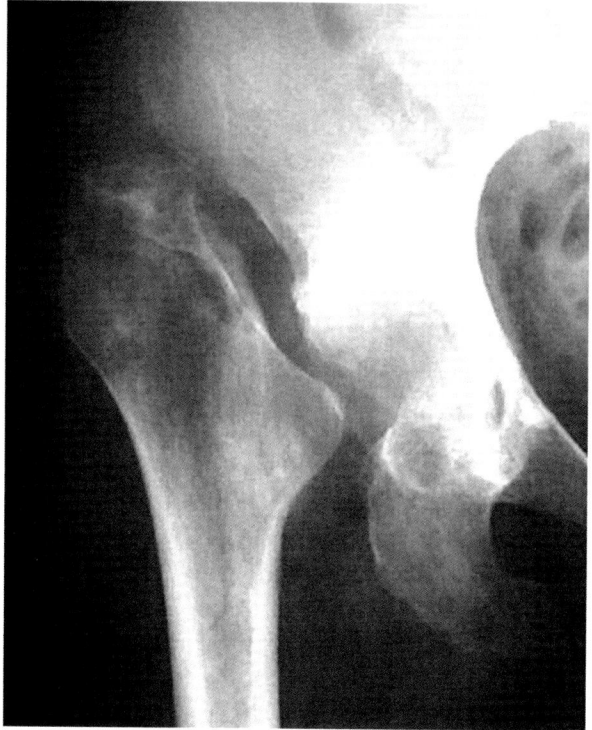

During surgery, it is important to perform a meticulous debridement, to remove all foreign material, and to perform temporary transfixion with wires to achieve proper apposition of distal femur to proximal tibia and the axis of the extremity. After surgery, the knee is immobilized for 6 months with weight bearing allowed [11]. The results achieved are poor. Among 26 patients with knee resection arthroplasty, the infection was cured in 89 %, and only 15 were able to ambulate with aids. Only five were able to walk without external support over the knee [21].

20.5 Two-Stage Exchange of an Infected Arthroplasty

Implant exchange in two stages represents the traditional form of PJI treatment (Fig. 20.14). It is far the most common form of treating infections associated with implants worldwide. The probability of germ eradication is high, though it is associated with decreased limb function due to multiple operative interventions, long-term ambulation difficulties, long-term antimicrobial therapy, higher complication rates, and higher treatment costs [22, 23]. Any clinical presentation of arthroplasty-related infections can be treated in a two-stage manner, although it is contraindicated in a severely debilitated patient, not being able to cope with potentially

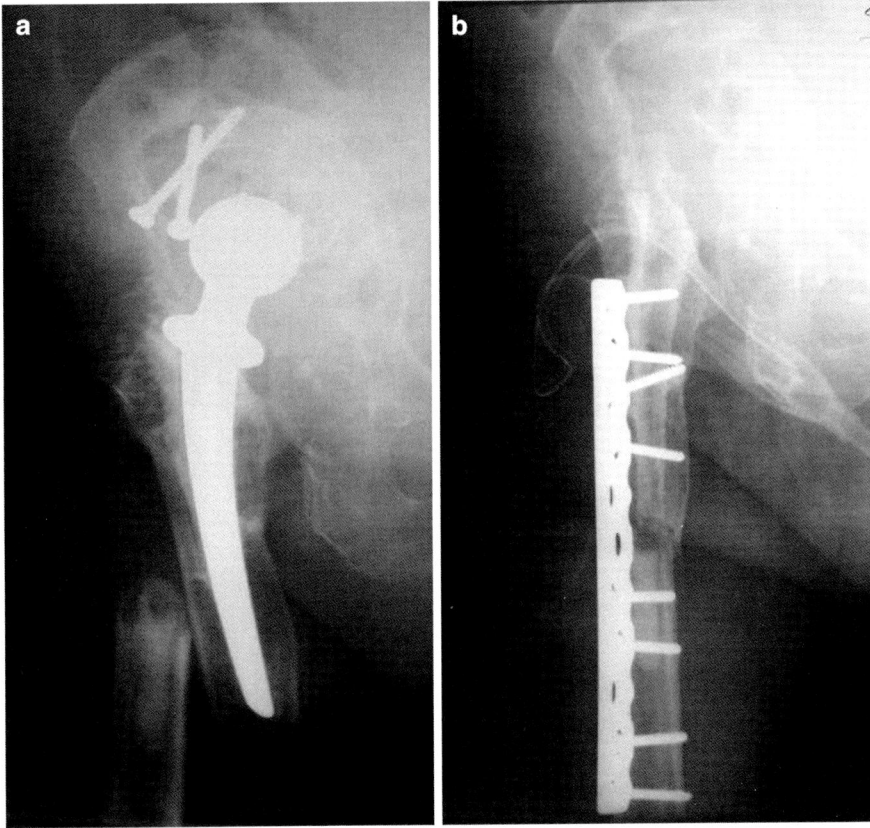

Fig. 20.8 (a) Deficient bone stock in elderly patient with poor general conditions, PJI, socket loosening, and periprosthetic fracture is an indication for permanent resection arthroplasty. (b) In this case, the implant was removed and an ostheosynthesis was performed

multiple surgical procedures. It is also contraindicated in i.v. drug abusers, due to frequent bacteremia and subsequen hematogenous spread to new or old infection sites. It is less frequently recommended in a severely immunocompromised host because antimicrobial therapy itself is not enough to eradicate the pathogens alone with no help of the host immune system. The type of microbes also influences the decision about two-stage implant exchange. Small colony variants *staphylococci*, nutritionally deficient *streptococci*, and other difficult to treat organisms represent a relative contraindication due to higher recidivism in spite of radical surgical and antimicrobial therapy.

The most appropriate indication for a two-stage exchange is a chronic infection with a virulent pathogen and a loose implant [24]. Antibiotic susceptibility does not play a key role with these infection types. Other treatment types are insufficient in this specific setting, will not work, and should be avoided. Soft tissue defects, sinus tracts, abscesses, and poor skin quality are not contraindications. Treatment is

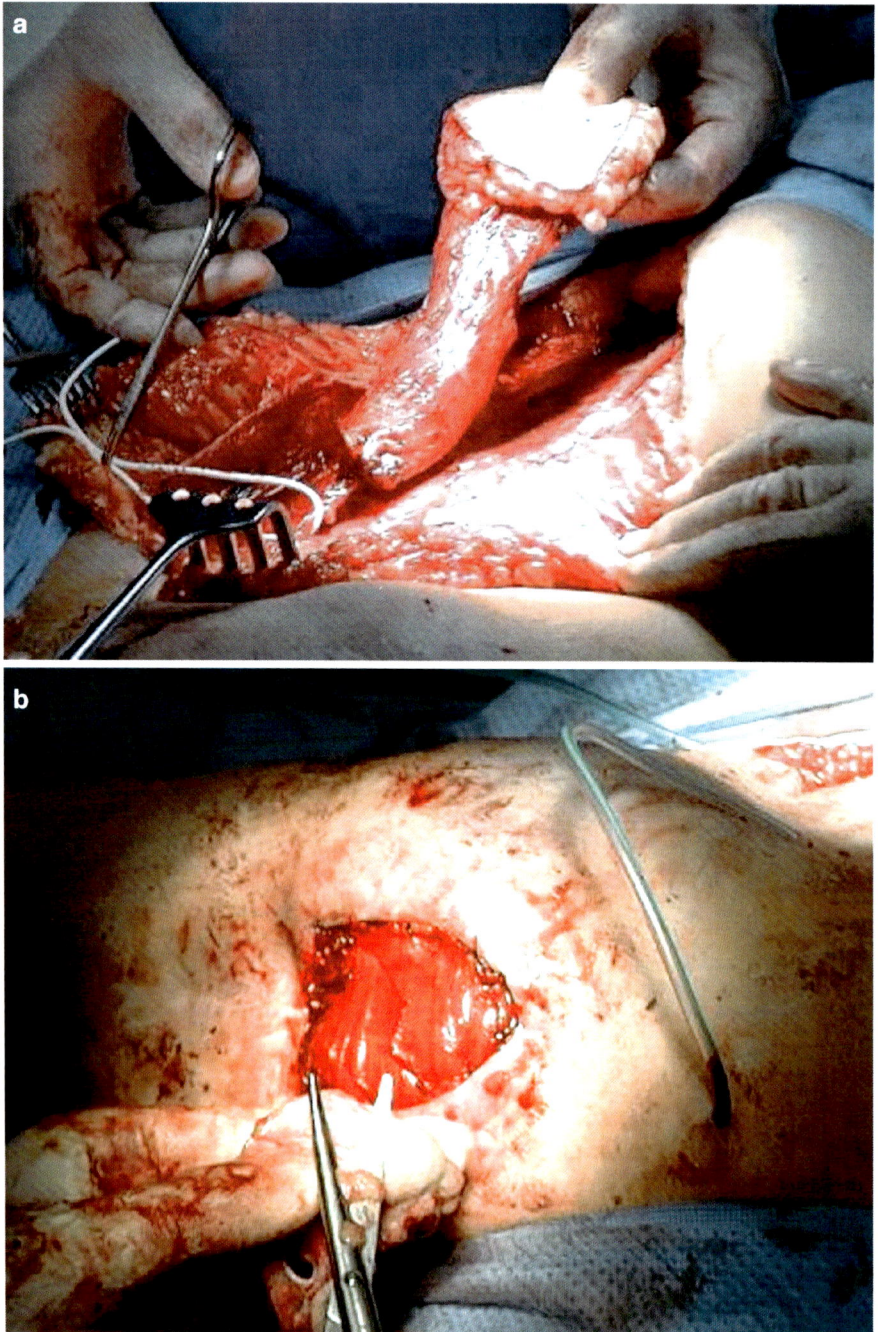

Fig. 20.9 (**a**) and (**b**) Rectus abdominis flap filling the infected sinus space after unsuccessful hip Girdlestone procedure

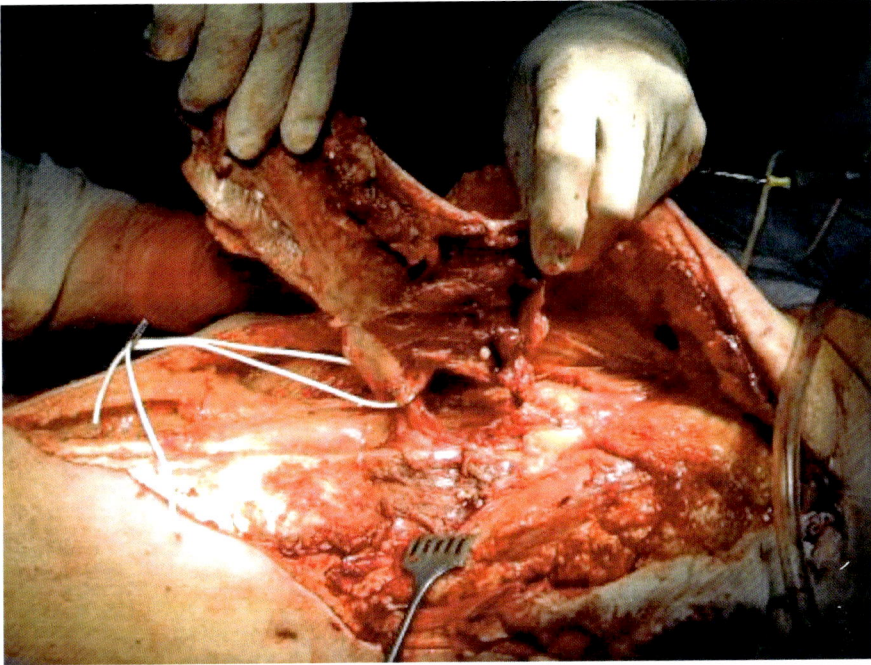

Fig. 20.10 Vastus lateralis flap for dead space filing in the hip region

successful and indicated at most arthroplasty sites, except at the ankle, where fusion is the key option in this setting.

Independently on the type of infected implant, the first stage of treatment is removal of all implants, including broken screws, K-wires, broken drill bits, and any PMMA particles if present. It is important to perform a thorough debridement and remove all inflamed or necrotic soft tissues or bone sequesters. Tissues samples are collected for synovial fluid analysis, microbiological analysis, histopathology, and gram specimens. Antimicrobial therapy should be stopped at least 2 weeks before surgery (if general condition of the patient allows) and should only be given during surgery when tissue samples are collected if preoperative diagnostics has been unsuccessful to identify the causative pathogen. The collection of tissue samples for microbial analysis is probably not needed if a sonication device is available. Postoperative wound drainage is always performed in a septic revision, although its use in a primary aseptic case is abandoned in many centers. Most surgeons decide to leave the drains anywhere between a few days and a few weeks; however, there is no consensus how long should the drains be left in place. We generally apply them up to a week, possibly less if there is little or no secretion. Antimicrobial therapy is started after all tissue samples (minimum six) are collected and is continued after surgery according to the protocol regime if the pathogenic organism is known or in an empirical manner if no organism has been preoperatively identified until the susceptibility tests are available for the organisms isolated. The most frequent

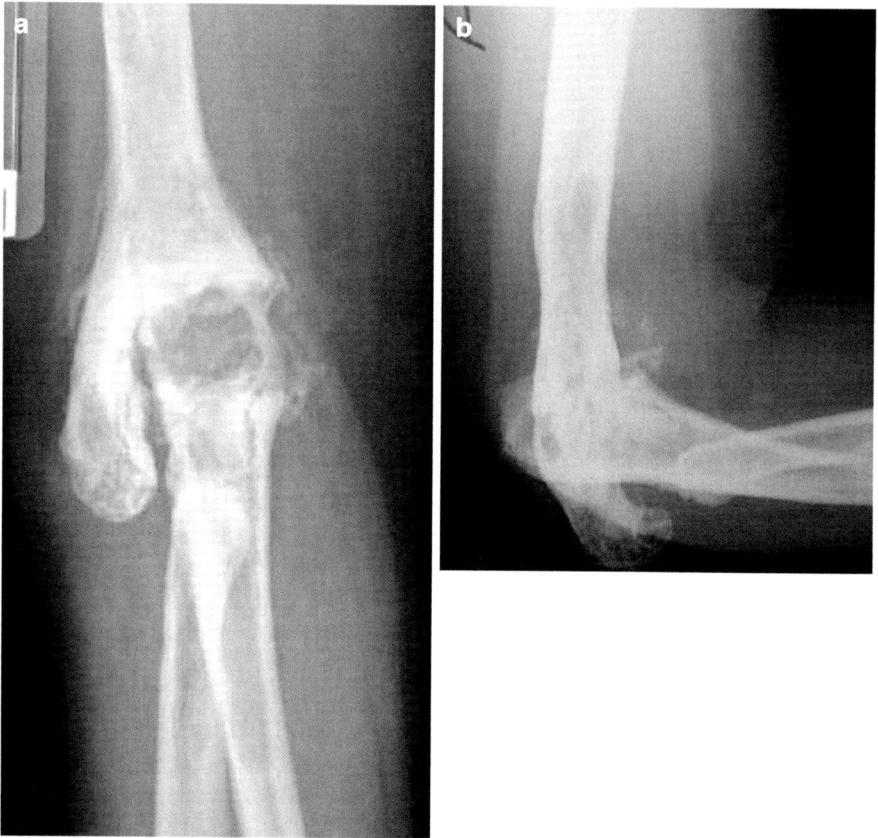

Fig. 20.11 Temporary resection arthroplasty of the elbow. (**a**) AP view (**b**) Lateral view

choice of antibiotics is a combination of a broad-spectrum beta-lactam antibiotic and an aminoglycoside. Gram stain is available within 24 h and helps in narrowing the antibiotic selection in the case organisms are noticed under the microscope. Gram staining is nearly 100 % specific but with very low sensitivity. It is invaluable when positive but of no help when negative. If, for example, gram-negative pathogens have been seen in the Gram-stained samples, quinolone therapy is started, until the final susceptibility tests are available.

There is, unfortunately, not a single gold standard protocol for the treatment activities after the first stage has been performed. Three scenarios of the second stage replantation have been described: an early reimplantation during the first couple of weeks after implant extraction [25], delayed reimplantation after 6 weeks of i.v. antibiotics and up to 3 months after the first stage [26], and a late replantation 3 months or more after the first stage after parenteral/oral combination has been administrated, the most frequently observed protocol in the past [27]. No official consensus exists, and various treatment protocols are published.

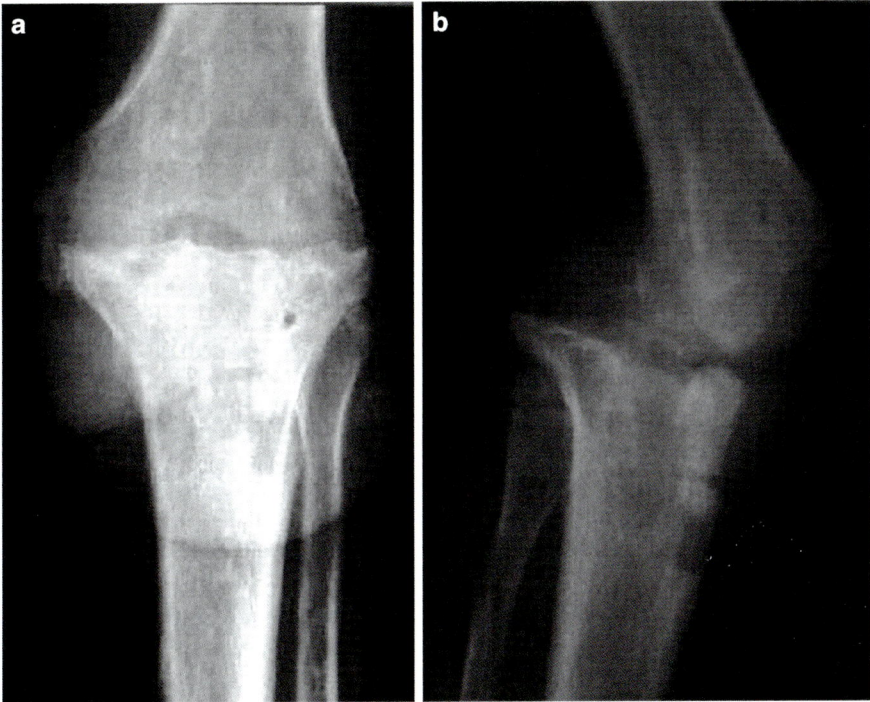

Fig. 20.12   X-ray showing a temporary resection arthroplasty of the knee. (**a**) AP view (**b**) Lateral view

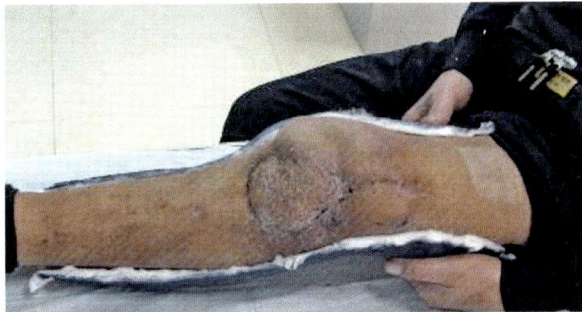

Fig. 20.13   Clinical appearance of the knee from the Fig. 20.12. Plastic surgery (gastrocnemius flap) was necessary to close the defect in the anterior part of the knee. Later the patient underwent a knee fusion due to quadriceps insufficiency

The timing of reimplantation is highly variable and can be performed just 2–4 weeks after implant explantation or 8 weeks when troublesome organisms have been isolated (MRSA; VRE, multidrug resistant microbes or fungi) [25, 28]. Shorter interval duration allows for reimplantation to be performed in the same hospitalization. One study shows, surprisingly, a higher reinfection rate when interval has been

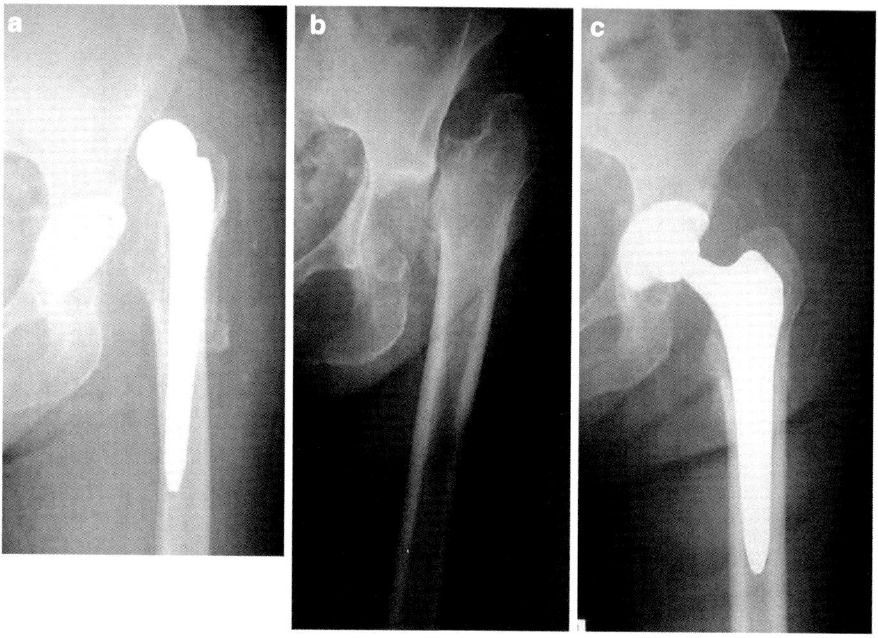

Fig. 20.14 (a) Chronic discharging infection in a patient with repeat dislocations. (b) and (c) The most reliable surgical option in such cases is a two-stage exchange arthroplasty as in this figure.

prolonged: 22 % reinfection rate after 22 months and 14 % reinfection rate within a period of 6 week or less [29].

Reimplantation is most commonly performed after 6 weeks of i.v. antibiotics, though it is not uncommon to wait for months or even years before reimplanting. In the USA, surgeons typically wait in average for 6 weeks before reimplanting [30]. During this interval, antimicrobial therapy is administered. Replantation is performed thereafter if CRP and ESR are within normal limits, and a negative needle aspirate is obtained 14 days after treatment ends.

When selecting an early reimplantation, this is performed before antimicrobial therapy is complete. In case of a longer interval before reimplanting, patients are administered antimicrobial therapy for a few weeks intravenously. Three to six months of oral antibiotics are subsequently administered before arthrography is performed and samples obtained for retesting. If cultures are negative, reimplantation is performed. If cultures are positive and there is a spacer, a revision is needed to remove it; otherwise, antimicrobial therapy is continued for 6 months in accordance with tissue cultures identification and antibiogram [25]. The value and importance of arthrocenthesis with cultivation of synovial fluid before reimplantation of a prosthetic joint has been published. In one study, there was only a 3 % relapse of infection after reimplantation if cultivation of synovial fluid step was performed before the second stage, compared to a 14 % relapse if no cultivation step was accomplished [31]. Several studies have shown that reimplantation is safer in terms of reinfection rates when using antibiotic-impregnated bone cement for implant fixation in the second stage. A study from Hospital for Special Surgery, that included 40 patients, has shown 95 % success rate after 5 years of follow-up in a subgroup of 16 patients treated with Palacos with gentamicin [32]. A direct comparison study showed 82 % success rate when using ordinary bone cement compared to a 90 % success rate with use of antibiotic-impregnated cement [5]. Older studies have shown less favorable results in terms of infection eradication (82 %) when using cementless implants at reimplantation and also a higher rate of aseptic loosening [27]. More recent studies with contemporary implants (50 two-stage procedures [33], 25 two-stage procedures [34]) show more favorable results with 8 % reinfections and no aseptic loosenings.

Aseptic loosening of joint replacement surgery is often associated with severe bone loss which may involve large segments that disappear as a consequence of the osteolytic process. To substitute for such bone loss either artificial bone from various manufacturers is used or, more often, bone from bone banks. A very similar or sometimes even worse scenario is seen when treating bone infections and septic loosenings – severe segmental bone loss (Fig. 20.15). The use of bone transplants is still doubtful in these cases because of the potential infection relapse. Two studies have shown a 7.5 and 0 % reinfection rates when using milled and impacted cancellous bone [35] and structural allografts [36], respectively.

Two-stage reimplantation has always been a gold standard in treating infected artificial joints and has given the highest cure rates with over 90 % success [5, 25, 37–39]. This holds true when treating infected total knee replacements [40–44], infected hip replacements [24, 29, 30, 45, 46], as well as in treating infected shoulder and elbow replacements (Fig. 20.16). Results are less favorable if multidrug resistant bacterias are isolated. A comparison study done by Volin on 46 patients has shown a 94.6 % cure rate with two-stage reimplantation when nonresistant bacterias where identified, compared to 88.9 % curing rate when MRSA was identified as the cause of infection [24]. Kilgus showed an unusually high relapse rate in a large series of 70 patients with 52 % of relapses in multidrug resistant bacteria (MRSA, MRSE) in infected total hip arthroplasties and 16 % relapses in infected knee arthroplasties. The success rates when dealing with nonresistant bacterias were also somewhat lower, 81 % for hips and 89 % for knees. The treatment, however, did not include two-stage revisions only, but some single-stage exchange and debridement with retention of the implant as well [47].

The disadvantage of two-stage reimplantation treatment protocol is the following. After implant extraction, the empty space remains that is prone to fibrous tissue formation. It is poorly vascularized or is completely avascular with low antibiotic penetration and thus ideal for bacterial focus. In addition, limb shortening and contractures develop Reimplantations performed long after implant extraction are demanding surgical procedures, and limb function is inferior compared to single-stage exchange. Many surgeons therefore decide to use "spacers" (Figs. 20.17, 20.18, and 20.19) made of cement to retain joint space for later easier reimplantation [48, 49]. Spacer also functions as a vehicle to release antibiotic in high concentrations in areas that are most affected by infection. A faster rate of sterilizing the pseudojoint and infection control is achieved this way, and the efficiency has been proven in clinical trials [50–52]. Spacers can be made by the surgeon himself intraoperatively from the cement. In case of a hip, the cement is strengthened with a metal reinforcements, or it is molded over a femoral stem (Fig. 20.17). Prefabricated, commercially available cement spacers are an alternative option, and special models are available for cement molding intraoperatively. The disadvantages of prefabricated cement spacers are that you need many sizes, and frequently, they do not fit well and already weak bone must be shaped in form to fit the spacer. The complications related to cement spacers use are frequent [53]: most commonly dislocations, especially

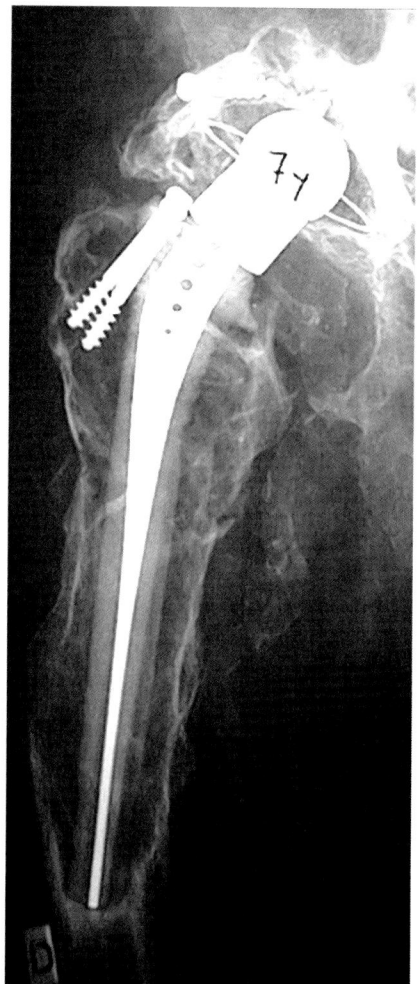

Fig. 20.15 Extreme bone loss due to chronic low-grade PJI caused by CNS 7 years after implantation. The presence of a periprosthetic fracture is hardly visible

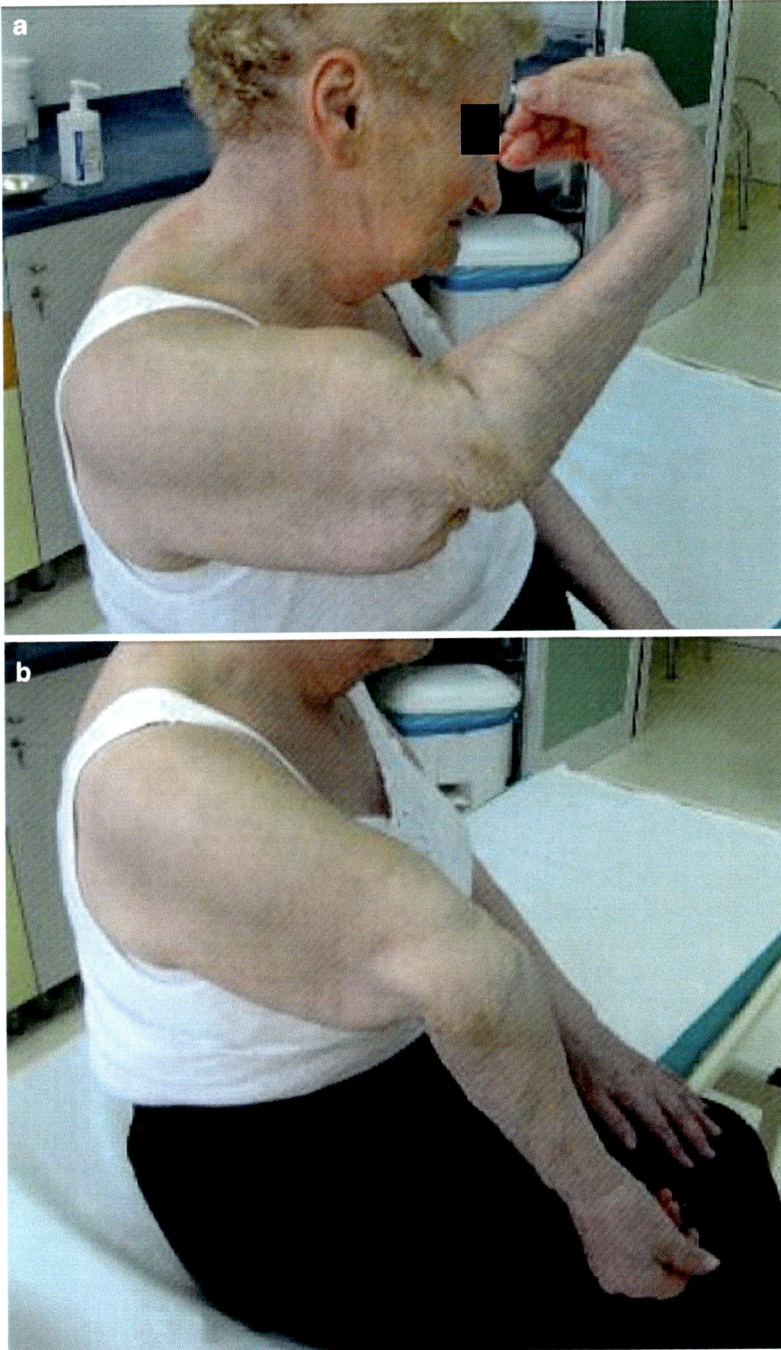

Fig. 20.16 Clinical appearance after removal of an infected elbow arthroplasty: (**a**) flexion
(**b**) extension

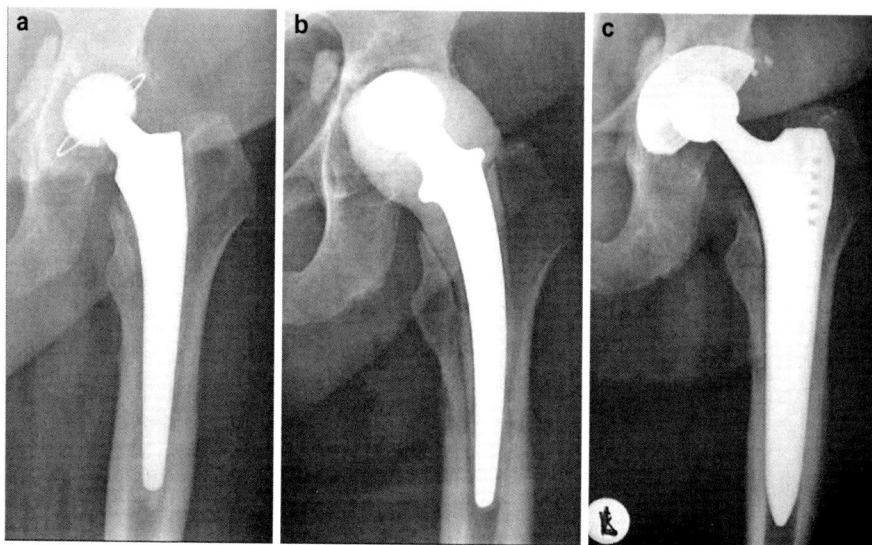

Fig. 20.17 Two-stage replacement of a total hip arthroplasty with a handmade cemented spacer (**a**) infected THA (**b**) molded around a femoral component to bridge the interval between the stages (**c**) Final result

when using handmade spacers and hip spacers with low offsets. Another complication is mechanical failure of the spacers itself, i.e., spacer fracture [52].

Use of gentamicin and other antibiotics in cement has been known for 40 years and is clinically well accepted [50, 54–57]. Palacos R has been shown to have excellent characteristics in terms of antibiotic excretion [50, 55, 56]. Changes of antibiotic susceptibility in pathogens causing bacterial implant infections, becoming multidrug resistant for antibiotics including gentamicin [50, 57], have encouraged the use of vancomycin in antibiotic spacers and beads in two-stage implant exchanges. Vancomycin is thermostabile and has favorable eluting properties, resulting in high local tissue concentrations days after implantation and has been shown efficient in clinical use [57]. Clinical studies where no systemic antibiotics were used, just cement loaded with antibiotics, showed a high rate of success in terms of efficiency to prepare bacteria-free field for reimplantation (97 %) even when virulent strains where isolated [58]. Some researchers used extremely high doses of antibiotics, most commonly vancomycin and gentamicin, without systemic side effects except transient increase of serum creatinine in 1 out of 36 cases [59]. Likewise, other studies have not been able to show serious side effects or allergies [58]. Other antibiotics have also been used in cement spacers, most commonly clindamycin [50] as well as penicillin, methycillin, lincomycin, nafcillin, fusidic acid, ceftriaxone, erythromycin, amikacin, and daptomycine.

A serious but frequently overlooked problem of antibiotic loaded cement is the appearance of multidrug resistant bacterial strains because of therapeutic and prophylatic use of antibiotics in cement and the possibility of infection of the cement spacer itself.

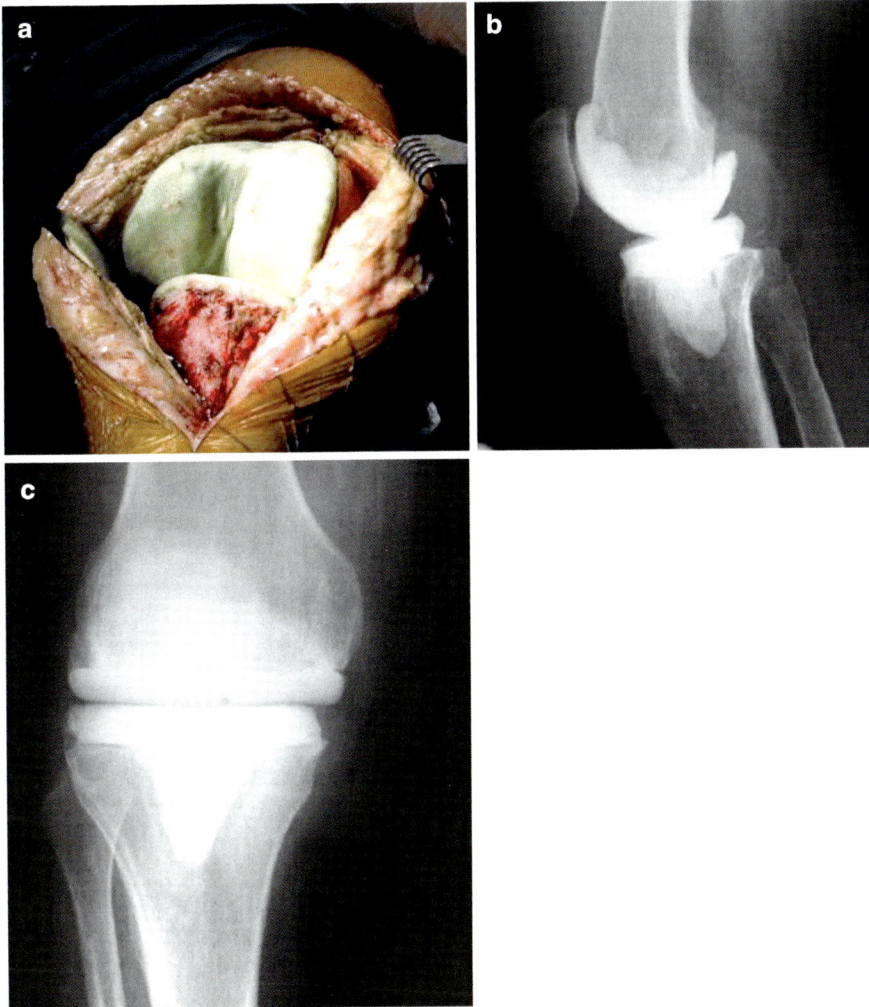

Fig. 20.18 Two-stage replacement of a total knee arthroplasty with a handmade cemented spacer (**a**) to bridge the interval between the stages. Good range-of-motion (see Fig. 20.19) in the interval between the stages allows for better function restoration after the second stage (**b**) Lateral view, (**c**) AP view

Other potential problems are unrecognized infected loose implants where prophylactic antibiotics were used in previous surgeries and are falsely diagnosed as negative due to high antibiotic concentrations eluding from cement when cracking and fracturing at the time of revision [50, 60]. Resistance development is probably less common with use of antibiotic cement like spacers and beads because they are subsequently removed, whereas prophylactic cement once implanted eludes low concentrations of antibiotics for a long period which makes it suitable to promote resistance development [57].

A concise review of laboratory properties and clinical success of antibiotic bone cements was published by van de Belt [50].

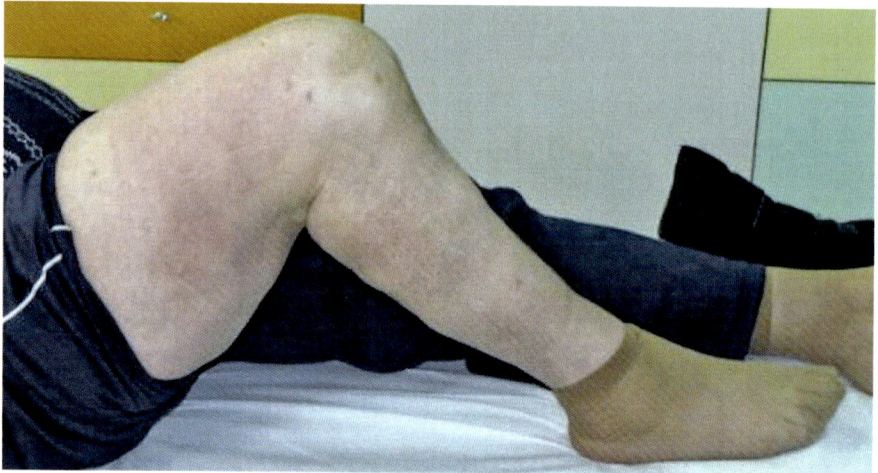

Fig. 20.19 Knee flexion in a female patient (Fig. 20.18) during spacer implantation

Many questions are still unanswered in spite of widespread use of two-stage implant exchange. It is still not known when is the best time for reimplantation, whether the use of antibiotic loaded cement spacers is always beneficial and in when it is not, what is the optimal dose of antibiotics in cement, how long should the antibiotic treatment last and in what form should be applied, whether allografts are to be used for bone reconstruction in the second stage, and whether cement with antibiotics is superior to cementless fixation in second stage or not.

20.6   One-stage Implant Exchange

One-stage implant exchange is a form of treatment where in one stage the infected implant is removed, precise, and radical debridement is performed nearly as in oncological surgery, and a new implant is inserted. This form of infection treatment originated from Europe. Bucholz, from Endo-Klinik in Hamburg, was among the originators [3]. The advantages include faster mobilization, lower morbidity, and lower expenses [61]. The disadvantages include higher reinfection rates, radical debridement with scarification of functionally important tissue, and obligatory use of antibiotic cement, which is mechanically inferior to ordinary cement. It is generally accepted that even if mechanically uncompromised cement (without antibiotics) is used, the survival curve after revision with cemented implants is inferior to un-cemented implants. The results are thus even more compromised and unpredictable if mechanically weaker antibiotic loaded cement is used for revision.

An important prerequisite for successful one-stage implant exchange is good general condition of the patient, preoperatively identified causative organism with a favorable antibiogram (no resistance for fluoroquinolones with gram-negative bacteria and no resistance for rifampicin for gram-positive bacteria). Another important prerequisite is the possibility for radical extraction of all infected implant parts. One-stage exchange is contraindicated if parts of bone cement, screws or other implants in the pelvis, or at some other site with difficult access cannot be removed or it is too dangerous to remove them. It is the primary method to treat orthopedic implant infections and performed in the majority of presented cases at some institutions. If not selectively applied it is, however, only successful if onco-logic surgery principles are strictly followed which seriously compromises func-tionality in many patients. It is rationale to choose one-stage exchange when soft tissues are intact or only mildly infected with no sinus tracts. In these cases, even radical debridement leaves functional tissues like muscles and tendons intact. Traditionally, one-stage exchange has been performed with cemented implants, with antibiotics mixed into cement according to the organism isolated and suscep-tibility tests in the operating theater without applying parenteral antibiotics postop-eratively. Nowadays, one-stage exchange is performed in different ways, mostly with cemented implants, although non-cemented implants are used as well. (Fig. 20.20) Use of intravenously administered antibiotics in the postoperative period is common, depending on the algorithm used by a particular hospital or the surgeon. Treatment success varied between 84 and 100 % [61–63].

In a large study including 183 patients treated with one-stage exchange in the United Kingdom, the total cure rate at 7 years follow-up was 84.2 %. Pain in the early postoperative period was proven as a sensitive indicator of long-term success [62]. Another study including 20 patients with staphylococcal and streptococcal prosthetic hip infections treated with one-stage exchange was initiated in the 1980s [61]. Antibiotic loaded bone cement as well as systemic antibiotic treatment was applied. Patients were followed for 3–17 years. All patients were cured (100 %), two patients developed aseptic loosening at 9 and 17 years. Another study including 72 patients with infected cemented prosthetic hips, caused exclusively by coagu-lase-negative *staphylococci* (CNS), treated with one-stage exchange, showed 87 % cure rate. The interesting finding was the presence of various strains of CNS, resis-tant to previously applied antibiotics, especially gentamicin when it was mixed in the cement during one-stage revision procedure [63].

One-stage exchange protocol was tried at Endo Klinik also with multiresistant organisms, such as MRSA [64]. Twenty patients with 15 infected hip arthroplasties and 5 infected knee arthroplasties were treated between 1996 and 1997. At 16 months follow-up, 61 % treatment success was achieved, confirmed with postoperative arth-rocenthesis. Mixing ofloxacin and vancomycin in metyl-methacrylate cement (Refobacin Palacos R) in this setting was advised by the study group.

In a series of 305 elbow prosthesis, six implant infections developed. All six were treated with one-stage implant exchange with antibiotic-loaded cement, and permanent infection eradication was achieved in five cases, whereas the unsuccess-ful one was treated with resection arthroplasty [65].

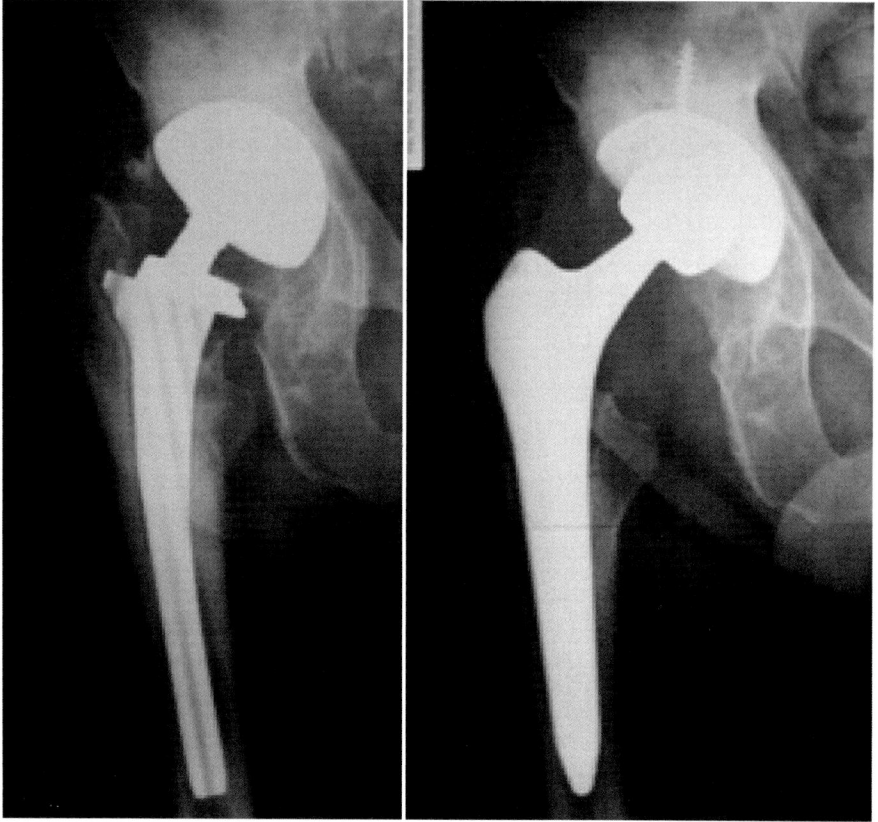

Fig. 20.20 Successful cementless one-stage exchange after 5 years of follow-up. The causative agent was a CNS

20.7 Debridement and Retention

Implant associated infections have been a very bothersome companion from the very early stages of joint arthroplasty era. Orthopedic surgeons have been fighting them from the very beginning as well. Artificial joint replacement is by definition an iatrogenic disease, and among the different treatment protocols that have evolved, implant retention is the least invasive and the most functional. The natural history of an infected implanted endoprosthesis is very diverse. Interestingly some proven infections seem to have healed even without any medical treatment at all [4] on the other hand patients have died due to sepsis. Reports on success of debridement and retention vary a lot ranging from only 15 % to [4, 66] up to 95–100 % cure rates [67–69]. Implant retention cure rates before 1992 were around 30 % [7, 82] but encouragingly, more recent reports on success of treatment of PJI with implant retention are significantly better, suggesting that our knowledge in this area is improving.

20.7.1   Diversity of surgical treatment protocols

Treatment protocols vary greatly in detail, yet they all have certain features in common: an early debridement, with or without perfusion, suction or passive drainage of different lengths, and subsequently additional antibiotic therapy starting intravenously and continuing later orally. Some authors tried arthroscopic debridement in artificial knee infections [70, 71] with 38 and 28 % success rates, respectively. Arthroscopic hip debridement is rarely used, and literature is scant. Hyman reported achieving 100 % cure rate in eight infected joints, respecting a very rigorous postoperative antibiotic protocol [72]. The Oxford group, however, although achieving 82 % success rate in a large series (100 cured cases from 120 treated) of infected hip implants treated with retention, report arthroscopic debridement as a negative predictor of cure [73]. Patients were treated with antibiotics for quite a long interval – 1.5 years in this study.

A special protocol was designed by Este in which infected orthopedic implants were treated in two or more stages but without implant removal. A thorough surgical debridement was followed by implantation of antibiotic beads close to the implant, followed by another revision later, for replacing or removing beads [68, 74]. Reported cure rates were high, 90 and 100 %, respectively. However, patient follow-up was relatively short (1–4 years). Kelm [75] reported treating patients with infected hip implants with a vacuum pump (V.A.C.). Successful infection eradication was achieved in 92 % (26 out of 28 patients) with implants retained and two patients remaining on lifelong antibiotic suppression therapy.

Some authors bravely attempted treating PJI with no provisional debridement at all, just antibiotics [2, 76–78], some even with just orally given antibiotics [76], removing or replacing loose implants after 5 months of treatment [76, 77]. Treatment lasted for up to 9 months with successful eradication rates reported ranging from 50 to 60 %.

20.7.2   Drainage

The role of postoperative drainage as predictor of successful outcome is currently unknown, as there have been no large randomized controlled studies done in this area. All surgeons performing open debridement also drain the wounds, with drains in place from just a few days up to many weeks, with or without perfusion.

20.7.3 Implant Stability

Retention is usually attempted only in stable implants. An interesting exception was shown by the Marseille group. Their protocol included antimicrobial therapy for 5 months and later a one-stage exchange with reported outcomes ranging from 50 up to 70 %, with long and precise patient follow-up [76–78].

20.7.4 Symptom Duration

Symptom duration seems one of the most important predictive factors for successful implant retention. Debridement performed early after symptom onset showed consistently higher successful treatment rates in all studies [30, 66, 72, 79]. Even in studies with no clearly defined antibiotic protocol, the results were better when treatment was started in the first days after symptom onset [66, 79].

It is not yet known at which point after symptom onset stands the time limit, when implant retention is still reliably successful. It also remains to be elucidated if symptoms follow microbial biofilm formation, the main cause of treatment failures. Some authors proposed a critical time value of 2 days [66, 72, 79], others up to 1 week [80, 81], again others have set the limit up to a few weeks [82, 83–85], or even a few months [98]. The latter showed a 33 % success rate even in chronic infections in patients with 30 % MRSA share. In studies where special "antibiofilm" antibiotic therapy was used, the treating teams allowed longer symptoms duration, compared to in studies with no such antibiofilm therapy, where they were successful only if time frame from beginning of symptoms was shorter. The logical explanation is that eradication without antibiofilm therapy is possible only if bacterial biofilm is not yet fully developed.

We can conclude that the more intense and acute the PJI is, the sooner and more aggressively must we react with debridement, lavage, and antibiotic therapy, if we are to achieve long lasting cure. This favorable time frame is probably longer in low-grade infections, where even diagnosing infection and isolating the responsible pathogenic agent is frequently challenging and time consuming. The acceptable time period for successful debridement and retention in acute infections is probably weeks after the onset of symptoms and in low-grade infections probably months if antibiofilm agents are used. Early infections with early treatment most probably need shorter treatment duration compared to long lasting, difficult to diagnose late infections.

20.7.5 Pathogenic Agents

In the majority of mainly older reports, the studies regarding PJI did not stratify the results according to the pathogens but included all of them as one entity. Gram-positive bacteria are, however, somewhat more thoroughly and separately discussed in many reports, as they represent the majority of causes of implant associated infections. In some studies, the exact microbial species was used as an inclusion criterion. Rifampicin-based algorithms showed consistently predictable results in more recent era, specific eradication rates for staphylococci have increased up to 80–100 % [69, 83, 85] and for streptococci as high as 90–100 % [72, 81, 86]. Everts successfully treated 15 out of 16 patients, although 4 of them were treated for a long time with suppressive antibiotics. Martinez-Pastor and his coworkers treated 47 patients with gram-negative implant associated infection with implant retention, 40 % of isolated organisms were *Enterococci* and 20 % *Pseudomonas* spp. The final infection eradication rate of 74 % was achieved at 1.5 year follow-up. Another author reports about treatment success rate as high as 82 % in treating enterococcal implant associated infections [87]. Even polymicrobial infections were treated successfully with implant retention in up to 66 % [84] of cases.

20.7.6   Antibiotic Therapy

Antibiotic therapy protocols are the most variable part of papers reporting about treating implant associated infections either with removal or retention of the implant. Some progress has been recently achieved. Most authors do not report about the types of antibiotics used, or reports are incomplete, i.e., only duration of treatment and application mode are presented with no details about which antibiotics were used and the dosing regimen. Most reports show variable duration of antibiotic application within the study among the patients included and typically depending on the decision of the treating surgeon – parenteral (intravenous) application commonly lasted from 0 to 8 weeks, most often from 3 to 6. Some authors have applied antibiotic treatment for up to 1.5 years [73]. In the early 1990s, the research group around Zimmerli and Widmer confirmed rifampicin as a unique drug for treatment of staphylococcal PJI. It has become the standard part of most treatment protocols. Improved study outcomes in recent years are probably at least partly reflecting the increased rifampicin use. It should not be used as monotherapy because of the danger of inducing emerging resistant bacterial strains. It is most often used in combination with quinolones [69, 85, 88, 89] but also with beta-lactams [76, 85], fusidic acid [76, 90], and minocycline [2]. Favorable results have also been obtained in monotherapy with high-dose cotrimoxazol [77]. Quinolones are drugs of choice in treating gram-negative infections and together with ceftazidime for *Pseudomonas* [78]. Linezolid has also been shown to have good results in treating implant associated infections, as well as in implant retention protocols [91] with 72 % success rate in acute and 42 % success rate in chronic infections. Anemia and thrombocytopenia have been noticed in 5 % of patients.

20.7.7   Protocols

Predictable success in treatment of PJI with retention of the implant according to a predefined algorithm was not widely practiced until recently. The main contributor in this area is W. Zimmerli, who published the cornerstone article in the *Journal of American Medical Association* (*JAMA*) in 1998 [69]. In a prospective randomized study, the efficacy in treating staphylococcal PJI with a ciprofloxacin/rifampicin combination was compared to ciprofloxacin in monotherapy. The group receiving ciprofloxacin/rifampicin combination was far more successful (12 out of 12 patients; 100 % were cured) compared to patients treated just with ciprofloxacin (7 out of 12 patients; 58 % were cured). The study protocol anticipated: staphylococcal infections, stable implants, early debridement, and a predefined antibiotic therapy. The same protocol became widely publicized after the same research group published a review article in the *New England Journal of Medicine* (*NEJM*) in 2004 [25]. Before and after Zimmerli's paper, most studies reported only about retrospective patient series treated in different ways but shearing some common features. Besides the only randomized article [25], there are a few prospective but nonrandomized ones [77, 83, 85] favoring the same conclusions. Berdal from Norway included 29 patients in his study, 12 with infected total hip arthroplasty, 6 with infected knee endoprosthesis, 8 with a partial hip endoprosthesis, and 3 were revision cases. After only 7 days of parenteral therapy, oral treatment started with lower dose ciprofloxacin (500 mg bid.) in combination with rifampicin. Altogether, the treatment lasted for 3 months independently on the joint involved. It was unsuccessful in 5 out of 29 (17.2 %) patients.

Until recently our knowledge about PJI with implant retention was based on a retrospective analysis of hospital patient records [7] and only recently have specific protocols emerged that are far from perfect and do not include all aspects of the selection criteria, diagnostics, and treatment. Further, well-designed RCT (randomized controlled trials) are necessary in this area.

20.7.8   Cost Issue

In a clinically not validated model of cost efficiency comparing implant exchange and retention, it was demonstrated that revision surgery with implant exchange was less expensive in younger patients and debridement/retention in older patients [46].

20.8   Permanent Antibiotic Suppression (PAS)

With permanent antibiotic suppression, the treatment plan is not to eradicate the infection, but rather to relieve patients' symptoms, hopefully keeping them fully asymptomatic. Lifelong suppression therapy is appropriate in selected patients that are not life threatened by PJI and are not at risk for sepsis but would be at high risk in case of a radical surgical procedure due to their comorbidities. There are other conditions supporting the decision for PAS: to avoid extremely demanding and dangerous surgical procedures (Fig. 20.21) or surgery that could on one hand cure the

Fig. 20.21 Low-grade
infection in ambulating
patient with low pain scores.
Radical surgery would have
been associated with
increased risk for
perioperative complications
and unpredictable functional
outcome

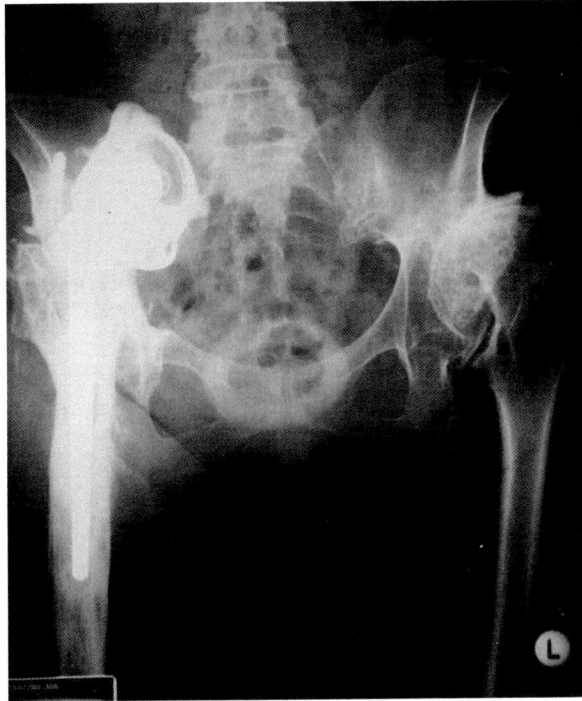

septic process but on the other seriously hamper patient functionality. It is important to balance the advantages and disadvantages of the potential complete eradication of infection on the costs of the impaired functionality of the (elderly) patient.

PAS is only possible if the causing organism is of low virulence and susceptible for planned oral antibiotics. The prescribed antibiotics must have low long-term toxicity and low incidence of side effects to be tolerable on lifelong basis. Suppression therapy is occasionally the only choice in patients who decline another surgical procedure.

The most common indications for lifelong suppression therapy are PJI in older patients with many comorbidities and patients with poor general medical health, very large bone defects, especially on the pelvis.

John Charnley was the first to propose chronic suppression therapy in the 1970s for selected patients [92]. A Swedish multicenter study showed a 21 % success rate (47 out of 225 knees). A New York group has shown a 63 % success rate with or without preliminary surgery and different antimicrobial protocols [92]. Rand analyzed the results of suppression therapy before 1993 and presented a mean 27 % success rate [7]. A decade later, Rao has shown an 86 % success rate after 5 years follow-up in 35 patients [93]. Patients were first surgically treated, with thorough debridement followed by many weeks of intravenous therapy as well as oral therapy with rifampicin in gram-positive organisms, and only later they were treated with chronic suppressive therapy. Segretti has also shown a similarly high success rate of

Fig. 20.22 Face
hyperpigmentation due to
chronic antibiotic
suppression with
minocycline

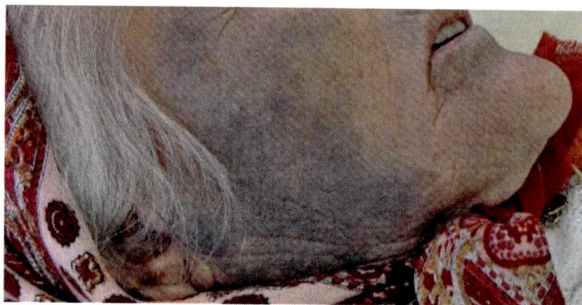

77 % [94] with a treatment protocol of preliminary surgery, parenteral therapy, and subsequent switch to chronic suppression for an average of 60 months. Fourteen patients were successfully treated: five with rifampicin+minocycline, one with rifampicin+cotrimoxazol, and all the other patients [8] with another antibiotic.

Suppression therapy is most commonly performed using minocycline, cotrimoxazol, cephalexin, cefadroxil, oxacillin, dicloxacillin, levofloxacin, penicillin, ampicillin, amoxicillin/clavulanic acid, clindamycin and linezolid [92–94], and the following combinations: minocycline/rifampicin, cotrimoxazol/rifampicin [94].

Good therapeutic concentration inside bony tissue has also been shown for certain newer antimicrobials, all also acting on MRSA [95]. They are already in clinical use for treating bone infections and in suppression protocols, but no large studies have been published considering their use in bone infections and implant associated infections. *Tigecycline* (Tigacyl), a glycylcycline, a novel promising drug, achieved 100 % therapeutic success rate in animal models in combination with rifampicin. *Daptomycin* (Cubicin) belongs to the cyclic lipopeptide family. Animal studies proved high efficiency in treating bone infections, although its bone concentration is low. *Linezolid* is a synthetic compound belonging to the oxazolidine group, which has been available for some time and has a broad spectrum against gram-positive pathogens, including MRSA, MRSE, and VRE, achieving high bone concentrations and efficient in PJI, too. It has also been used for chronic suppressive treatment.

It is not yet clearly proven which antibiotics are most efficient for suppressive therapy. Minocycline is most often used for staphylococcal device associated infections.

It is also not yet clear how long should suppressive therapy be administered and when is the appropriate time for discontinuation of the therapy. It is commonly given for many years or even for life. Side effects are common, at best between 8 and 22 % [93, 94, 96], most commonly enterocolitis, allergic, and toxic skin eruptions.

In author's own series of six patients on chronic suppressive therapy with tetracycline (minocycline) lasting for many years, only one patient has failed with infection reactivation. Three patients had side effects: facial and surgical scar area skin hyperpigmentation and systemic skin darkening (Fig. 20.22). These are rare side effects known in dermatology with acne treatment [97]. These side effects have not been yet described in orthopaedics.

References

1. SooHoo NF, Zingmond DS, Ko CY. Comparison of reoperation rates following ankle arthrodesis and total ankle arthroplasty. J Bone Joint Surg Am. 2007;89:2143–9.
2. Isiklar ZU, Darouiche RO, Landon GC, Beck T. Efficacy of antibiotics alone for orthopaedic device related infections. Clin Orthop. 1996;332:184–9.
3. Buchholz HW, Elson RA, Engelbrecht E, Londenkamper H, Rottger J, Siegel A. Management of infection of total hip replacement. J Bone Joint Surg Br. 1981;63:342–53.
4. Hunter G, Dandy D. The natural history of the patient with an infected total hip replacement. J Bone Joint Surg Br. 1977;59:293–7.
5. Hanssen AD, Rand JA. Evaluation and treatment of infection at the site of a total hip or knee arthroplasty. Instr Course Lect. 1999;48:111–22.
6. Rand JA. Alternatives to reimplantation for salvage of the total knee arthroplasty complicated by infection. J Bone Joint Surg. 1993;75:282–9.
7. Rand JA. Sepsis following total knee arthroplasty. In: Rand JA, editor. Total knee arthroplasty. 1st ed. New York: Raven; 1993. p. 349–75.
8. Hintermann B, Schneiderbauer MM, Trampuž A, Widmer A. Infection rate after primary ankle replacement: a cohort study of 386 consecutive ankle replacements. #74. In: Presented at the American Academy of Orthopaedic Surgeons 74th Annual Meeting, San Diego; 14–18 February 2007.
9. Pring DJ, Marks L, Angel JC. Mobility after amputation for failed total knee arthroplasty. J Bone Joint Surg Br. 1988;70:770–1.
10. Blom AW, Brown J, Taylor AH, Pattison G, Whitehouse S, Bannister GC. Infection after total knee arthroplasty. J Bone Joint Surg Br. 2004;86:688–91.
11. Leone JM, Hanssen AD. Management of infection at the site of a total knee arthroplasty. Instr Course Lect. 2006;55:449–61.
12. Knutson K, Hovelius L, Lindstrand A, Lindgren L. Arthrodesis after failed knee arthroplasty: a nationwide multicenter study investigation of 91 cases. Clin Orthop. 1984;191:201–11.
13. Wiedel JD. Salvage of infected total knee fusion: the last option. Clin Orthop. 2002;404: 139–42.
14. Nichols SJ, Landon GC, Tullos HS. Arthrodesis with dual plates after failed total knee arthrodesis. J Bone Joint Surg Am. 1991;73:1020–4.
15. Morrey BF, editor. The elbow and its disorders. 4th ed. Philadelphia: Elsevier-Sounders; 2009.
16. Lew DP, Waldvogel FA. Osteomyelitis. N Engl J Med. 1997;336:999–1007.
17. Suda AJ, Hepperd V. Vastus lateralis muscle flap for infected hips after resection arthroplasty. J Bone Joint Surg Br. 2010;92B:1654–8.
18. Bourne RB, Hunter GA, Rorabeck CH, Macnab JJ. A six-year follow-up of infected total hip replacement managed by Girdlestone's arthroplasty. J Bone Joint Surg Br. 1984;66:340–3.
19. Castellanos J, Flores X, Llusa M, Chiriboga C, Navarro A. The Girdlestone pseudoarthrosis in the treatment of infected hip replacements. Int Orthop. 1998;22:178–81.
20. Clegg J. The results of the pseudoarthrosis after removal of an infected total hip prosthesis. J Bone Joint Surg Br. 1977;59:298–301.
21. Falahee MH, Matthews LS, Kaufer H. Resection arthroplasty as a salvage procedure for a knee with infection after a total arthroplasty. J Bone Joint Surg Am. 1987;69:1013–21.
22. Morrey BF, editor. Reconstructive surgery of the joints. 2nd ed. New York: Churchill-Livingstone; 1996.
23. Sculco TP. The economic impact of infected total joint arthroplasty. Instr Course Lect. 1993;42:349–51.
24. Volin SJ, Hinrichs SH, Garvin KL. Two-stage reimplantation of total joint infections. Clin Orthop. 2004;427:94–100.
25. Zimmerli W, Trampuž A, Ochsner P. Prosthetic joint infections. N Engl J Med. 2004;351: 1645–54.

26. Lieberman JR, Callaway GH, Salvati EA, Pellicci PM, Brause BD. Treatment of the infected total hip arthroplasty with a two-stage reimplantation protocol. Clin Orthop. 1994;301: 205–12.

27. Nestor BJ, Hanssen AD, Ferrer-Gonzalez R, Fitzgerald RH. The use of porous prostheses in delayed reconstruction of total hip replacements that have failed because of infection. J Bone Joint Surg Am. 1994;76:349–59.

28. Trampuž A, Zimmerli W. Prosthetic joint infections: update in diagnosis and treatment. Swiss Med Wkly. 2005;135:243–51.

29. Colyer RA, Capello WN. Surgical treatment of the infected hip implant. Two-stage reimplantation with a one-month interval. Clin Orthop. Relat.Res. 1994;298:75–9.

30. Tsukajama DT, Estrada R, Gustilo RB. Infections after total hip arthroplasty: a study of the treatment of one hundred and six infections. J Bone Joint Surg Am. 1996;78:512–23.

31. Mont MA, Waldman BJ, Hungerford DS. Evaluation of preoperative cultures before second stage reimplantation of a total knee prosthesis complicated by infection. J Bone Joint Surg Am. 2000;82:1552–7.

32. Garvin KL, Evans BG, Salvati EA, Brause BD. Palacos gentamicin for the treatment of deep periprosthetic hip infections. Clin Orthop. 1994;298:97–105.

33. Haddad FS, Muirhead-Allwood SK, Manktelow AR, Bacarese-Hamilton I. Two stage uncemented revision hip arthroplasty for infection. J Bone Joint Surg Br. 2000;82:689–94.

34. Fehring TK, Calton TF, Griffin WL. Cementless fixation in 2-stage reimplantation for peripros-thetic sepsis. J Arthroplasty. 1999;14:175–81.

35. English H, Timperley AJ, Dunlop D, Gie G. Impaction grafting of the femur in two-stage revision for infected total hip replacement. J Bone Joint Surg Br. 2002;84:700–5.

36. Alexeeff M, Mahomed N, Morsi E, Garbuz D, Gross A. Structural allograft in two-stage revisions for failed septic hip arthroplasty. J Bone Joint Surg Br. 1996;78:213–6.

37. Steckelberg JM, Osmon DR. Prosthetic joint infection. In: Bisno AL, Waldvogel FA, editors. Infections associated with indwelling medical devices. 3rd ed. Washington, DC: American Society for Microbiology; 2000. p. 173–209.

38. Fitzgerald Jr RH, Arthroplasty ITH. Diagnosis and treatment. J Am Acad Orthop Surg. 1995;3:249–62.

39. Zimmerli W, Ochsner PE. Management of infection associated with prosthetic joints. Infection. 2003;31:99–108.

40. Windsor RE, Insall JN, Urs WK, Miller DV, Brause BD. Two-stage reimplantation for the salvage of total knee arthroplasty complicated by infection. Further follow-up and refinement of indications. J Bone Joint Surg Am. 1990;72:272–8.

41. Lonner JH, Barrack R, Fitzgerald Jr RH, Hanssen AD, Windsor ER. Infection in total knee arthroplasty: part II. Treatment. Am J Orthop. 1999;28:592–7.

42. Bengtson S, Knutson K. The infected knee arthroplasty. A 6-year follow-up of 357 cases. Acta Orthop Scand. 1991;62:301–11.

43. Hirakawa K, Stulberg BN, Wilde AH, Bauer TW, Secic M. Results of 2-stage reimplantation for infected total knee arthroplasty. J Arthroplasty. 1998;13:22–8.

44. Teeny SM, Dorr L, Murata G, Conaty P. Treatment of infected total knee arthroplasty. Irrigation and debridement versus two-stage reimplantation. J Arthroplasty. 1990;5:35–9.

45. Langlais F. Can we improve the results of revision arthroplasty for infected total hip replacement? J Bone Joint Surg Br. 2003;85:637–40.

46. Fisman DN, Reilly DT, Karchmer AW, Goldie SJ. Clinical effectiveness and cost-effectiveness of two management strategies for infected total hip arthroplasty in the elderly. Clin Infect Dis. 2001;32:419–30.

47. Kilgus M. Results of periprosthetic hip and knee infections caused by resistant bacteria. Clin Orthop. 2002;404:116–24.

48. Hsieh PH, Shih CH, Chang YH, Lee MS, Yang WE. Two-stage revision hip arthroplasty for infection: comparison between the interim use of antibiotic-loaded cement beads and a spacer prothesis. J Bone Joint Surg. 2004;86:1989–97.

49. Yamamoto K, Miyagawa N, Masaoka T, Katori Y, Shishido T, Imakiire A. Clinical effectiveness of antibiotic-impregnated cement spacers for the treatment of infected implants of the hip joint. J Orthop Sci. 2003;8:823–8.
50. van de Belt H, Neut D, Schenk W, van Horn JR, van de Mei HC, Busscher HJ. Infection of orthopedic implants and the use of antibiotic-loaded bone cements. A review. Acta Orthop Scand. 2001;72:557–71.
51. Fang-Yao C, Chuan-Mu C, Chien-Fu JL, Wai Hee L. Cefuroxime-impregnated cement in primary total knee arthroplasty. A prospective randomized study of three hundred and forty knees. J Bone Joint Surg Am. 2002;84:759–62.
52. Leunig M, Chosa E, Speck M, Ganz R. A cement spacer for two-stage revision of infected implants of the hip joint. Int Orthop. 1998;22:209–14.
53. Jung J, Schmid NV, Kelm J, Schmitt E, Anagnostakos K. Complications after spacer implantation in the treatment of hip joint infections. Int J Med Sci. 2009;2:265–73.
54. Buchholz HW, Engelbrecht H. Depot effects of various antibiotics mixed with palacos resins. Chirurg. 1970;41:511–5.
55. Marks KE, Nelson CL, Lautenschlager EP. Antibiotic impregnated acrylic bone cement. J Bone Joint Surg Am. 1976;58:358–64.
56. Kuechle DK, Landon GC, Musher DM, Noble PC. Elution of vancomycin, daptomycin, and amikacin from acrylic bone cement. Clin Orthop. 1991;264:302–8.
57. Tunney MM, Ramage G, Patrick S. Antimicrobial susceptibility of bacteria isolated from orthopedic implants following revision hip surgery. Antimicrob Agents Chemother. 1998; 42:3002–5.
58. Taggart T, Kerry M, Norman P, Stockley I. The use of vancomycin-impregnated cement beads in the management of infection of prosthetic joints. J Bone Joint Surg Br. 2002;84:70–2.
59. Springer BD, Lee GC, Osmon D. Systemic safety of high-dose antibiotic-loaded cement spacers after resection of an infected total knee arthroplasty. Clin Orthop. 2004;427:47–51.
60. Wininger DA, Fass RJ. Antibiotic-impregnated cement and beads for orthopedic infections. Antimicrob Agents Chemother. 1996;40:2675–9.
61. Ure KJ, Amstutz HC, Nasser S, Schmalzried TP. Direct-exchange arthroplasty for the treatment of infection after total hip replacement. An average ten-year follow-up. J Bone Joint Surg Am. 1998;80:961–8.
62. Raut VV, Siney PD, Wroblewski BM. One-stage revision of total hip arthroplasty for deep infection. Long-term followup. Clin Orthop. 1995;321:202–7.
63. Hope PG, Kristinsson KG, Norman P, Elson RA. Deep infection of cemented total hip arthroplasties caused by coagulase-negative *staphylococci*. J Bone Joint Surg Br. 1989;71:851–5.
64. Kordelle J, Frommelt L, Klüber D, Seemann K. Results of one-stage endoprosthesis revision in periprosthetic infection cause by methicillin-resistant *Staphylococcus aureus*. Z Orthop Ihre Grenzgeb. 2000;138:240–4.
65. Gille J, Ince A, Katzer A, Loehr JF. Single-stage revision of peri-prosthetic infection following total elbow replacement. J Bone Joint Surg Br. 2006;88:1341–6.
66. Crockarell JR, Hanssen AD, Osmon DR, Morrey BF. Treatment of infection with debridement and retention of the components following hip arthroplasty. J Bone Joint Surg Am. 1998;80: 1306–13.
67. Laffer RR, Graber P, Ochsner PE, Zimmerli W. Outcome of prosthetic knee-associated infection: evaluation of 40 consecutive episodes at a single centre. Clin Microbiol Infect. 2006;12:433–9.
68. Tintle SM, Forsberg JA, Potter BK, Islinger RB, Andersen RC. Prosthesis retention, serial debridement, and antibiotic bead use for treatment of infection following total joint arthroplasty. Orthopedics. 2009;32:87.
69. Zimmerli W, Widmer AF, Blatter M, Frei R, Ochsner PE. Role of rifampin for treatment of orthopedic implant-related staphylococcal infections: a randomized controlled trial. Foreign-Body Infection (FBI) Study Group. JAMA. 1998;279:1537–41.
70. Waldman BJ, Hostin E, Mont MA, Hungerford DS. Infected total knee arthroplasty treated by arthroscopic irrigation and debridement. J Arthroplasty. 2000;15:430–6.

71. Dixon P, Parish EN, Cross MJ. Arthroscopic debridement in the treatment of the infected total knee replacement. J Bone Joint Surg Br. 2004;86-B:39–42.
72. Hyman JL, Salvati EA, Laurencin CT, Rogers DE, Maynard M, Brause DB. The arthroscopic drainage, irrigation, and debridement of late, acute total hip arthroplasty infections: average 6-year follow up. J Arthroplasty. 1999;8:903–10.
73. Byren I, Bejon P, Atkons BL, Anqus B, Masters S, McLardy-Smith P, Gindle R, Berendt A. One hundred and twelve infected arthroplasties treated with "DIAR" (debridement, antibiotics, and implant retention): antibiotic duration and outcome. J Antimicrob Chemother. 2009; 63:1264–71.
74. Estes CS, Beauchamp CP, Clarke HD, Spangehl MJ. A two-stage retention debridement protocol for acute periprosthetic joint infections. Clin Orthop Relat Res. 2010;468:2029–38.
75. Kelm J, Schmitt E, Anagnostakos K. Vacuum-assisted closure in the treatment of early hip joint infections. Int J Med Sci. 2009;6:241–6.
76. Drancourt M, Stein A, Argenson JN, Roiron R, Groulier P, Raoult D. Oral treatment of *Staphylococcus* spp. infected orthopaedic implants with fusidic acid or ofloxacin in combination with rifampicin. J Antimicrob Chemother. 1997;39:235–40.
77. Stein A, Bataille JF, Drancourt M, Curvale G, Argenson JN, Groulier P, Raoult D. Ambulatory treatment of multidrug-resistant *Staphylococcus*-infected orthopedic implants with high-dose oral co-trimoxazole (trimethoprim-sulfamethoxazole). Antimicrob Agents Chemother. 1998; 42:3086–91.
78. Brouqui P, Rousseau MC, Stain A, Drancourt M, Raoult D. Treatment of *Pseudomonas aeruginosa*-infected orthopedic prostheses with ceftazidime-ciprofloxacin antibiotic combination. Antimicrob Agents Chemother. 1995;39:2423–5.
79. Brandt CM, Sistrunk WW, Duffy MC, Hanssen AD, Steckelberg JM, Ilstrup DM, Osmon DR. *Staphylococcus aureus* prosthetic joint infection treated with debridement and prosthesis retention. Clin Infect Dis. 1997;24:914–9.
80. Tattevin P, Cremieux AC, Pottier P, Huten D, Carbon C. Prosthetic joint infection: when can prosthesis salvage be considered? Clin Infect Dis. 1999;29:292–5.
81. Meehan AM, Osmon DR, Duffy CT, Hanssen AD, Keating MR. Outcome of penicillin-susceptible streptococcal prosthetic joint infection treated with debridement and retention of the prosthesis. Clin Infect Dis. 2003;36:845–9.
82. Schoifet SD, Morrey BF. Treatment of infection after total knee arthroplasty by debridement with retention of the components. J Bone Joint Surg Am. 1990;72:1383–90.
83. Berdal JE, Skramm I, Mowinckel P, Gulbrandsen P, Bjornholt JV. Use of rifampicin and ciprofloxacin combination therapy after surgical debridement in the treatment of early manifestation prosthetic joint infections. Clin Microbiol Infect. 2005;11:834–55.
84. Van Kleunen JP, Knox D, Garino JP, Lee G-C. Irrigation and debridement and prosthesis retention for treating acute prosthetic infections. Clin Orthop Relat Res. 2010;468:2024–8.
85. Widmer AF, Gaechter A, Ochsner PE, Zimmerli W. Antimicrobial treatment of orthopedic implant-related infections with rifampin combinations. Clin Infect Dis. 1992;14:1251–3.
86. Everts RJ, Chambers ST, Murdoch DR, Rothwell AG, Mc Kie J. Successful antimicrobial therapy and implant retention for streptococcal infections of prosthetic joints. ANZ J Surg. 2004;74:210–4.
87. El Helou OC, Berbari EF, Marculescu CE, El Atrouni WI, Razonable RR, Steckelberg JM, Hanssen AD, Osmon DR. Outcome of enterococcal prosthetic joint infections: is combination systemic therapy superior to monotherapy? Clin Infect Dis. 2008;47:903–9.
88. Trebše R, Milošev I, Kovač S, Mikek M, Pišot V. The isoelastic total hip replacement: a fourteen to seventeen years follow-up study. Acta Orthop. 2005;76:169–76.
89. Berbari EF, Osmon DR, Duffy MC, Harmssen RN, Mandrekar JN, Hanssen AD, Steckelberg JM. Outcome of prosthetic joint infection in patients with rheumatoid arthritis: the impact of medical and surgical therapy in 200 episodes. Clin Infect Dis. 2006;42:216–23.
90. Aboltins CA, Page MA, Buising KL, Jenney AW, Daffy JR, Choong PF, Stanley PA. Treatment of staphylococcal prosthetic joint infections with debridement, prosthesis retention and oral rifampicin and fusidic acid. Clin Microbiol Infect. 2007;13:586–91.

91. Soriano A, Garcia S, Ortega M, Almela M, Gallart X, Vila J, Sierra J, Tomas X, Martinez JA, Mensa J. Treatment of acute infection of total or partial hip arthroplasty with debridement and oral chemotherapy. Med Clin. 2003;121:81–5.

92. Goulet JA, Pellici PM, Brause BD, Salvati EM. Prolonged suppression of infection in total hip arthroplasty. J Arthroplasty. 1998;3:109–16.

93. Rao N, Crossett LS, Sinha RK, Le Frock JL. Long term suppression of infection in total joint arthroplasty. Clin Orthop. 2003;414:55–60.

94. Segreti J, Nelson JA, Trenholme GM. Prolonged suppressive antibiotic therapy for infected orthopedic implants. Clin Infect Dis. 1998;27:711–3.

95. Venugopalan V, Martin CA. Selecting anti-infective agents for the treatment of bone infections: new anti-infective agents and chronic suppressive therapy. Orthopedics. 2007;30:832–4.

96. Sin JG, Berbari EF, Karchmer AW. Prosthetic joint infections. Infect Dis Clin North Am. 2005;19:885–914.

97. Patel K, Cheshire D, Vance A. Oral and systemic effects of prolonged minocycline therapy. Br Dent J. 1998;185:560–2.

98. Marculescu CE, Berbari EF, Hanssen AD, Steckelberg JM, Harmsen SW, Mandrekar JN, Osmon DR. Outcome of prosthetic joint infections treated with debridement and retention of components. Clin Infect Dis. 2006;42(4):471–8.

Chapter 21
Total Ankle Replacement Infections

Michaela Maria Schneiderbauer

Abstract Total ankle replacements have some peculiarities in comparison to other artificial joints. The workout and the algorithm to evaluate a suspicion of an artificial ankle infection is presented and discussed in the chapter.

Keywords Total ankle replacement • Complications • Infections • Algorithm

21.1 Total Ankle Replacements

Total ankle replacements of various designs (Fig. 21.1) are becoming more common since many patients and doctors assume a superiority of ankle replacements over ankle fusions over time. Ankle replacements might have the advantage of protecting adjacent joints from early arthritis since range of motion in the ankle is somewhat preserved. So far larger studies and a literature review have failed to demonstrate a superior outcome of total ankle replacements over ankle fusions [1–3]. The infection rates of ankle replacements seem to be higher than in ankle fusions [3]. This is most likely caused by wider surgical exposure and larger foreign body. Of note it is often easier to revise an infected fusion than an infected ankle replacement. With an infection fusion suppression of the infection until the fusion heals and then removal of the hardware (usually a few screws) is a valid option. This is not a choice in infected ankle replacements.

21.2 Scope of Problem

Recent studies have shown that the rate of infection in total ankle replacements is significantly higher than in total knee and total hip replacements with rates published as high as 6 % [3]. There are multiple reasons why this might be the case.

M.M. Schneiderbauer, M.D., Ph.D.
Miller School of Medicine, University of Miami,
1400 NW 12th Avenue, Miami, FL 33136, USA
e-mail: mschneiderbauer@gmail.com; mschneiderbauer@med.miami.edu

R. Trebše (ed.), *Infected Total Joint Arthroplasty*,
DOI 10.1007/978-1-4471-2482-5_21, © Springer-Verlag London 2012

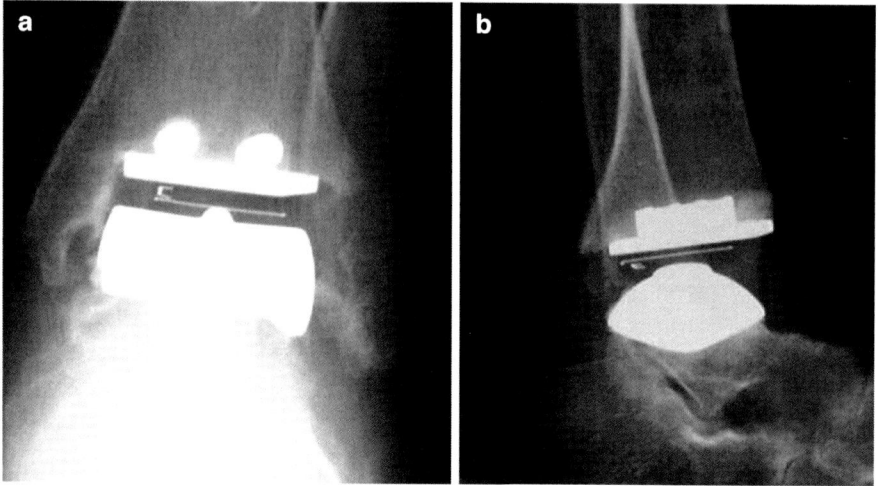

Fig. 21.1 Scandinavian total ankle replacement (STAR) (R. Trebše archive). (**a**) a.p. view, (**b**) lateral view

Many patients who are candidates for total ankle replacements have an underlying diagnosis of posttraumatic arthritis often with multiple previous surgeries, multiple surgical scars, and therefore compromised soft tissues. Additionally, many patients have comorbidities including diabetes and peripheral vascular disease that can cause poor blood supply due to microangiopathy as well as macroangiopathy. Overall the soft tissue coverage over the prosthesis is scarce, even scarcer than in total knee replacements. Limited soft tissue coverage is an argument why the rate of infection in total knee replacements is higher than in total hip replacements. Down at the ankle, this problem is even more pronounced.

21.3 Diagnostic Problems

Many patients with major surgery around their ankle will have a significant degree of soft tissue swelling and even some warmth and erythema. These signs do not necessarily indicate an infection. They could just reflect a prolonged healing process. In the immediate postoperative period, it is hard to distinguish. Sequential CRP, ESR, and white blood cell monitoring are good indicators with rising parameters after a few days postoperatively constituting a warning sign. Drainage that persists past 7 days after surgery is certainly a reason for concern. In case of doubt, it is better to intervene early and do an appropriate irrigation and debridement with liner exchange and harvest of intraoperative cultures. Antibiotics should only be started at the time of this surgery. Starting antibiotics randomly without surgical intervention might suppress the infection subclinically for some time but in the end lead to a more resistant infection in the total ankle prosthesis with a patient that is often in chronic pain.

Rise of CRP and
or WBC 5 days
after surgery

• Irrigation and
debridement
• Liner exchange

• Persistent drainage
• Fever (with other
sources excluded)
• Increase In redness
and swelling

?

Infection likely →

• Intraoperative
cultures
• Antibiotic therapy

Drainage > 7 days
after surgery

Dry, unremarkable wound ⟶ Infection unlikely → Monitor clinically

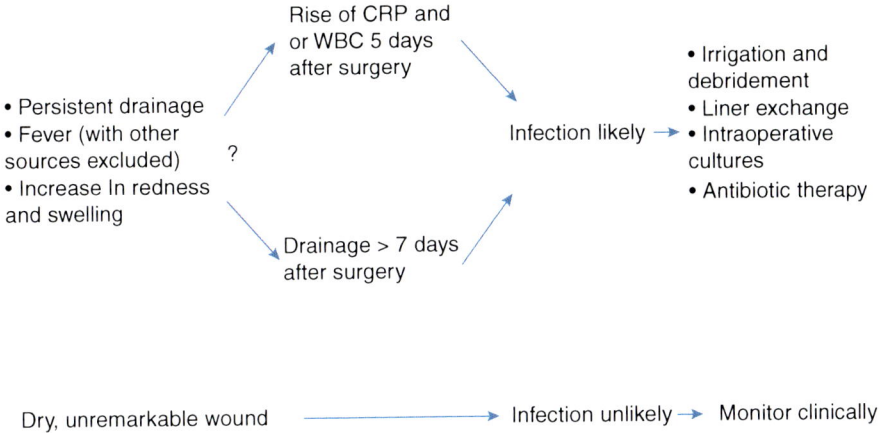

Fig. 21.2 Suggested diagnostic and treatment algorithm if symptoms last less than 3 weeks

Infection rates of total ankle arthroplasties in registry-based data are stated as less than 1 % with significantly higher aseptic loosening complication rates [4–6]. A doubt arises if all aseptic loosenings in the literature are truly aseptic or if they might encompass some septic loosenings with low-grade or suppressed pathogens that were not properly diagnosed. An important question to clarify in the patient's history is if he or she received oral antibiotics at any time after implantation for a presumed cellulitis in the area of surgery. Well-meaning primary care physicians often initiate antibiotic therapy for this kind of clinical picture. In order to guarantee the best long-term outcome for patients with loose ankle replacements or suspicious soft tissues, all efforts should be undertaken to rule in or rule out an infection with the help of the diagnostic algorithms presented in this chapter (Figs. 21.2 and 21.3). Oral antibiotics that are given without the proper diagnosis of an infection should be stopped and determination of the pathogen should be attempted after discontinuation of antibiotics for at least 5 days.

21.4   Treatment Problems

Many patients with infected total ankle replacements do present with a significant soft tissue problem and even dehiscence and large defects around the prosthesis. Along with the necessary orthopedic surgery and antibiotic treatment, these patients often do require coverage with flaps and skin grafts. It is recommendable to involve plastic surgery early in the treatment course of infected ankle replacements in order to improve the outcomes. Vacuum seals are very popular in wound infections and to treat soft tissue defects. They can be used for wound management where the fascia is closed over the implant or no implant is in place. Vacuum seals are not recommended directly on bone or on an implant, since they will maintain the colonization

Clinical suspicion of infection (any one of sings):
- Redness
- Swelling
- Persistent pain

Joint aspiration

CRP,ESR,WBC in blood

Negative   Any one
            elevated
            (without other
            source)

Cell count and
differential,
CRP

Culture and
sensitivity

Infection
unlikely

Normal

Elevated   Growth   No growth

1 or 2 stage exchange surgery
Cultures at time of surgery
Antibiotic treatment

- Monitor
- Reassess
- Protect ankle for some weeks
    - Restricted weight bearing
    - Brace/cast

+

With large defects consider
- Additional plastic surgery procedure
- Arthrodesis
- Amputation

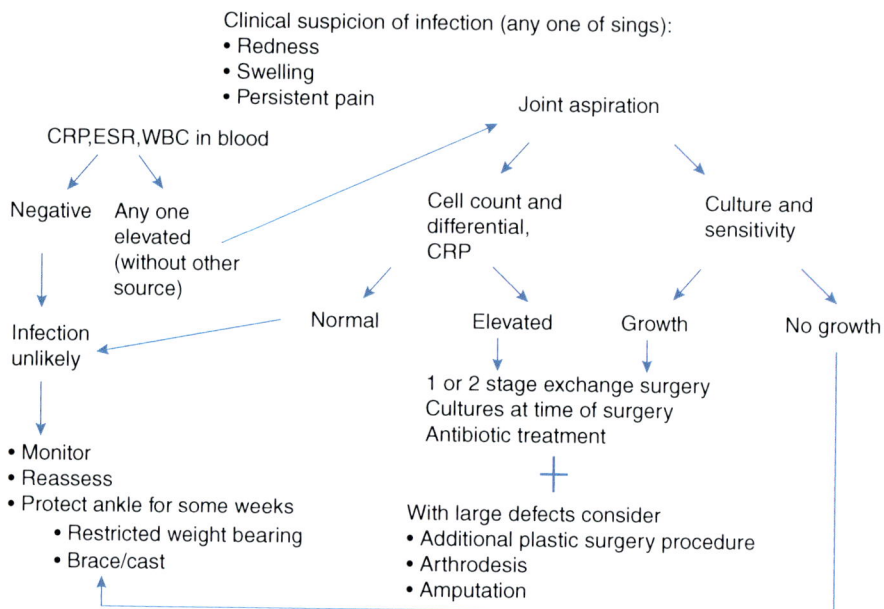

Fig. 21.3 Suggested diagnostic and treatment algorithm if symptoms last more than 3 weeks

Fig. 21.4 The defect after the removal of the prosthetic ankle (R. Trebše archive)

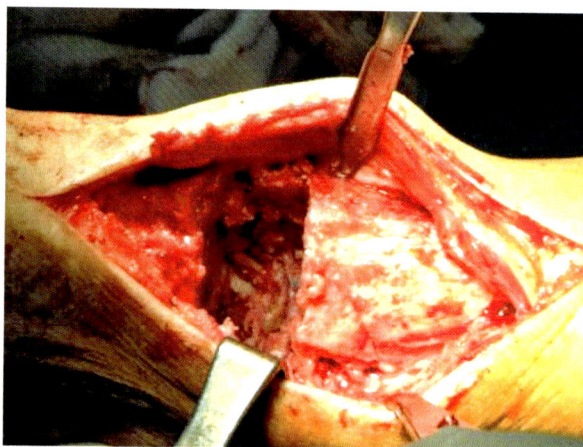

with skin bacteria on foreign materials or bradytrophic tissue and lead to resistant bacteria on these structures if used with antibiotic therapy. In some patients, the joint is not salvageable, and an arthrodesis, often with large osseous defects (Figs. 21.4 and 21.5), will have to be attempted. Rarely even below the knee amputation will be necessary if multiple revision surgeries and targeted antibiotics do not render the ankle infection free.

Fig. 21.5 The defect after
the removal of the prosthetic
ankle filled with femoral head
bone graft (R. Trebše archive)

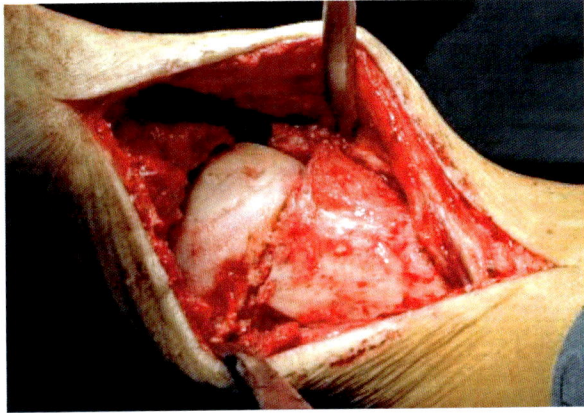

References

1. Haddad SL, Coetzee JC, Estok R, Fahrbach K, Banel D, Nalysnyk L. Intermediate and long-term outcomes of total ankle arthroplasty and ankle arthrodesis. A systematic review of the literature. J Bone Joint Surg Am. 2007;89:1899–905.
2. Thomas R, Daniels TR, Parker K. Gait analysis and functional outcomes following ankle arthrodesis for isolated ankle arthritis. J Bone Joint Surg Am. 2006;88:526–35.
3. Krause FG, Windolf M, Bora B, Penner MJ, Wing KJ, Younger ASE. Impact of complications in total ankle replacement and ankle arthrodesis analyzed with a validated outcome measurement. J Bone Joint Surg Am. 2011;93:830–9.
4. Fevang BT, Lie SA, Havelin LI, Brun JG, Skredderstuen A, Furnes O. 257 ankle arthroplasties performed in Norway between 1994 and 2005. Acta Orthop. 2007;78:575–83.
5. Henricson A, Skoog A, Carlsson A. The Swedish ankle arthroplasty register: an analysis of 531 arthroplasties between 1993 and 2005. Acta Orthop. 2007;78:569–74.
6. Hosman AH, Mason RB, Hobbs T, Rothwell AG. A New Zealand national joint registry review of 202 total ankle replacements followed for up to 6 years. Acta Orthop. 2007;78:584–91.

Chapter 22
Periprosthetic Infection Issues with Osseointegrated (OI) Implant Technology in Amputees

Catherine Loc-Carrillo, Alec C. Runyon, and James Peter Beck

Abstract The emerging technology of percutaneous osseointegrated skeletal attachment of artificial limbs, for the amputee population, presents new research and clinical challenges for preventing and treating infections at the implant/skin interface and the deep bone/implant attachment. The goal of this chapter is to review the current literature and to identify the challenges and possible solutions to these challenges that would ultimately allow wider introduction of this technology, particularly for the benefit of patients with multiple short stump amputations not amenable to current socket prosthetic docking systems.

Keywords Amputees • External osseointegrated implant • Complications

22.1 Introduction

For centuries, stump socket prosthetic docking technologies have been the only means for the attachment of artificial limbs to patients with limb loss. This grasping of the residual limb through the stump skin, underlying soft tissues, and boney prominences has always been a source of problems that can prevent the truly

C. Loc-Carrillo, Ph.D.
Department of Orthopedics, VA SLC Health Care System,
500 Foothill Drive, 151F, Salt Lake City, UT 84148, USA
e-mail: c.loc.carrillo@hsc.utah.edu

A.C. Runyon, M.S.
University of Nevada School of Medicine,
1664 North Virginia Street, Mail Stop 0357, Reno, NV 89557, USA
e-mail: arunyon@medicine.nevada.edu

J.P. Beck, M.D. (✉)
Department of Orthopaedics, The University of Utah,
Salt Lake City, UT, USA

George E. Wahlen Department of Veterans Affairs Medical Center,
VA Salt Lake City Health Care System,
Salt Lake City, UT 84148, USA
e-mail: james.beck@hsc.utah.edu

R. Trebše (ed.), *Infected Total Joint Arthroplasty*,
DOI 10.1007/978-1-4471-2482-5_22, © Springer-Verlag London 2012

255

effective use of prosthetic arms and legs. In spite of advances in biomaterials and socket designs, including suction sockets and harness attachment, these difficulties, which are intrinsic to the biology of the amputation stump and the physics of the stump/socket attachment system, are unlikely to have a timely solution. When put into the perspective of the activity expectations and the physical demands of modern day patients, particularly young and otherwise healthy patients with short stumps and multiple limb amputations, like those resulting from the wars in Iraq and Afghanistan, the limitations of socket technology become glaringly obvious.

22.2   Issues with Current Socket Technologies

In even the most advanced socket technologies, maintaining proper stump/socket fit is very difficult and very expensive. Stump volumes fluctuate due to soft tissue edema and muscle and soft tissue atrophy. Muscle atrophy and bone mineral loss occur from failure to mechanically load these tissues. Improper fit results in pressure sores, skin breakdown, and sometimes infection. Resultant stump pain prevents socket use and some otherwise optimally fitted sockets, in even single-limb amputees, allow only several hours of prosthesis use each day. Between 62 and 95 % of all amputees experience skin breakdown [1; Todd Kuiken – personal communication]. Because socket-induced pain can result in halting and inefficient and antalgic gait patterns, patients experience back pain, early osteoarthritic changes in the joints of the opposite intact extremity, and greater metabolic and oxygen demands compared to individuals with normal gait patterns. Upper extremity prostheses also produce skin breakdown and the inability to lift weight and maneuver complex robotic arms. Suspensory systems such as straps and socket flanges impinge upon the shoulder girdle and breasts. Socket impingement on the pelvis and groin, particularly in bilateral short stump amputees, prevents sitting with prostheses attached. As "donning and doffing" of lower limb prostheses is a lengthy and time-consuming process that requires undressing, exertive physical effort, and the common need for assistance, "walking" in sockets is difficult and inconvenient and becomes more and more infrequent. Adding to these limitations, situations of multiple short stump amputations (of both upper and lower extremities), heterotopic ossification seen particularly with the military victims of improvised explosive device (IED) blast injuries, and the problems of obesity and psychological depression, it is no wonder that practical locomotion eventually devolves to the use of a wheelchair.

Short of limb regeneration, the attachment of exoprostheses directly into the bone of the residual limb, offers an ideal solution to the problems of socket technology. Direct skeletal docking obviates the need for sockets, allows muscle function and bone loading, eliminates skin breakdown, reduces pain, and improves gait [2]. Ideal for multiple extremity limb loss and short residual limbs, this technology allows implantation into as little as 10–12 cm of remaining bone. There is no socket to impinge upon proximal joints and shoulder or pelvic girdles, and any underlying heterotopic ossification is essentially bypassed [3]. As the residual limb bone retains proprioceptive innervation, patients utilizing skeletal prosthetic attachment experience "osseoperception," which is an ability to perceive underlying terrain changes and limb position in space [4]. There is little to no restriction on the length of time the prosthesis is worn, short of discomfort at the attachment site. The process of "donning and doffing" exoprosthetic limbs is effortless and takes only seconds. Patients can repeatedly sit and stand, and unlimited sitting with attached prostheses even with bilateral short limb amputations is no longer a problem [5]. Finally, skeletal attachment is ideal for the secure docking of advanced exoprostheses, such as the DEKA arm, Utah arm, and powered knee prostheses, as well as robotic devices with neural and myoelectric control systems.

22.3 Percutaneous Osseointegrated Prostheses

It is beyond 20 years since Rickard Brånemark first introduced skeletal exoprosthetic attachment in human patients [6]. There are now three systems of percutaneous osseointegrated prosthesis (POP) attachment currently in use in European amputee volunteers [2, 7, 8]. As would be anticipated, a major complication facing this technology is that of infections at the implant stoma and the deep bone-implant interface. The deep infections may begin with primary bacterial contamination occurring during initial implantation surgery or later due to the hematogenous spread of bacteria from the skin, mouth, or urogenital tract as in conventional total joint arthroplasty infections [8–10]. Percutaneous osseointegrated devices, however, bear the additional vulnerability of ascending infection with ingress along the tract of the stomal linkage that begins with a superficial stomal infection and can conclude with deep periprosthetic infection and osteomyelitis.

Historically, the infection rates in POP devices, including deep and superficial infection, range from 18 to 30 % [8, 11] (Astrid Clausen and Horst Heinrich Aschoff – presentation at the First International Endo-Exo Meeting, May 2009, Lubeck, Germany). While these historic infection rates are significantly higher than those experienced in total joint arthroplasty (between 1 and 2 %), it is interesting that most patients, perhaps greater than 70–80 %, experience no significant problems from infection and indeed are infection-free for periods of years [8]. This is quite remarkable in that it would be intuitively anticipated that 100 % of devices would become infected because the bone/implant interface communicates with the outside microbial environment. While it appears that through modification of implant designs and postoperative strategies these infection rates have decreased [7; Horst-Heinrich Aschoff – personal communication], percutaneous systems face the same problems inherent to any implanted device, i.e., those of microbial resistance to antibiotics [12, 13], biofilm [14–17], and persister cell [18, 19] infection, and sometimes the ultimate need to remove devices to control infection [7, 8, 20, 21].

Percutaneous-bone-attached prostheses, by definition, have two structural requirements with biological implications. The first is an osseointegrated bone/implant interface involving viable bone growing into or attaching onto a metal

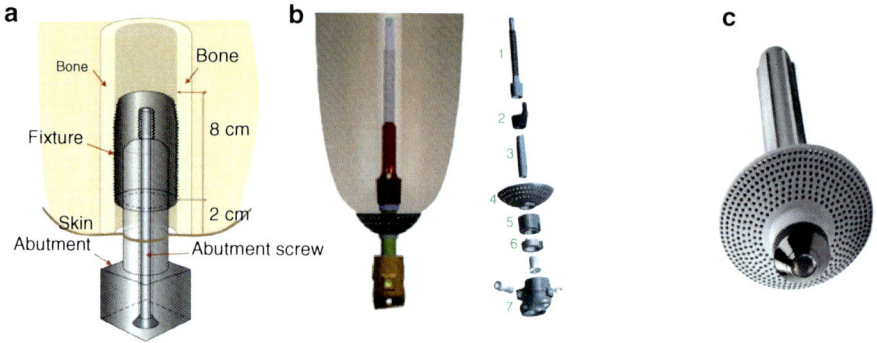

Fig. 22.1 Representative European percutaneous OI implant designs. (**a**) Brånemark design by integrum AB Sweden. (**b**) ESKA endo-exo prothesis Germany. *1* femurstem, *2* sleeve (optional), *3* dual cone adapter, *4* silicone cap, *5* sleeve, *6* rotating disc, *7* knee connecting adapter. (**c**) ITAP prothesis UK

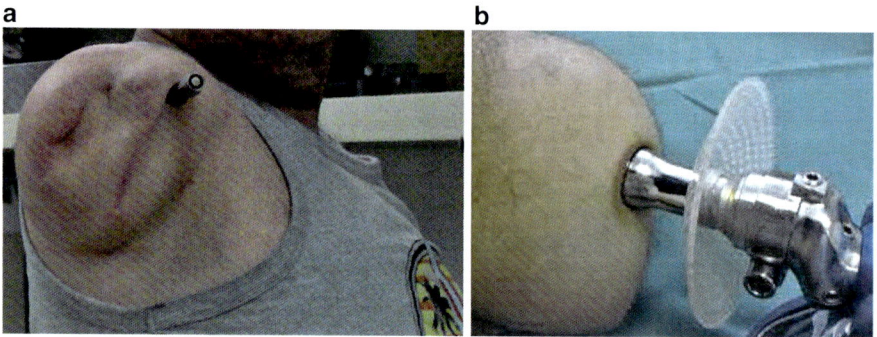

Fig. 22.2 European percutaneous osseointegrated implants in human subjects in clinical trials. (**a**) Brånemark implant in humerus. (**b**) Endo-exo implant in femur

implant. Current systems have either a "cancellous" structured surface in intimate initial contact with endosteal bone [7, 8] or a smooth implant with the configuration of a large screw, which, after tapping the medullary canal, is screwed in place into the canal [2]. These systems, unlike total joint replacements, have no moving parts subject to wear and in theory are free from the risk of particle debris and resultant particle-induced osteolysis. As they have the potential to last a lifetime, the stable biological attachment provided by osseointegration (OI) is, in theory, a much better attachment option than that of bone cement. The second "biostructural" requirement is a skin-implant interface or stoma, the exit point of the POP that permits the linkage between the stump bone and the exoprosthesis. Again, in current European models, this interface is handled by different strategies. In the Brånemark titanium alloy fixture and abutment system (see Figs. 22.1a and 22.2a), the defatted skin is attached and grows onto the distally resected surface of the vascular cortical stump bone, limiting skin motion at the stoma. Thus, the distance from the outside microbial environment to the endosteal bone is only millimeters [2].

The endo-exo system of Aschoff uses medullary canal press fit and has a cast-structured cobalt chrome steel shaft and an expanded section that caps the end of the stump bone (see Figs. 22.1b and 22.2b). In the third generation of the endo-exo device, the second stage surgical procedure uses a core to penetrate the skin, intentionally leaving a 2 cm depth of skin and underlying healthy soft tissue to "separate" the outside microbial environment from the cap of the device. This cap is itself distal to the resected bone surface and thus protects against bacterial entry to the endosteal bone [7]. The soft tissue tract along the connecting shaft, in theory, fills with granulation tissue from the deep regions of the initial surgical wound and simultaneously re-epithelializes, i.e., the surface skin grows down into the granulation tissue in the soft tissue tunnel. It is assumed that, as the wound matures, this epithelialized surface attaches in the deep granulations, providing a biological barrier to microbial ingress.

The ITAP device, designed by Blunn's group [22] at the University College London, is in essence a hybrid of the two previously described devices in that it employs a press-fit titanium alloy stem and a porous subcutaneous titanium flange (see Fig. 22.1c), the latter with novel surface features that attempt to mimic the boney anatomy at the skin/bone interface in deer antlers [23]. With the skin showing secure attachment to this hydroxyapatite-coated flange, the investigators designate this system to be one of "osseocutaneous integration" or one where both the bone and the skin become integrated with the implant.

22.3.1 Infection Associated with Current OI Implants

The incidence of infections associated with the current percutaneous skeletal attachment systems appears to be changing as the systems and techniques themselves have undergone improvement iterations over time. Brånemark's group, as of September 2009, had treated over 100 patients with femoral titanium implants: 3 with tibial implants, 15 with humeral implants, and 20 with implants in the radius or ulna of the forearm [5]. In order to allow for improvements in technique established from 1990 to 1999, once a standard treatment protocol was defined, Tillander et al. [8] evaluated a cohort of 39 patients previously treated with 45 transcutaneous osseointegrated titanium implants, selected during a 6-month period in 2005, and then identically reevaluated the cohort after 3 years. Their aims were to describe the frequency of clinical infections and the bacterial flora at the stoma and its relation to the development of local and implant-related infection as well as antibiotic use. Intramedullary titanium "fixtures" had been implanted a mean of 54 months earlier than the first study (range 3–132 months). The cohort randomly captured 33 femoral, 1 tibial, 4 ulnar, 4 radial, and 3 humeral implant patients returning for routine clinical follow-up in that 6-month window. There were three more men than women, and mean age was 49 years (range 28–74 years). Implants were considered osseointegrated when they were stable upon clinical examination and pain-free when loaded and radiography showed no radiolucent zone around the implant, indicating loosening. It was assumed that these patients were a representative sample of the entire population [8].

In the Tillander study, routine patient follow-up included an evaluation for pain, implant stability, and the condition of the skin and soft tissues. Radiographs were taken for evidence of implant loosening or deep infection ("osteolysis with or without periosteal sclerosis"). A questionnaire determined any infectious complications and antibiotic use during the 6 months preceding evaluation. At the beginning of the study and at 2.5–3 years follow-up, microbial samples were taken from the native, unprepared skin-implant interface with a sterile cotton swab and "cultured on routine agar plates for at least 2 days." No mention was made of the use of enrichment culture media, modified growth conditions, or extended incubation periods, which would be required to detect fastidious, anaerobic, or slow growing bacteria, respectively. However, it was mentioned that it was unfortunate that genetic typing of the bacteria was not done.

Clinical degrees of infection were defined as:

1. *Definite implant infection*: Clinical symptoms and radiographic signs of deep implant infection and three of five intraoperative cultures with the same pathogen.
2. *Probable implant infection*: Same criteria but with a "positive relevant culture."
3. *Possible implant infection*: Same criteria but no relevant cultures.
4. *Local infection in the skin penetration area*: Local signs and symptoms of infection including inflammation, with or without secretions, but no evidence of deep infection including negative radiographs but positive *or* negative relevant stomal cultures.
5. *Bacterial colonization around the skin-implant interface*: No inflammation or symptoms of infection with or without secretion, negative radiographs but positive bacterial cultures.

From their results, infection frequencies for definite/probable/possible implant infections at inclusion were 5 % (2 of 39), while the questionnaire revealed that 6 months prior to inclusion, seven patients had experienced local infections at the stoma, and of these, four were successfully treated with short-term antibiotics. At the study's 2.5–3 year endpoint, the investigators reported 18 % (7 of 39) of the patients had infections; however, it is worth noting that due to some dropouts and poor compliance, only 30 patients had cultures taken. The "results" for the limbs of the remaining nine patients were reported to be infection-free by local physicians. During the 6 months preceding the last data points, 11 of the 39 patients had local infections, six of whom had been treated with short-term antibiotics. Fourteen patients had secretion from the "skin pocket," and of these, ten patients had purulent secretions.

The seven infected cases involved six patients with femoral implants and one with a humeral device. Two femoral patients had chronic skin fistulas for 5 years prior to and throughout the study but with no pain, fever, or implant loosening and no antibiotic therapy. They were listed as implant infections and grew group B

Streptococcus (GBS) from the fistula and GBS and *Proteus mirabilis* from the skin penetration site in one-patient and coagulase negative staphylococci (CNS) from the fistula and *Staphylococcus aureus* at the stoma, in the other. Two other infected patients had "poor primary osseointegration," which assumes preexisting micromotion at the bone-implant interface. One had the femoral device extracted and grew a mixed flora of CNS, alpha streptococci, and *Peptostreptococcus* sp. The humeral implant had a stomal culture of CNS, but an *Escherichia coli* infection was verified by deep culture at biopsy and was treated for 6 months with ciprofloxacin. One year later there were no signs of relapse. Two of the remaining patients had good primary osseointegration but bone and soft tissue infection, one with *S. aureus* and CNS and the other with *S. aureus* and *Enterococcus faecalis*. Each had a revision and prolonged antibiotic treatment and was listed as "on-going." Finally, one femoral implant patient had acute osteomyelitis at the mid-fixture level and grew CNS and *S. aureus*. The functional summary of these six patients with salvaged devices stated that in two patients "prosthetic use was not affected at any time, three patients were affected only briefly during the time around surgical intervention, and for the patient with acute osteomyelitis the treatment outcome is still pending."

The most common bacteria at the stoma in all patients (those with and without infection) were *S. aureus* > CNS > GBS > group G Strep > group A Strep. Other bacteria cultured at the interface, in single uninfected patients, were *Citrobacter* sp., *Serratia* sp., *Pseudomonas* sp., other Gram-negative rods, aerobic *Streptococci*, alpha *Streptococci*, and Coryneforms. Eight of the inclusion stomas showed no bacterial growth, but none of the final cultures, at the end of the study, were negative, and all grew at least colonizing bacteria. There were no methicillin-resistant *Staphylococcus aureus* strains detected during the study.

Brånemark's group speculated that bacteria ascending from the stoma, facilitated by loose devices, likely accounted for infections in two of their patients. No patients appeared to develop infection from residual contamination resulting from the initial surgical procedures as infections were commonly delayed beyond 2 years, and were more likely the result of hematogenous spread similar to those seen in late infections common to the arthroplasty experience. Approximately half of the patients were colonized with *S. aureus* at the skin interface; however, only three patients suffered from a *S. aureus* infection. The investigators felt that titanium oxide is more biocompatible than stainless steel and cobalt chrome alloys and that the tight junction at the bone/implant interface might help prevent bacterial adhesion, deep colonization and subsequent biofilm formation, and infection.

In 1999, ESKA Implants of Lubeck, Germany, produced the first generation endo-exo femur prosthesis, and it was implanted into the femur of a young motorcyclist with a transfemoral amputation. In 2010, Aschoff et al. [7] reported on a population of 37 patients, mostly male (30 of 37) trauma victims using the first and second generations of this device. In a first stage procedure, the stable amputation stump is revised of redundant soft tissue, the medullary canal prepared with "cold" rasps, and the implant impacted into the femoral canal. The femur is cut proximally to 16 cm from the knee axis to allow for the joint mechanism of the prosthetic limb. Six to eight weeks later, using a sharp circular coring tool with a diameter intentionally greater than the diameter of the connecting coupler, the skin is entered and the prosthesis coupler is attached to the intramedullary implant. Once the coupler is attached, "the skin heals around it in a few days." The skin will epithelialize around the stoma channel from the outer skin margin, and granulating connective tissue will fill in the gap from the femoral cortex out, "in a manner similar to how a dental implant heals." Full weight bearing occurs in 4–6 weeks of this procedure [7].

Analysis of Aschoff's patients showed, as with Brånemark, better results with increasing experience with surgical and rehabilitative procedures and advancing implant design changes. Twenty of the 37 patients underwent further revisions and four required implant removal, of the latter, one for chronic intramedullary infection, two for "chronic soft-tissue problems at the dermal interface" (not defined as infection), and one with mechanical implant failure at 7 years (the metal exit point broke). Two of these patients had successful reimplantation at a later date. Fourteen patients had problems with the rough subcutaneous surface of the first generation implant, and 12 of these had replacement with a smooth polished coupler solving the problem of skin irritation. These revisions were not due to infection.

In May of 2009, Drs. Astrid Clausen and Horst Aschoff presented a summary of the microbiological analysis from the endo-exo femur prosthesis (EEFP) experience, at a meeting in Lubeck, Germany. Apparently, they used "conventional agar plate culture techniques," presumably implying the isolation of bacteria capable of growing under aerobic conditions only. At this stage of implant development, they reported ten "clinically relevant" infections in 30 patients. The bacterial populations were very similar to those reported by Brånemark and included five patients with *S. aureus*, three with *Peptostreptococcus*, three with Bacteroides, and one each with multiresistant *Staphylococcus epidermidis*, *Enterobacter*, *Proteus mirabilis*, and beta-hemolytic *Streptococcus viridans*. As these numbers total greater than ten bacterial strains, they indicate that some patients had mixed infections. Of these ten patients, five were classified as early infections linked with implantation of the EEFP and five were late infections. While the infecting bacteria were presumed pathogens, many of the same species were cultured at the stoma of uninfected patients and many stomas showed polymicrobial colonization. The quantity of bacterial colonization included 13 with *S. aureus*, 3 Bacteroides, 3 *Enterococcus faecalis*, 3 *Escherichia coli*, 3 *Peptostreptococcus* sp., and 3 group B *Streptococci*, with the number of bacterial species colonizing any given stoma 0–7 species. The spectrum of colonizing bacteria included, in addition to those mentioned, *Acinetobacter* sp., MRSA, *Staphylococcus haemolyticus* and *S. anginosus*, *Pseudomonas aeruginosa*, *Proteus* sp., and *Peptostreptococcus* sp. Of note was that the patients done earliest in the series and, still free of infection, had a more varied polymicrobial colonizing flora, including aerobic and anaerobic bacteria, than patients operated later in the series.

Aschoff's conclusions pertaining to the microbiology of his initial experience were:

"Bacterial colonization of the stoma is unavoidable." (and we might add, may be beneficial.)
"Bacterial colonization does not correlate with infection."

"Pathogenicity and virulence of bacteria does not correlate with the appearance of infections."

"Disinfection and antibiotic treatment of colonizing bacteria are counterproductive."

In 2010, the Stanmore group [24] reported the 2-year follow-up of their experience with "osseocutaneous integration" of a press-fit, intraosseous transcutaneous implant in a transhumeral amputee. Surgery was done as a single-stage procedure. As mentioned previously, their system is a hybrid of the devices used in the two larger series. The defatted skin with its' subdermal vascular plexus intact attaches to a parasol-shaped subcutaneous porous and perforated titanium expansion (flange) of the intramedullary attachment. The surface, that is intended to mimic the exit region of the deer antler and that allows bone and skin attachment, is coated with hydroxyapatite. On the flange this coating ends at the central exit shaft that is then further coated with diamond-like carbon. The skin is held against the flange surface with a Poron washer during the time the cutaneous integration occurs. At the time of publication, this was the only patient to receive this device. There had been no episodes of infection, and with a fairly large expansion for attachment of skin and soft tissue, they reported that the "skin-implant interface remains stable, with no serous discharge or pain."

22.3.2   Prevention of OI Implant Infection

Avoidance of deep and superficial infection, in the situation of a percutaneous device interface, is a complex problem, and clinical investigators working with human volunteers and some with translational animal experimentation have approached the problem in various ways. There seems to be a general consensus that the skin-implant interface should ultimately become micromotion-free and that a solid device/bone interface is essential. Brånemark found that preexisting implant loosening resulted in deep infection, and in a sheep amputation implant system, we found that implant loosening resulted in the only deep infections in the series. Immediate and continued, tight and stable implant "fit and fill," in the medullary canal, is absolutely essential when weight bearing is begun if osseointegration rather than fibrous attachment is to be achieved. Fibrous attachment leads to ultimate loosening and infection.

The time it takes for osseointegration to occur varies with device design. In human designs impacted (press fit) into the medullary canal, weight bearing is begun generally at about 12 weeks from the first stage surgery [7]. In patients with good bone, this period is sometimes shortened to allow partial weight bearing several weeks after the second stage percutaneous attachment is placed. Using a cancellous structured titanium implant surface, our press-fit sheep amputation model showed that very stable osseointegration occurs by 3 months and continued to

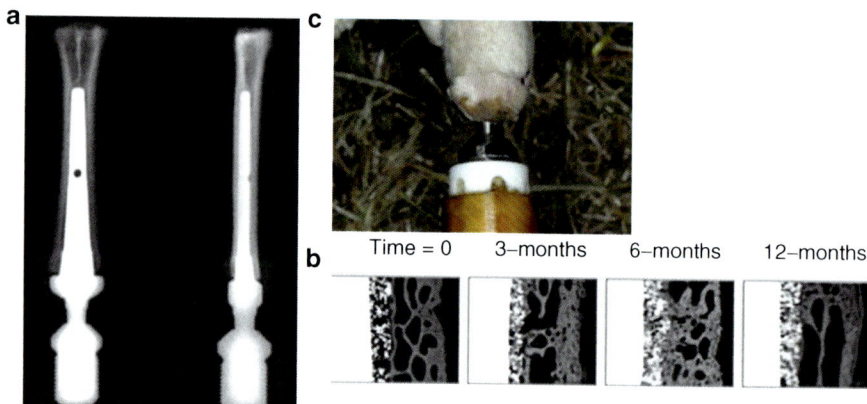

Fig. 22.3 Translational animal model of osseointegration and skin seal in sheep with porous structured titanium. (**a**) X-ray showing medullary "fit and fill." (**b**) SEM-back scatter image showing bone integrating with porous implant at various times post surgery. (**c**) BJRL implant in a sheep forelimb (2 weeks post surgery)

increase out to 1 year, as verified by scanning electron microscopy and Instron pull-out studies [25]. Interestingly, in this translational model, the sheep bore weight immediately after the single-stage procedure. The Brånemark system uses a titanium screw that is placed into the tapped medullary canal [5]. Since weight bearing puts non-impacting forces on the interface, they delay weight bearing until presumed osseointegration occurs based upon past clinical experience and pain felt by the patient at the attachment site with weight bearing. This can delay full weight bearing for much longer periods of time out to 12–18 months. It appears that osseointegration can occur with either a structured cobalt chrome interface or with titanium implants. There has been discussion that the biocompatibility of titanium may be an asset to a tight interface attachment and that this solid bond excludes bacterial biofilms from the interface once the race for the implant surface, a race between potentially infecting bacteria and ingrowing bone, is won by the bone [5]. Tight and precise initial "fit and fill" apposition of the implant to the medullary bone (see Fig. 22.3a) with less than 50 μm separating the two surfaces favors rapid osseointegration (see Fig. 22.3b) and lessens a fibrous tissue interface and probably the chance of infection [26, 27].

Having a "cap" on the entrance to the medullary canal may prevent deep bacterial ingress, assuming healthy skin and soft tissues surround the cap. All devices other than the Brånemark system have this feature and, in our sheep model, an immediate skin seal, and cap separation (see Fig. 22.3c) probably contributed to our sheep remaining infection-free out to 1 year, in a barnyard environment [25, 28, 29].

The design of the surface structure of the shaft connecting the implant to the outside environment has been approached in several ways. The Brånemark design is an abutment of titanium that in theory has minimal soft tissue surrounding it as it exits the bone surrounded by defatted skin attached to the bone portal. The endo-exo femur prosthesis has eliminated the aggressive subcutaneous structure of the first generation (which eroded through the skin) and the smooth cobalt chrome steel of the second generation, in favor of a third generation, low energy, ultra smooth surface of "oxy-nitrate" that prevents biofilm adhesion by a "lotus effect" (Horst Aschoff - personal communications). These patients wash their interfaces once or twice daily with a mild soap and a soft washcloth or shaving brush and wrap a sterile sponge around the shaft to absorb any serous drainage. In most patients, there is little or no drainage, and with this third generation device, there have been no infections in 24 of 24 patients, with some of the patients possessing implants for almost 3 years. Aschoff avoids disturbing colonizing bacteria with disinfectants and rigorously avoids antibiotics for fear of bacterial evolution to resistant forms and superinfection.

22.4   The Skin Microbiome and Its Implications

As previously mentioned, it is remarkable that 70–80 % of patients with skeletal docking of their prosthetic limbs remain infection-free for years, and it seems likely that the biology of the skin-implant interface holds the clue to this improbable success. Recent advances in molecular identification of bacteria have shown that only 3 % of the resident bacteria populating the human skin can be found with conventional culturing techniques.

The Human Microbiome Project (HMP) [http://nihroadmap.nih.gov/hmp], initiated by the National Institutes of Health in 2007, has sought by molecular means, to determine all of the genomes of the myriad bacteria that defy cultivation but populate the human [30]. The skin and four other body sites are being characterized (mouth, vagina, gut, and nasal/lung). The intent of the HMP is to determine if changes in the human microbiome are associated with human health or human disease states and if it will "also define parameters needed to design, implement and monitor strategies for intentionally manipulating the human microbiota, to optimize its performance in the context of an individual's physiology" [30]. The skin microbiome [31] has been found to vary with skin sampling sites on the individual (axilla, groin, nares, chest, forearm, etc.) but correlate with specific sites in multiple individuals [32]. There is also temporal variability that is somewhat site specific in individuals; although generally individuals remain more like themselves, over time, than like other tested subjects [33]. Although the relationships are complex, there is strong evidence to suggest that microbes that can live commensally on the skin, i.e., from the genera *Staphylococcus*, *Corynebacterium*, *Propionibacterium*, *Streptococcus*, and *Pseudomonads*, may directly benefit the host (mutualism) and only rarely will they become pathogens [34]. They indeed can inhibit other pathogenic bacteria and combine to maintain healthy skin by helping to promote the skin bacterial barrier and enhance innate immunity. In fact a product of *Pseudomonas fluorescens* has been used as a topical antibiotic (mupirocin) against staphylococcal and streptococcal pathogens, and *Pseudomonas* itself inhibits the growth of many fungal species [34].

The history of bone and joint infection has amply shown that bone is particularly vulnerable to *S. aureus* [12, 13] and that it is less susceptible to Gram-negative bacterial invasion, although not completely so [35, 36]. It seems highly likely that serendipitous variation in the colonizing bacteria comprising the stomal microbiotas of the 70–80 % of individuals who tolerate percutaneous bone docking systems plays an unrecognized role in implant survival. Further molecular studies of the stoma and surrounding skin may open the door to manipulating them to the advantage of the individual. Perhaps, the unrecognized polymicrobial communities of bacteria colonizing the skin-implant interface are indeed the guard dogs at the gate.

References

1. Levy SW. Skin problems in the amputee. In: Smith DG, Michael JW, Bowker JH, editors. Atlas of amputations and limb deficiencies surgical, prosthetic, and rehabilitation principles. 3rd ed. Rosemont: American Academy of Orthopaedic Surgeons; 2004. p. 701–10.
2. Frossard L, Hagberg K, Haggstrom E, Gow DL, Branemark R, Pearcy M. Functional outcome of transfemoral amputees fitted with an osseointegrated fixation: temporal gait characteristics. J Prosthet Orthot. 2010;22(1):11–20.
3. Hagberg K, Haggstrom E, Uden M, Branemark R. Socket versus bone-anchored trans-femoral prostheses: hip range of motion and sitting comfort. Prosthet Orthot Int. 2005;29(2):153–63.
4. Hagberg K, Haggstrom E, Jonsson S, Rydevik B, Branemark R. Osseoperception and osseointegrated prosthetic limbs. In: Gallagher P, Desmond D, MacLachlan M, editors. Psychoprosthetics. London: Springer; 2008. p. 131–40. doi:10.1007/978-1-84628-980-4_10.
5. Hagberg K, Branemark R. One hundred patients treated with osseointegrated transfemoral amputation prostheses – rehabilitation perspective. J Rehabil Res Dev. 2009;46(3):331–44.
6. Brånemark R, Brånemark PI, Rydevik B, Myers RR. Osseointegration in skeletal reconstruction and rehabilitation: a review. J Rehabil Res Dev. 2001;38(2):175–81.
7. Aschoff HH, Kennon RE, Keggi JM, Rubin LE. Transcutaneous, distal femoral, intramedullary attachment for above-the-knee prostheses: an endo-exo device. J Bone Joint Surg Am. 2010;92 Suppl 2:180–6. doi:10.2106/JBJS.J.00806. PII:92/Supplement_2/180.
8. Tillander J, Hagberg K, Hagberg L, Branemark R. Osseointegrated titanium implants for limb prostheses attachments: infectious complications. Clin Orthop Relat Res. 2010;468(10):2781–8. doi:10.1007/s11999-010-1370-0.
9. Arciola CR, An YH, Campoccia D, Donati ME, Montanaro L. Etiology of implant orthopedic infections: a survey on 1027 clinical isolates. Int J Artif Organs. 2005;28(11):1091–100.
10. Pulido L, Ghanem E, Joshi A, Purtill JJ, Parvizi J. Periprosthetic joint infection: the incidence, timing, and predisposing factors. Clin Orthop Relat Res. 2008;466(7):1710–5. doi:10.1007/s11999-008-0209-410.1016/j.jbiomech.2011.08.020.
11. Clausen A, Aschoff H-H. Microbiology of the endo- exo-femur prosthesis (EEFP) experience. In: First International Endo-Exo Meeting, Lubeck. May 2009.
12. Ellington JK, Harris M, Hudson MC, Vishin S, Webb LX, Sherertz R. Intracellular *Staphylococcus aureus* and antibiotic resistance: implications for treatment of staphylococcal osteomyelitis. J Orthop Res. 2006;24(1):87–93. doi:10.1002/jor.20003.
13. Wright JA, Nair SP. Interaction of staphylococci with bone. Int J Med Microbiol. 2010;300 (2–3):193–204. doi:10.1016/j.ijmm.2009.10.003. PII:S1438-4221(09)00121-0.
14. Gristina AG, Costerton JW. Bacterial adherence to biomaterials and tissue. The significance of its role in clinical sepsis. J Bone Joint Surg Am. 1985;67(2):264–73.
15. Donlan RM, Costerton JW. Biofilms: survival mechanisms of clinically relevant microorganisms. Clin Microbiol Rev. 2002;15(2):167–93.

16. Costerton JW. Biofilm theory can guide the treatment of device-related orthopaedic infections. Clin Orthop Relat Res. 2005;437:7–11.
17. Fitzpatrick F, Humphreys H, O'Gara JP. The genetics of staphylococcal biofilm formation – will a greater understanding of pathogenesis lead to better management of device-related infection? Clin Microbiol Infect. 2005;11(12):967–73. doi:10.1111/j.1469-0691.2005.01274.x. PII:CLM1274.
18. Oliver JD. The viable but nonculturable state in bacteria. J Microbiol. 2005;43:93–100. PII:2134.
19. Lewis K. Persister cells. Annu Rev Microbiol. 2010;64:357–72. doi:10.1146/annurev.micro.112408.134306.
20. Mittal Y, Fehring TK, Hanssen A, Marculescu C, Odum SM, Osmon D. Two-stage reimplantation for periprosthetic knee infection involving resistant organisms. J Bone Joint Surg Am. 2007;89(6):1227–31.
21. Diwanji SR, Kong IK, Park YH, Cho SG, Song EK, Yoon TR. Two-stage reconstruction of infected hip joints. J Arthroplasty. 2008;23(5):656–61. doi:10.1016/j.arth.2007.06.007. PII:S0883-5403(07)00360-9.
22. Kim HJ, Fernandez JW, Akbarshahi M, Walter JP, Fregly BJ, Pandy MG. Evaluation of predicted knee-joint muscle forces during gait using an instrumented knee implant. J Orthop Res. 2009;27(10):1326–31. doi:10.1002/jor.20876.
23. Pendegrass CJ, Goodship AE, Price JS, Blunn GW. Nature's answer to breaching the skin barrier: an innovative development for amputees. J Anat. 2006;209(1):59–67.
24. Kang NV, Pendegrass C, Marks L, Blunn G. Osseocutaneous integration of an intraosseous transcutaneous amputation prosthesis implant used for reconstruction of a transhumeral amputee: case report. J Hand Surg Am. 2010;35(7):1130–4. doi:10.1016/j.jhsa.2010.03.037. PII:S0363-5023(10)00384-9.
25. Beck JP, Bloebaum RD, Jeyapalina S, Bachus KN. A single-stage ovine amputation model for developing a safe osseointegrated implant system. In: Proceedings of the 27th Army Science Conference, Orlando. 30 November 2010. p. KO-03, 01–08.
26. Bloebaum RD, Mihalopoulus NL, Jensen JW, Dorr LD. Postmortem analysis of bone growth into porous-coated acetabular components. J Bone Joint Surg Am. 1997;79-A(7):1013–22.
27. Bloebaum RD, Bachus KN, Jensen JW, Scott DF, Hofmann AA. Porous-coated metal-backed patellar components in total knee replacement. J Bone Joint Surg Am. 1998;80-A(4):518–28.
28. Bloebaum RD, Beck JP, Olsen R, Norlund L, Bachus KN. Development of a single stage surgical model for percutaneous osseointegrated implants for amputees. In: 55th Annual Meeting of the Orthopaedic Research Society. Trans. Orthopaed. Res. Soc., Las Vegas. 22–25 February 2009. p. 2255.
29. Shelton TJ, Beck JP, Bloebaum RD, Bachus KN. Percutaneous osseointegrated prostheses for amputees: Limb compensation in a 12-month ovine model. J Biomech. 2011;44(15):2601–6. PII:S0021-9290(11)00580-X.
30. Turnbaugh PJ, Ley RE, Hamady M, Fraser-Liggett CM, Knight R, Gordon JI. The human microbiome project. Nature. 2007;449(7164):804–10. doi:10.1038/nature06244. PII:nature06244.
31. Grice EA, Segre JA. The skin microbiome. Nat Rev Microbiol. 2011;9(4):244–53. doi:10.1038/nrmicro2537. PII:nrmicro2537.
32. Gao Z, Tseng CH, Pei Z, Blaser MJ. Molecular analysis of human forearm superficial skin bacterial biota. Proc Natl Acad Sci USA. 2007;104(8):2927–32.
33. Grice EA, Kong HH, Conlan S, Deming CB, Davis J, Young AC, Bouffard GG, Blakesley RW, Murray PR, Green ED, Turner ML, Segre JA. Topographical and temporal diversity of the human skin microbiome. Science. 2009;324(5931):1190–2. doi:10.1126/science.1171700. PII:324/5931/1190.
34. Cogen AL, Nizet V, Gallo RL. Skin microbiota: a source of disease or defence? Br J Dermatol. 2008;158(3):442–55. doi:10.1111/j.1365-2133.2008.08437.x. PII:BJD8437.
35. Galanakis N, Giamarellou H, Moussas T, Dounis E. Chronic osteomyelitis caused by multi-resistant gram-negative bacteria: evaluation of treatment with newer quinolones after prolonged follow-up. J Antimicrob Chemother. 1997;39(2):241–6.
36. Meyers BR, Berson BL, Gilbert M, Hirschman SZ. Clinical patterns of osteomyelitis due to Gram-negative bacteria. Arch Intern Med. 1973;131(2):228–33.

Chapter 23
The Algorithm for Diagnostic Evaluation and Treatment

Rihard Trebše and Andrej Trampuž

Abstract The most important issue in treatment of PJI is the correct evaluation of the patients and the decision about the appropriate treatment strategy, namely, debridement and retention, one-stage exchange, two-stage exchange, permanent resection arthroplasty, and permanent antibiotic suppression. The chosen strategy determines the final functionality and clinical results but the probability of infection cure as well. In general, more aggressive treatment results in poorer functionality but better chance of eradication of infection. This is not true for all subsets of patients. The algorithm helps to discriminate which patients would have an acceptable probability for eradication with less invasive treatment strategy. The goal is to apply the strategy that gives the best function without trading-off the probabilities of permanent infection cure too much.

Keywords Algorithm • Diagnosis • Surgical strategy • Medical treatment

23.1 Introduction

Prosthetic joints can fail in many ways and the underlying reasons are numerous (Fig. 23.2). A PJI is an iatrogenic condition in which there is a conflict between organisms growing on a foreign material causing infection and host defense mechanism. The proprieties of the foreign material, the virulence of the invading organism, and the strength of the host defense mechanisms determine the clinical

R. Trebše, M.D., Ph.D. (✉)
Department for Bone Infections and Adult Reconstructions,
Orthopaedic Hospital Valdoltra,
Jadranska cesta 31, Ankaran SI-6286, Slovenia
e-mail: rihard.trebse@ob-valdoltra.si

A. Trampuž, M.D.
Division of Infectious Diseases & Septic Unit, University Hospital of Lausanne,
Rue du Bugnon 46, Lausanne CH-1011, Switzerland
e-mail: andrej.trampuz@chuv.ch

R. Trebše (ed.), *Infected Total Joint Arthroplasty*,
DOI 10.1007/978-1-4471-2482-5_23, © Springer-Verlag London 2012

269

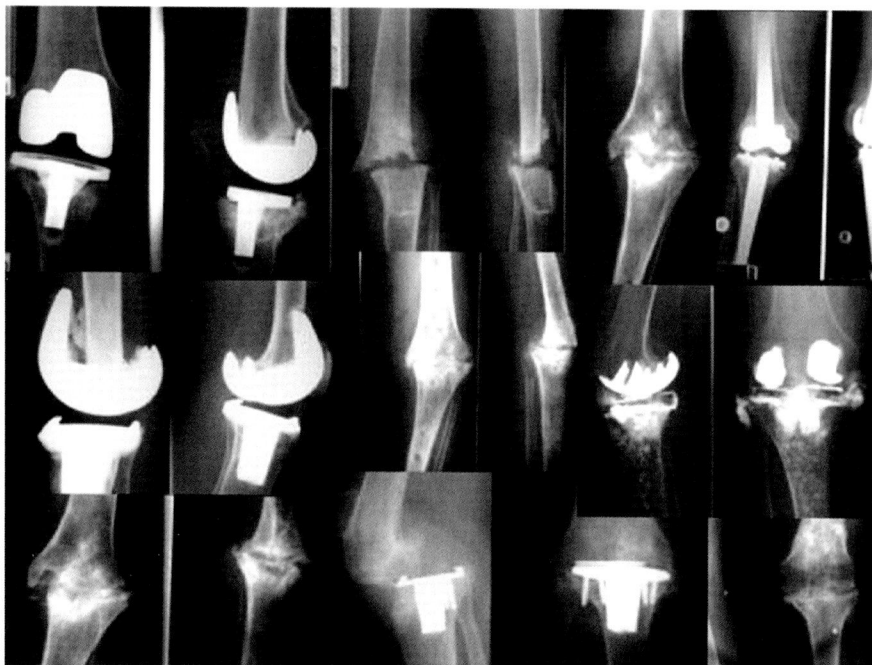

Fig. 23.1 High variability of clinical presentation patterns for prosthetic knee infections

manifestation of the disease (Fig. 23.1). It is thus easy to understand the whole variety of clinical manifestations that range from acute fatal sepsis to a fully asymptomatic course. The concept of asymptomatic infections is not widely accepted, but a lot of evidence supports it [7, 15, 23]. These infections are relevant because they can become clinically manifested in the case of sudden deterioration of immune status as after application of biological or other immunosuppressing drugs and in other conditions that influence host defense mechanisms.

The precise incidence of the device-related infections is thus not known, but the published incidence (refer to Chap. 6) is surely underestimated and depending on the working definition. The stronger the diagnostic tool used, the higher the incidence of the infection found.

As for the treatment of any disease, the most important issue in the evaluation of a problematic artificial joint is to find a correct diagnosis. Since the treatment of a septic and aseptic failure of an implant differs considerably the major challenge in revision surgery is to reliably diagnose infection preoperatively. Wrongly diagnosed PJI as an aseptic failure leads to high rate of subsequent failures.

Every symptomatic artificial joint with no obvious reason for the symptoms and also joints that failed prematurely are potentially infected and need assessment regarding infection.

The diagnostic evaluation consists of verification of the presence of an ongoing infection, isolation of the etiologic organism, and determination of its antibiotic susceptibility. It is of the utmost importance to perform the diagnostic evaluation

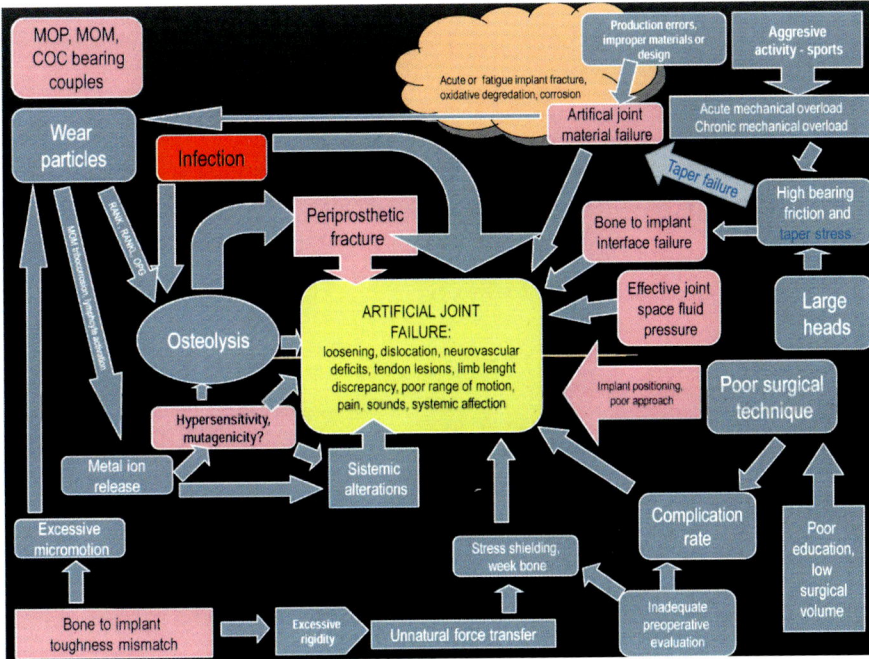

Fig. 23.2 A simplified overview of modes of failure affecting artificial joints

before starting with treatment activities. If it is not successful, the last chance to determine the presence of an infection and obtain the organisms with its antibiotic resistance pattern is during the surgical procedure. If we fail any treatment afterward is guesswork and the prognosis poor.

Diagnosing a PJI can be very easy in the case of high-grade infections but difficult in low-grade ones. Consequently, we need to build up the diagnosis by using staged system to confirm the suspicion and finally to fulfill one of the aforementioned criteria (refer to Chap. 4) that determine that an arthroplasty is infected. If more than 2 out of 3 or more tissue cultures grow the same organism (one positive is enough for synovial fluid culture taken by aspiration) or there is a direct communication with the implant or there is acute inflammation around the prosthetic joint in the form of pus, either macroscopic, cytological, or histological, the PJI is confirmed.

In order to institute an appropriate treatment, it is important to define the indications for evaluation for infection and the appropriate diagnostic workflow. Every patient with a problematic implant is a potential candidate for evaluation for infection if the reason for the problem cannot be readily established.

23.2 The Indications for Diagnostic Evaluation

Most frequently, patients with a diagnosis of PJI (or infected OS material that needs to be treated with a joint prosthesis) present before any attempt of treatment

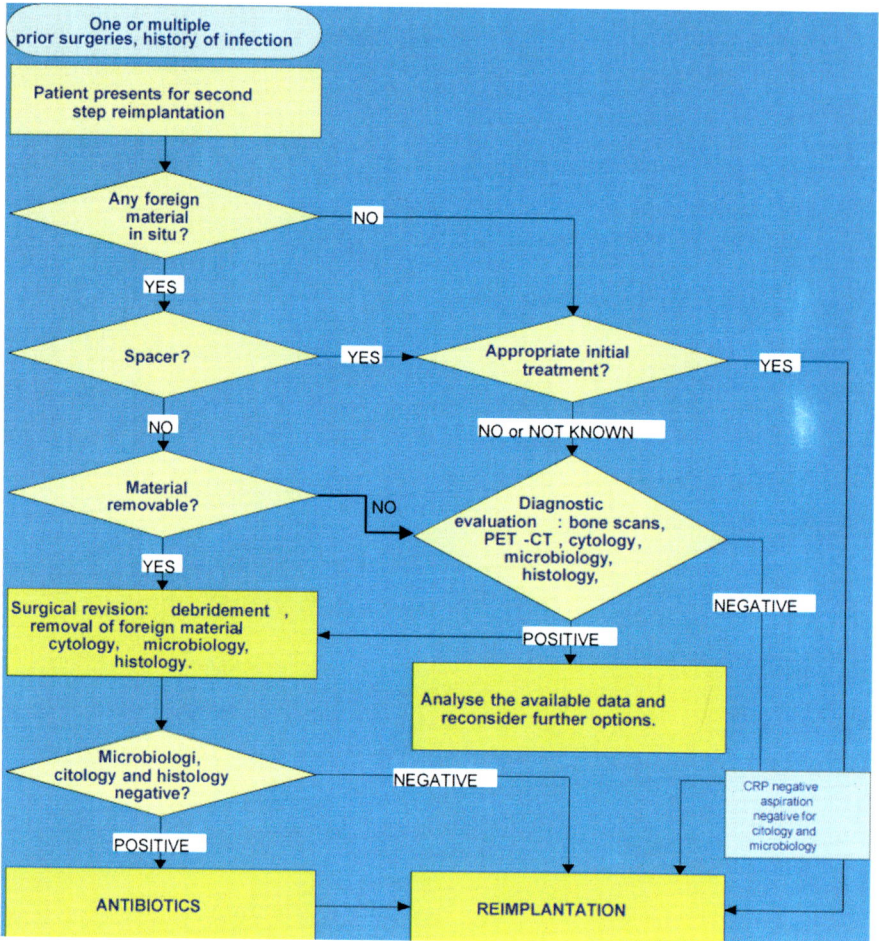

Fig. 23.3 The diagnostic algorithm for evaluation of patients presenting for a second step (re)implantation of an artificial joint

affected with one of the three classic types, namely, early, delayed, or late infection, or with a "low-grade" infection that can be of either early, delayed, or late onset.

There are, however, many patients presenting differently. They commonly have a history of PJI (or infected osteosinthesis) and have already been submitted to various attempts of treatment with doubtful success, or they may still have problems but it is not known if the symptoms are related to former infection or not.

Some of the patients present for a regular second stage after being primarily treated for PJI with removal of the artificial joint. It is helpful to follow an algorithm for evaluation of these patients to avoid errors, increase success rate, and repeatability (Fig. 23.3).

Fig. 23.4 Girdlestone situation with antibiotic-loaded beads still present

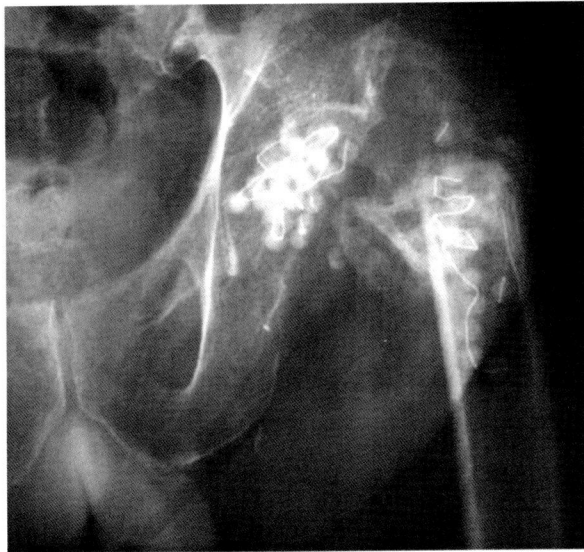

They are either with or without a spacer, frequently with some foreign material (screw, wire, antibiotic-loaded cement beads, or something else) left in the joint region (Fig. 23.4).

The prior surgical and/or medical treatment at the time of presentation could have been conducted properly, insufficiently, or it is unknown.

> Evaluation for possible infection is one of the necessary and the most important steps in the assessment of nearly any patient which presents with a problematic artificial joint despite the type of the problem besides those presenting with a periprosthetic fracture and aseptic loosenings more than 10 years after primary implantation.

Sometimes the reason for diagnostic workout to evaluate potential infection is an early failure of an implant (Fig. 23.5), unexplained pain, repeat dislocation, or stiffness. It is difficult to define an early failure. But since most of the contemporary implants have more than 90 % survival rate after 10 years with aseptic loosening as an end point [14], it seems reasonable to consider an early failure if it occurs less than 10 years after the implantation. There are many potential reasons for an early aseptic failure (Fig. 23.1) such as poor cementation [12], suboptimal component placement (Fig. 23.6), overuse, implant failure, allergy [10], soft tissue problems, trauma, and some others.

An important reason especially after the exclusion of the aforementioned reasons is infection.

Fig. 23.5 Cemented stem breakage 2 years after implantation. Excellent cement mantle

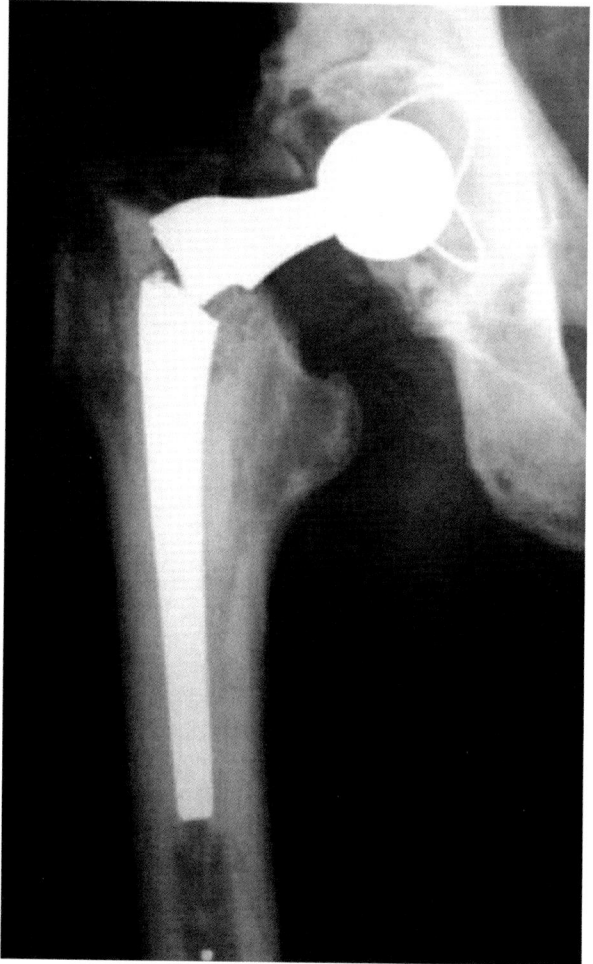

Of course, it is possible that even some of those patients that fail more than 10 years after primary implantation have a low-grade infection. It is, however, difficult to justify the complete evaluation since the probability that the cause of the failure is in fact an aseptic process is much higher. The history of long-term and early-onset problems such as pain, occasional chills, and unexplained fevers raises the suspicion that there is a hidden septic process around an artificial joint (or any other implant). In patients (especially immunodeficient) presenting with sepsis of unknown origin that have had implanted prosthetic joints or other devices, evaluation of these joints for sepsis is very important even if the joints seem asymptomatic. The presence of foreign material gives enough probability for a septic focus to allow for evaluation.

Stratification. In the first instance, it is important to stratify presenting patients according to the risk factors they carry to determine the probability of infection and

Fig. 23.6 Component malposition resulting in painful total knee arthroplasty. The infection was ruled out prior to revision in this patient

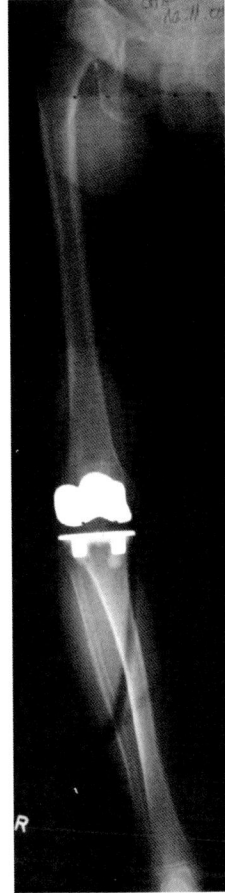

base the diagnostic treatment strategy accordingly [1]. In an immunocompromised patient, low-grade symptoms are more likely caused by an infection than in a normal subject, for instance. There are many studies that can be performed to increase or decrease the probabilities for correctly diagnosing a septic failure such as the following.

Laboratory evaluation. In a recent guideline published by the American Academy of Orthopaedic Surgeons (AAOS), screening for inflammatory markers like erythrocyte sedimentation rate (ESR) and C-reactive protein (CRP), has achieved strong level of recommendation especially for ruling out PJI. The recommendation is supported by excellent evidence [1]. Based on the analysis of the included papers, it seems, however, that the problem of low-grade infections was underestimated. In the recommendation number five regarding the repeat aspiration, the authors, however, acknowledged this potential inadequacy.

These low-grade CRP-negative PJI are actually the real challenge if we want to avoid early repeat, presumably aseptic, revisions. In our series of 150 + culture proven infections, 25 % have presented with CRP below 5 mg/L. The question is what would the failure rate be if those would have been treated as normal revisions. With combined ESR and CRP, we can successfully rule out inflammation but not infection. Other studies like peripheral white blood cell count and differential are neither specific nor sensitive enough to warrant consideration.

Imaging. It is important to perform x-ray studies in presumed PJI, mainly to rule out other causes for failure and to ascertain whether the implant is stable or loose. Other imaging studies to be considered are the arthrography and the fistulography. CT scan and MRI probably have no major additional role to discriminate between a septic and aseptic failure (see Chap. 14, [1]).

Bone scans. There are several nuclear imaging studies useful for diagnostic workout of potential PJI (see Chap. 14 for more detailed discussion), namely, bone or bone marrow scans, FDG-PET imaging, gallium imaging, or labeled-leukocyte imaging, and especially the combinations of the later with either bone or bone marrow scan. Their value is not yet fully determined (Chap. 14, [1]). They are useful to narrow the selection of patients that need further diagnostic studies.

In all cases, with no obvious aseptic reason for symptoms, it is necessary to perform an aspiration to try to obtain the pseudosynovial fluid. The sample is than cultured (Chap. 17, 18) and if the quantity of the aspirated liquid allows also analysed by a cytologist (see Chap. 15) and, especially in cases with low-grade symptoms, also by molecular methods (see Chap. 19). There is a general consensus to withhold the antibiotics for two weeks before the aspiration in patients without serious systemic signs of infections [1]. Since the sensitivity of the aspiration is about 70 % (Chapter 14, 17, 18) a repeat aspiration is justified in some patients, where clinical data and other previous evaluations like bone scans, laboratory evaluation etc. indicate high probability of a PJI.

The primary goal in the evaluation of PJI is to find out the germ(s) with its antibiotic susceptibility since this information guides further steps. If the treating team was able to diagnose the PJI with a high probability, but was not able to find the germ, the treatment method tend to be the most aggressive, namely, two-stage replacement with a long interval between steps.

23.2.1   The Allocation of Patients with PJI to Treatment Options

It is convenient to divide presenting patients with diagnosed PJI into categories with similar evaluation and treatment needs. The considered information retrieved from the previous chapter serves as the basis for development of the algorithm about the treatment options (Fig. 23.7).

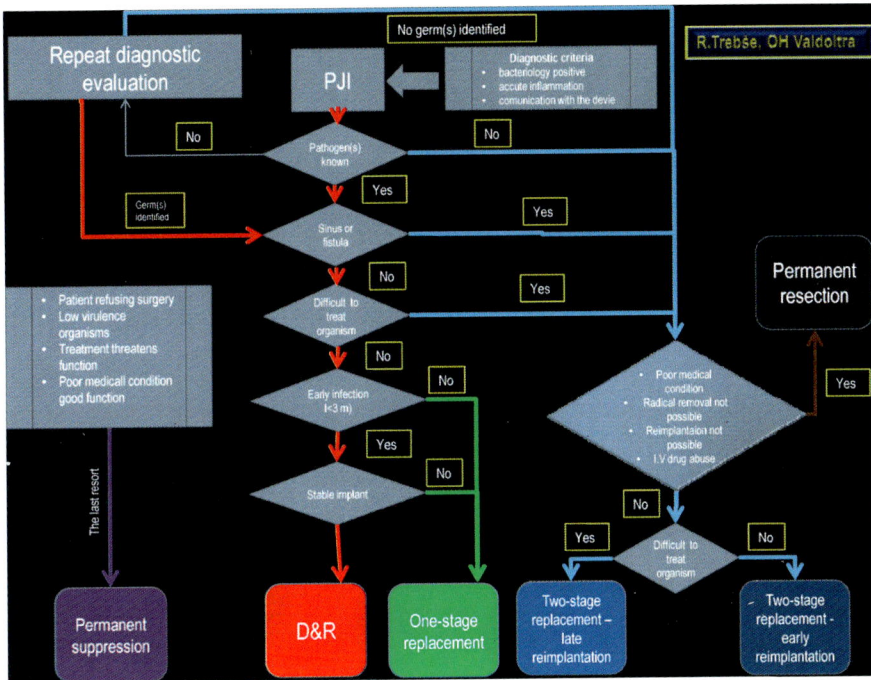

Fig. 23.7 The algorithm for patient allocation to treatment options

23.2.1.1 The Causative Agent

The most important element for the decision about which way to proceed in the treatment protocol is the causative agent with its characteristics especially the susceptibility against antibiotics. *If the treating team was not able to reliably identify the germ, a predictable treatment can only be a two-stage exchange* since the organism may not be responsive to any antibiotic treatment. In this case, it also seems reasonable to avoid spacers. They may act as a foreign body if the unidentified germ (or germs) is not reactive to the antibiotics loaded in the cement that forms the spacer. Unidentified agent may even be a fungus or another type of unusual pathogen with unknown antibiotic affinities like, for instance, those from the genus *Abiotrophia* or *Granulicatella* or mixed flora with diverse antibiotic susceptibility.

It is important to acknowledge that in general, *PJI caused by rifampicin-resistant staphylococci and Gram-negative bacteria resistant to quinolones should better be treated by a two-stage exchange*. If organisms, which are generally described as "difficult to treat" including MRSA, VRE, molds, yeasts, *Granulicatella*, *Abiotrophia*, and "small colony variants," are identified the patient should again only be treated by two-stage exchange. If bacteria that caused the PJI are not reactive to planned antibiotic regimens displayed in Table 23.1, it is better to avoid deb-

Table 23.1 Selection of antibiotics for systemic treatment of PJI [22, 24]

Causative agent	Antibiotic	Dose		Alternative	Dose	
Staphylococci (*S. aureus and CNS*) – penicillin sensitive	benzylpenicillin + rifampicin for 2 weeks, then ciprofloxacin + rifampicin	4 × 5 MU 2 × 450 mg 2 × 750 mg 2 × 450 mg	i.v. p.o. p.o. p.o.	cefamezin + rifampicin amoxicillin + rifampicin	3 × 2 g 2 × 450 mg 3 × 750 mg 2 × 450 mg	i.v. p.o. p.o. p.o.
Staphylococci (*S. aureus and CNS*) – methicillin sensitive	(flu) cloxacillin + rifampicin for 2 weeks, then ciprofloxacin + rifampicin	4 × 2 g 2 × 450 mg 2 × 750 mg 2 × 450 mg	i.v. p.o. p.o. p.o.	cefamezin + rifampicin amoxicillin + cla. + rifampicin	3 × 2 g 2 × 450 mg 2 × 1 g 2 × 450 mg	i.v. p.o. p.o. p.o.
Staphylococci (*S. aureus and CNS*) – methicillin resistant	vancomycin + rifampicin for 4–6 weeks, then	2 × 1 g 2 × 450 mg	i.v. p.o.	teicoplanin + rifampicin co-trimoxazole or fusidic acid, monocyclic and ciprofloxacin + rifampicin	1 × 400 mg 2 × 450 mg 3 × 1 DS tab 3 × 500 mg 2 × 100 mg 2 × 750 mg 2 × 450 mg	i.v., i.m. p.o. p.o. p.o. p.o. p.o. p.o.
Streptococcus sp.	benzylpenicillin for 4 weeks, then amoxicillin + rifampicin	4 × 5 MU 3 × 750 mg 2 × 450 mg	i.v. p.o. p.o.	ceftriaxone clindamycin	1 × 2 g 3 × 600 mg	i.v. p.o.
Enterococcus sp. – penicillin sensitive	benzylpenicillin + gentamicin for 4 weeks, then amoxicillin	4 × 5 MU 2 × 120 mg 3 × 750 mg	i.v. i.v. p.o.	vancomycin + gentamicin amoxicillin	2 × 1 g 2 × 120 mg 3 × 750 mg	i.v. i.v. p.o.
Anaerobes	clindamycin for 2–4 weeks, then clindamycin	3 × 600 mg 3 × 600 mg	i.v. p.o.	metronidazole	4 × 500 mg	p.o.
Enterobacteriaceae – ciprofloxacin sensitive	ciprofloxacin for 1 week, then ciprofloxacin	2 × 400 mg 2 × 750 mg	i.v. p.o	ceftriaxone	1 × 2 g	i.v.
Pseudomonas aeruginosa	ceftazidime + gentamicin for 2–4 weeks, then ciprofloxacin	3 × 2 g 1 × 240 mg 2 × 750 mg	i.v. i.v. p.o.	imipenem/ cilastatin + gentamicin	4 × 500 mg 1 × 240 mg	i.v. i.v.

Table 23.1 (continued)

Causative agent	Antibiotic	Dose		Alternative	Dose
Mixed infections (without methicillin resistant staphylococci)	imipenem/ cilastatin or	4 × 500 mg	i.v.	meropenem	3 × 1 g
	piperacillin/ tazobactam	3 × 4.5 g	i.v.	amox. + clav.	3 × 1.2 g
	for 2–4 weeks, then: individually (infectologist)		?		

Total length of treatment: 3 months (THR, TSR) or 6 months (TKR, TAR).

For patients older than 70, rifampicin doses can be reduced to 300 + 300 mg daily.

Doses must be adjusted depending on renal function, blood cell count, and serum creatinine level.

Methicillin-resistant *S. aureus* should not be treated with fluoroquinolones.

DS tablet equals 160 mg trimethoprim + 800 mg sulfametoxazole.

Vancomycin trough levels should be monitored to achieve the target concentrations 15–20 µg/ml

For *enterococci* and methicillin resistant *staphilococci* daptomincin 8–12 mg/kg can be used in special circumstances.

For gram-positive anaerobes penicillin G or ceftriaxone can be used and metronidazole for the gram-negative, rifampicin 2 x 450mg p.o. can be administrated in Propionibacterium acnes.

MU million units, *p.o.* per os, *i.v.* intravenous, *i.m.* intramuscular.

ridement and retention or one-stage revision and seek a consultation with an infectious disease specialist with experience in device-associated bone infections. The data about the success rates for treatment of PJI caused by these organisms is either not existing or too conflicting to recommend any other option but two-stage exchange (for details, refer to chap. 20).

23.2.1.2   The Duration of Symptoms

Another important element that influences the decision regarding the treatment type is the duration of the symptoms. For acute PJI that last up to 1 month, debridement and retention or one-stage replacement depending on soft tissue status is indicated if the causative agent is identified and the antibiotic susceptibility suitable. There is evidence that it is safe to extend this period to 3 months [21].

Especially in low-grade infections, it is, however, difficult to establish exactly the symptomatic period.

23.2.1.3   The Soft Tissue Quality

It is difficult to objectively visually grade the quality of the soft tissues or the degree of inflammation during the surgical procedure. The easiest way is to consider every wound with a discharging sinus as a contraindication for debridement and retention or one-stage exchange due to poor soft tissue envelope. With internal sinuses that do not communicate through the skin, the reasoning is a bit different. If the surgeon is able to dissect the entire inflamed joint capsule, the soft tissues might be considered acceptable for debridement and retention or one-stage procedure. If, however, there is a sinus extending into the pelvic cavity through an opening in the acetabular dome which cannot be dissected and removed or a similar situation in the popliteal region of the knee, the soft tissues must be considered inadequate for retention or one-stage replacement. In case where during surgical procedure it would be necessary to remove inflamed but viable muscles and tendons to achieve a healthy soft tissue environment, it is better to leave these tissues in place and proceed with a two-stage exchange; otherwise, the functionality could be severely impaired.

23.2.1.4 The Stability of the Implant

There are two levels of assessment of the stability of the implant. Preoperatively, we base our judgment on serial x-rays and arthrography. Occasionally the studies are supplemented with a CT scan (see chap. 14 on imaging).

On the radiographs, we are looking for implant shifting, tilting or subsidence, and radiolucent lines around prosthetic components.

In THA, radiographic acetabular loosening is considered when there is a complete radiolucent line >1 mm in all three zones of DeLee and Charnley, cup migration of more than 3 mm or more than 5° of cup inclination. The femoral component is considered loose if serial radiographs demonstrate a change in position of the femoral component (i.e., subsidence of more than 2 mm or varus or valgus tilt) as described by Engh [8]. Expansile osteolyses do not necessarily determine a loosened implant, but long-term stability might be questioned in their presence.

Despite fulfilling all the criteria described below for retention of the implant, considerable osteolyses (might be encountered in late hematogenous infections) indicate the need for exchange of the implant to avoid early re-revision for mechanical loosening.

The final assessment of stability is performed during surgery. Manual testing for stability of the implants shall be done and a try of removal with one strong blow with the hammer. If the implant does not change in position, it might be considered stable enough to warrant retention if all other prerequisites for retention are met as well.

23.2.2 Debridement and Retention of the Implant

Inclusion Criteria

- Acute early or late infection <1–3 months symptoms duration.
- Known pathogen; susceptible to predetermined antibiotics (Table 23.1) (i.e., *staphylococci* susceptible to rifampicin, Gram-negative organisms to quinolones).
- Good soft tissue envelop (no fistula or sinus tract).
- Stable implant (x-rays and intraoperative manual testing).
- No severe permanent immunosuppression (a relative contraindication).

23.2.3   One-Stage Exchange

Inclusion Criteria

- Symptom duration not limited.
- Known pathogen(s); Staphylococci susceptible to rifampicin, Gram-negative organisms to quinolones.
- Good soft tissue envelop (no fistula or sinus tract).
- No severe permanent immunosuppression (a relative contraindication).

23.2.4   Two-Stage Exchange

All the patients that do not fulfill the criteria for debridement and retention, one-stage reimplantation, or permanent resection arthroplasty are best treated with a two-stage exchange.
Inclusion Criteria

- Patients not suitable for debridement or one-stage exchange and not candidates for permanent resection arthroplasty

23.2.5   Two-Stage Exchange: Early Reimplantation

There is a subgroup of immuno competent patients that are candidates for early reimplantation – a fast track two-stage procedure. The candidates were not suitable for one-stage procedure due to the presence of the fistula or the causative agent was not known, but they were infected with low-grade pathogens, or pathogens with optimal antibiotic susceptibility. The prosthetic joint can be reimplanted during the same hospitalization within 2–4 weeks as soon as the skin has healed. Early results are promising but the long-term success is still to be assessed.

23.2.6   Permanent Resection Arthroplasty

Absolute and Relative Inclusion Criteria

- Patients not suitable for debridement or one-stage exchange.
- Patients with severe dementia.
- Bedridden patents (the reason not related to PJI).
- Intravenous drug abusers.
- Poor medical conditions (ASA 4).
- Retained and extremely difficult to remove foreign material (intrapelvic screws, cement, etc.).
- Patient not willing to attempt reimplantation.

- Severe permanent immunosuppression.
- Difficult-to-treat organisms.
- Repeat failed reimplantation.

23.2.7   Jiont fusion

Indications are the same as for one- or two-stage exchange. The only difference is instrumental fusion instead of implant exchange. The anatomic conditions do not allow for functional prosthetic reconstruction (i.e., no functional knee extensor mechanism etc.). For some PJI (i.e. total ankle arthroplasty infection) the results of fusion are more reliable than the results of the revision.

23.2.8   Amputation

Absolute and Relative Inclusion Criteria

- Life-threatening PJI not responding to resection arthroplasty and antibiotics.
- Repeat unsuccessful two-stage revisions with poor limb function and discharging wound.

23.2.9   Permanent Antibiotic Suppression

Inclusion Criteria

- Patient not willing to sustain further surgery.
- Low-virulence organism.
- Good function of the infected prosthetic joint that would potentially be lost after revision.
- Extremely technically demanding revision.
- Long-term antibiotic tolerance.

23.3   The Surgery

Surgical revision is a necessary step in PJI treatment independently on the treatment option chosen (Except for the antibiotic suppression). During the surgical procedure, extensive debridement is performed by which all necrotic soft tissue and bone are removed. Retained necrotic material is avascular and if it is not completely removed serves as growth medium and a reservoir for pathogenic organisms from where they spread again around the joint after the procedure. In the avascular necrotic tissues, the antibiotic concentrations are very low because the drug can only reach the area by diffusion from the surrounding vascularized tissues. After

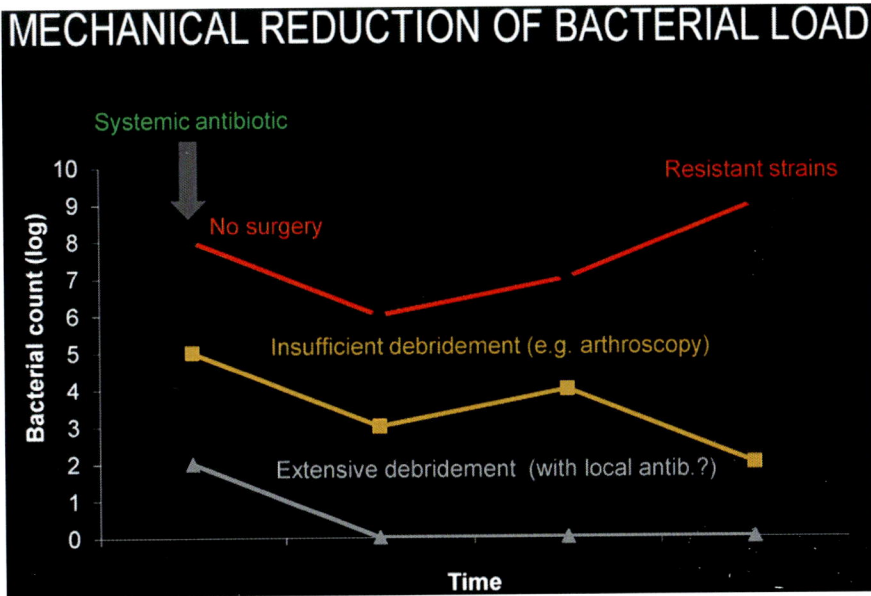

Fig. 23.8 Mechanical reduction of bacterial load

thorough debridement and lavage with large amounts (5 L) of saline, the vast majority of bacteria is removed and the probability for emergence of resistant strains during subsequent antibiotic therapy is considerably reduced (Fig. 23.8).

23.3.1 The Surgical Technique

Depending on the joint involved, it is advisable to choose an extendible approach (Figs. 23.9, 23.10, and 23.11). There is no place for limited approaches in revision total joint arthroplasty being septic or aseptic in nature because unexpected findings or events are frequent. The surgery starts with excision of the previous skin scar (and dissection of the fistula if there is one), and the procedure continues with dissection and removal of infected subcutaneous tissues. Dissection of the joint pseudo-capsule follows. At this point, it is helpful to dissect as much as possible around the pseudo-capsule before entering the joint space. Aspiration of the liquid releases the capsule and provides the sample for cytological, microbiological investigation and Gram staining. After opening the capsule, the joint cavity is thoroughly rinsed with saline and inspected for hidden sinuses and pockets that may not have been seen on preoperative arthrography. The capsule is then removed as well as all pockets that were found (Fig. 23.12). At this stage, three to six tissue biopsies are taken for microbiological investigations as well as one for histopathology. The best samples are pseudomembranes in contact with the implant. If muscles, tendons, major vessels, and nerves are inflamed but seem viable, it is better to debride their surface but

Fig. 23.9 Extended approach for knee revision surgery. Revision of failed hinged total knee arthroplasty

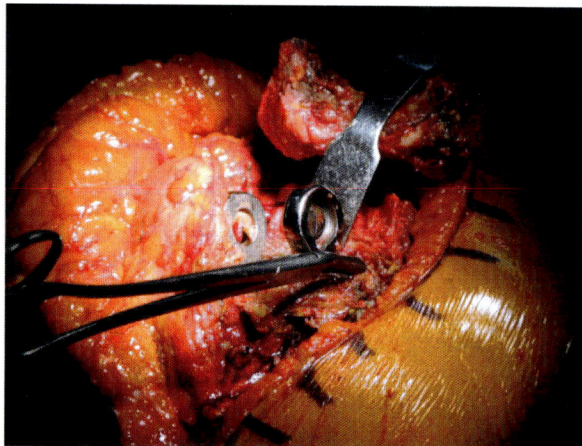

Fig. 23.10 Approach with tibial tubercle osteotomy (Courtesy of S. Kovač, MD)

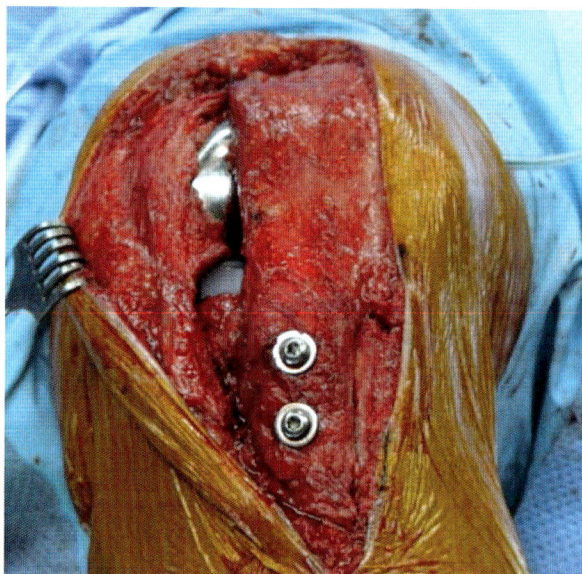

Fig. 23.11 Reimplantation of a revision total hip arthroplasty. A transfemoral approach was needed for removal of the femoral component

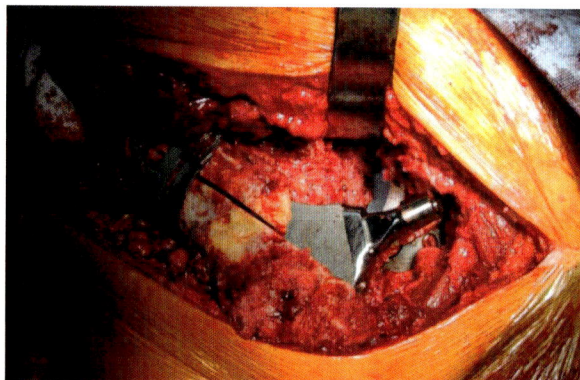

Fig. 23.12 Severe degree of tissue destruction due to PJI at the knee. Tibial component still in situ

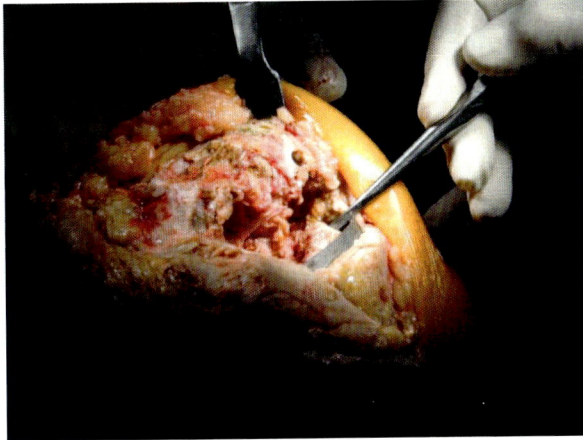

leave these important structures in place. These structures will be necessary for reinstitution of function afterwards.

All dead bone needs to be removed as well as the inflamed bone. The exemption is the bone of the insertion region of a major muscle complex such as tibial tuberosity, trochanter, and similar. It is important to preserve bony attachment of major muscles to retain the function after reconstruction.

In case the criteria for retention are fulfilled, the joint is dislocated and all the exchangeable parts are removed and sonicated. The parts of the joint cavity behind the implant are inspected and debrided if necessary. In case of one- or two-stage exchange, the implant is removed together with all the screws, wires, pins, and bone cement. Every possible effort is needed to remove all pieces of foreign material in the joint proximity. The description of procedures for removal of a stable implant is beyond the scope of this book. The technique is demanding and, besides the necessary experience with revision surgery, necessitates a large variety of revision tools including chisels of many different shapes and thicknesses. The removed implants are placed in boxes for sonication. The bony bed is then checked and the remaining interface membranes removed. After extensive lavage with several liters of saline the bones are prepared for reimplantation, spacer, or being left as such depending on the protocol chosen preoperatively (Fig. 23.13). The wound is meticulously closed in layers and a drain is left in situ. We usually leave the drain closed for 3 h. After that, the drain is opened to release 50 mL of blood once every 4 h (night excluded), until the drainage stabilizes. The drain should be left in situ for up to 7 days depending on the circumstances.

The eventuality of a plastic surgeon's help for wound closure should have already been considered and planned in advance.

After the perioperative prophylaxis has been administrated, the antibiotics are prescribed as planned in accordance with susceptibility of the causative agent if it is known. If the agent is not known, a broad spectrum beta-lactam antibiotic in combination with an aminoglycoside is administered until the results of cultures are available. Other antibiotics might be indicated empirically in case of a particular local microbiological environment.

Fig. 23.13 Debrided soft tissues and bone prepared for one-stage reimplantation of a total knee arthroplasty

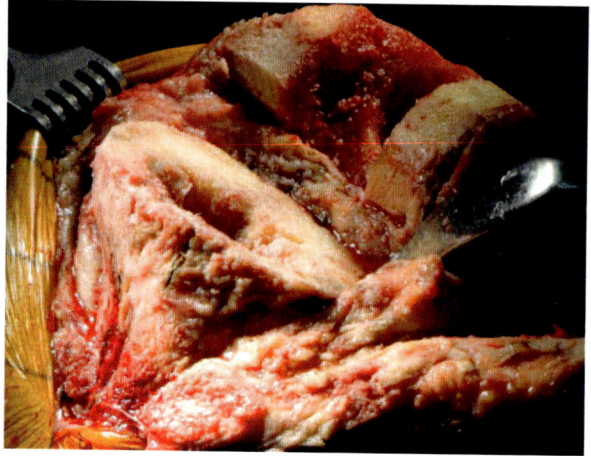

Among the most challenging procedures in PJI surgery is the reimplantation of a total hip arthroplasty after a long-lasting Girdlestone situation with 5 cm or more of shortening. Soft tissue contractions encountered during surgery make it look, at first instance, very difficult or nearly impossible to achieve the correct leg length. We developed a technique that helps in this situation. In the first instance, it is necessary to remove all the fibrous tissue that has formed in place of the former hip joint. The bone in the acetabular region is then prepared and the socket implanted. The selection of the surgical technique and the implant for socket reconstruction depend on the bone loss present. After the socket is securely fixed in the acetabular cavity, the proximal femur is exposed and prepared according to the preoperative plan and then the largest trial rasp is left in situ and the femur is reduced with a short head. If this is readily performed, larger rasps are tried until the reduction with short trial head is hardly possible. With the trial femoral component in situ gentle movements through the range of motion forcing flexion, extension, abduction, and adduction are performed for 5 min, and then the short head is exchanged for the medium one. The procedure is then repeated until we are able to reduce the trial femoral component with the longest head. If the leg length is not yet correct, the rasp is exchanged for a larger one and the steps repeated. It is usually possible to lengthen the leg more than 2 cm from the starting point achieved with the first trial forceful reduction.

23.4   The Systemic Antibiotic Treatment

The antibiotics that are suitable for treatment of PJI must obtain elevated concentrations in bone and be active against adherent bacteria. Bone concentration is dependent on bone vascularity, chemical features of the antimicrobial, lipid solubility, and pH value.

Just after the surgical debridement has been performed, the antibiotic treatments start according to the susceptibility pattern and the protocol from Table 23.1 where

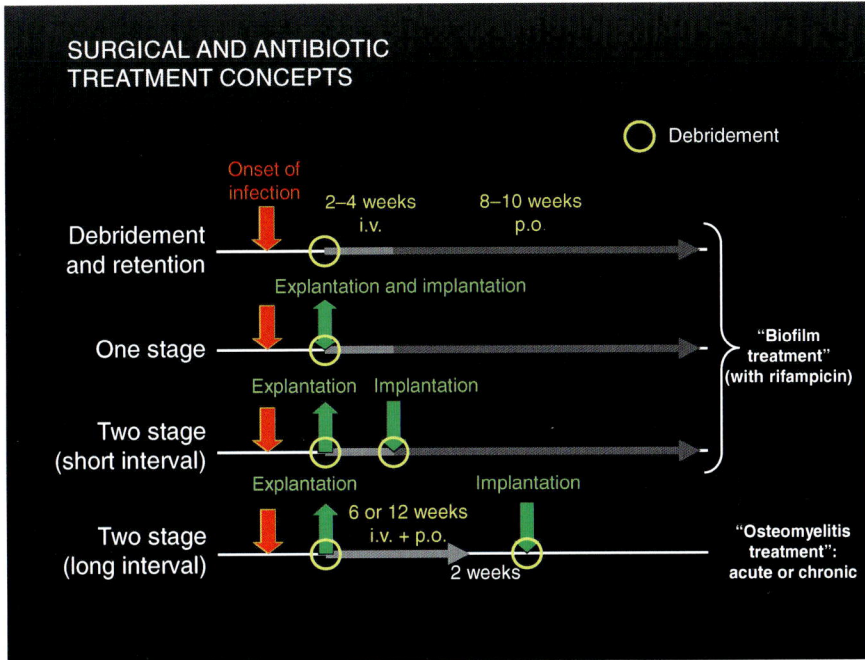

Fig. 23.14 Timetable of surgical intervention and antibiotic treatment

antibiotic dosages are displayed as well. In the case causative agents were not identified before surgery, empirical antibiotic should be administrated based on local bacterial susceptibility pattern. A combination of broad spectrum β-lactam antibiotic (i.e., amoxicillin/clavulanic acid) combined with an aminoglycoside is indicated in institution with low incidence of MRSA.

In case of debridement and retention or one-stage exchange, anti-biofilm antibiotic regimes are administrated (Table 23.1) including rifampicin. *For two-stage exchange or permanent resection, an osteomyelitis antibiotic treatment is administrated for 6 or 12 weeks* for acute (<3 months) or chronic (>3 months) PJI, respectively (Fig. 23.14). *For osteomyelitis treatment, rifampicin is not indicated.*

Staphylococcus aureus PJI systemic antibiotic treatment is the most studied and well supported by in vitro and in vivo studies [25]. Rifampicin is the drug of choice [20] but it, cannot be administered alone because of rapid development of resistance. For early parenteral application, a β-lactam antibiotic like cloxacillin, nafcillin, or cefazolin is suitable for methicillin-sensible and vancomycin or alternatively linezolid [17] for methicillin-resistant *S. aureus*. Linezolid is active against Gram-positive cocci including methicillin-resistant *S. aureus* (MRSA) and vancomycin-resistant *enterococci* (VRE). The utility of the drug is hindered by its toxicity which includes central and peripheral neuropathy and myelosuppression. Daptomycin

(Cubicin®) has the potential of becoming the drug of choice for MRSA and VRE PJI, especially in combination with aminoglycosides, and rifampicin [4, 9].

Initial intravenous treatment should last for 2 weeks for cloxacillin (β-lactam) and 4 weeks for vancomycin. The initial intravenous treatment serves for rapid killing of the planktonic bacteria that were left in the wound after meticulous debridement and lavage. Because of good ability to penetrate the biofilm, and synergistic activity with β-lactams, aminoglycosides can be added [5]. Rifampicin has shown good activity on adhered and slow-growing staphylococci in vitro in animal models and in vivo [2, 21, 25] and should be added to the therapy as soon as the wound dries. To prevent the development of resistant strains, it must not be applied alone but only in combination. After the initial parenteral therapy has been administrated and the infection has dwindled, as confirmed by serial CRP measurements, the oral antimicrobial therapy is prescribed. Optimally rifampicin is combined with a quinolone (ciprofloxacin or levofloxacin). Ciprofloxacin activity does not change within the biofilm in contrast with other antibiotic agents [16]. Depending on the susceptibility profile, rifampicin can be used also in combination with fusidic acid [6], minocycline [11, 18] or co-trimoxazole [19]. As for chronic osteomyelitis treatment in two-stage or permanent resection, the total length of antimicrobial treatment should last for 3 months but for total knee and ankle arthroplasty even 6 months of oral treatment is recommended.

For coagulase-negative staphylococci (CNS), the same antibiotic protocol applies as for *S. aureus*.

Streptococcal PJI are best treated with benzylpenicillin, alternatively with ampicillin, amoxicillin, or ceftriaxone [13, 24] for 4 weeks and after that amoxicillin orally for 2 months (6 months for the knee and ankle replacement).

Enterococcus species PJI treatment typically is initiated with a combination of benzylpenicillin and aminoglycosides (if the bacteria is susceptible), for 2–4 weeks, and continued with amoxicillin orally till the end of the third month (sixth months for the knee and ankle replacement).

Enterobacteriaceae: Not a lot of studies are available reporting clinical results of PJI caused by Gram-negatives. According to bone penetration studies, ease of application and susceptibility profiles quinolones are the treatment of choice for 3 months (or 6 months for total ankle and knee PJI).

Pseudomonas aeruginosa PJI systemic treatment starts with a combination of ceftazidime and aminoglycosides for 2–4 weeks and continues with ciprofloxacin orally till the end of the third month (sixth months for the knee and ankle replacement). This combination was clinically used with success [3].

Anaerobes PJI can be initially treated intravenously with benzylpenicillin or clindamycin for 2–4 weeks and continued orally with clindamycin for the same time span as for the other causative agents. For Propionibacterium acnes rifampicin should be added initially.

Mixed infections (no MRSA or MRCNS included) are better not treated with debridement and retention or one-stage replacement. In case it happens, the possible initial intravenous antimicrobials include imipenem or piperacillin/tazobactam and followed orally according to the antibiotic susceptibility.

References

1. AAOS (American academy of orthopedic surgeons). The diagnosis of periprosthetic joint infections in the hip or knee. Guideline and evidence report. 1st ed. Rosemont: AAOS; 2010. http://www.aaos.org/research/guidelines/guide.asp.
2. Berdal JE, Skramm I, Mowinckel P, Gulbrandsen P, Bjornholt JV. Use of rifampicin and ciprofloxacin combination therapy after surgical debridement in the treatment of early manifestation prosthetic joint infections. Clin Microbiol Infect. 2005;11:834–55.
3. Brouqui P, Rousseau MC, Stain A, Drancourt M, Raoult D. Treatment of *Pseudomonas aeruginosa*-infected orthopedic prostheses with ceftazidime-ciprofloxacin antibiotic combination. Antimicrob Agents Chemother. 1995;39:2423–5.
4. Carpenter CE, Chambers HF. Daptomycin: another novel agent for treating infections due to drug-resistant gram-positive pathogens. Clin Infect Dis. 2004;38:994–1000.
5. Ceri H, Olson ME, Stremick C. The Calgary biofilm device: new technology for rapid determination of antibiotic susceptibility of bacterial biofilms. J Clin Microbiol. 1999;37:1771–6.
6. Drancourt M, Stein A, Argenson JN, Roiron R, Groulier P, Raoult D. Oral treatment of *Staphylococcus spp.* infected orthopaedic implants with fusidic acid or ofloxacin in combination with rifampicin. J Antimicrob Chemother. 1997;39:235–40.
7. Dupont JA. Significance of operative cultures in total hip arthroplasty. Clin Orthop. 1986;211:122–7.
8. Engh CA, Massin P, Suthers KE. Roentgenographic assessment of the biologic fixation of porous-surfaced femoral components. Clin Orthop. 1990;257:107–28.
9. Furustrand Tafin U, Majic I, Zalila Belkhodja C, Betrisey B, Corvec S, Zimmerli W, Trampuz A. Gentamicin improves the activities of daptomycin and vancomycin against *Enterococcus faecalis* in vitro and in an experimental foreign-body infection model. Antimicrob Agents Chemother. 2011;55:4821–7.
10. Hallab N, Merritt K, Jacobs JJ. Metal sensitivity in patients with orthopedic implants. J Bone Joint Surg Am. 2001;83-a:428–36.
11. Isiklar ZU, Darouiche RO, Landon GC, Beck T. Efficacy of antibiotics alone for orthopaedic device related infections. Clin Orthop. 1996;332:184–9.
12. Kovac S, Trebše R, Milošev I, Pavlov i V, Pišot V. Long-term survival of the straight titanium stem. J Bone Joint Surg Br. 2006;88-B:1567–73.
13. Meehan AM, Osmon DR, Duffy CT, Hanssen AD, Keating MR. Outcome of penicillin-susceptible streptococcal prosthetic joint infection treated with debridement and retention of the prosthesis. Clin Infect Dis. 2003;36:845–9.
14. Milosev I, Trebše R, Kovač S. Materials development and latest results of various bearings. In: Aoi T, Toshida A, editors. Hip replacements, approaches, complications and effectiveness. New York: Nova Science Publishers Inc; 2009.
15. Moojen DJ, van Hellemondt G, Vogely HC, Burger BJ, Walenkamp GH, Tulp NJ, Schreurs BW, de Meulemeester FR, Schot CS, van de Pol I, Fujishiro T, Schouls LM, Bauer TW, Dhert WJ. Incidence of low-grade infection in aseptic loosening of total hip arthroplasty. Acta Orthop. 2010;81:667–73.
16. Ramage G, Tunney MM, Patrick S, Gorman SP, Nixon JR. Formation of *Propionibacterium acnes* biofilms on orthopaedic biomaterials and their susceptibility to antimicrobials. Biomaterials. 2003;24:3221–7.
17. Razonable RR, Osmon DR, Steckelberg JM. Linezolid therapy for orthopedic infections. Mayo Clin Proc. 2004;79:1137–44.
18. Segreti J, Nelson JA, Trenholme GM. Prolonged suppressive antibiotic therapy for infected orthopedic implants. Clin Infect Dis. 1998;27:711–3.
19. Trampuz A, Zimmerli W. Prosthetic joint infections: update in diagnosis and treatment. Swiss Med Wkly. 2005;135:243–51.

20. Trampuz A, Zimmerli W. Antimicrobial agents in orthopedic surgery. Drugs. 2006;66:1089–105.
21. Trebše R, Pisot V, Trampuz A. Treatment of infected, retained implants. J Bone Joint Surg Br. 2005;87-B:249–56.
22. Trebše R. Treatment of orthopedic device related infection with device retention and defined antibiotic therapy. Thesis. University of Ljubljana, Ljubljana. 2010.
23. Tsukajama DT, Estrada R, Gustilo RB. Infections after total hip arthroplasty: a study of the treatment of one hundred and six infections. J Bone Joint Surg Am. 1996;78:512–23.
24. Zimmerli W, Trampuž A, Ochsner P. Prosthetic joint infections. N Engl J Med. 2004;351:1645–54.
25. Zimmerli W, Widmer AF, Blatter M, Frei R, Ochsner PE. Role of rifampin for treatment of orthopedic implant-related staphylococcal infections: a randomized controlled trial. Foreign-Body Infection (FBI) Study Group. JAMA. 1998;279:1537–41.

Chapter 24
Bone Grafts and Bone Graft Substitutes in Infected Arthroplasty

Martin Clauss and Thomas Ilchmann

Abstract Prosthetic joint infections are associated with various degrees of bone loss. Different procedures and materials are available to fill bone defects in this setting. This chapter overviews the indications for use of bone and bone substitutes in two- and one-stage procedures, their benefits, and disadvantages. Differences in bone defect treatment in septic and aseptic revisions are discussed as well.

Keywords Bone grafts • Bone graft substitutes • Revision surgery • Infection

24.1 Introduction

Bone grafts are increasingly used to fill bone defects in orthopedic and trauma surgery [18]. Autologous, fresh cancellous bone grafts are typically harvested from the iliac crest and transplanted as *fresh* bone grafts during the same operation [12], but due to the limited amount of material, they are seldom used in arthroplasty surgery. Alternatively, allogeneic cancellous bone grafts can be harvested from femoral heads during primary hip replacement surgery and stored as so-called *fresh-frozen* bone grafts in a bone bank [16, 27]. During implantation of the artificial joint, they can be either used as structural grafts [20, 22, 40] or morselized for impaction grafting [3, 5, 23]. The combination of both preparations is possible; if necessary, additional reinforcement rings can be used in combination [34].

Another strategy to fill bone defects is the use of *processed cancellous bone grafts (human or bovine)* or *artificial bone grafts* such as β-tricalcium phosphate (β-TCP) or hydroxyapatite (HA) [3, 6]. Some authors also investigated mixing both fresh-frozen human and artificial bone grafts [5, 17]. *Bone graft substitutes* (such as poly(methyl methacrylate)[PMMA]) loaded with antibiotics [8] are a third option in the reconstruction

M. Clauss, M.D. (✉) • T. Ilchmann, M.D., Ph.D.
Department of Orthopedic Surgery, Kantonsspital Basel land Liestal,
Rheinstrasse 26, Liestal, CH-4410, Switzerland
e-mail: martin.clauss@ksli.ch; thomas.ilchmann@ksli.ch

R. Trebše (ed.), *Infected Total Joint Arthroplasty*,
DOI 10.1007/978-1-4471-2482-5_24, © Springer-Verlag London 2012

of bony defects in revision arthroplasty. The fundamental difference between the two latter groups is that bone grafts get incorporated by the host bone and are substituted either completely (fresh-frozen cancellous bone, processed cancellous bone, β-TCP) or partially (HA), while bone graft substitutes are not biodegradable and, thus, remain permanently incorporated in the bone unchanged.

The majority of infections associated with artificial joints are caused by staphylococci (70–90 %) [15, 24, 25], which are typically growing attached on the surface as a specialized structure known as biofilm [11, 24]. Biofilm is recognized as the main challenge in treatment of infections associated with implants and bone surgery [18, 37]. Infections associated with biofilms on foreign material are more difficult to treat than the ones caused by bacteria growing in free-living (planktonic) form. Susceptibility of bacteria growing in biofilm against antibiotics is about 1,000-fold decreased to planktonic counterparts [4, 35, 36, 38, 39]. Eradication of biofilm infections is therefore often only possible by complete removal of the foreign body (arthroplasty) and long-term antimicrobial treatment [13, 18].

In case of infected artificial joints, there are various treatment concepts which are described in detail in this book. In brief, treatment options can be described as either a one-stage or two-stage exchange of the artificial joint. Both concepts have shown reasonable success rates exceeding 90 % curing implant-associated infection [1, 8, 14, 19, 33, 39]. Additionally, debridement and retention of the implant has also shown reasonable results under well-defined circumstances [7, 26, 37, 39]. Alternative treatment options would be a lifelong antibiotic suppression or a girdlestone procedure [37]; both options are not to be discussed in this chapter.

The fundamental difference between two-stage exchange (i) on the one hand and one-stage exchange or debridement and retention (ii) is the treatment of an osteomyelitis in absence of an implant (i) or the treatment of the infection in presence of an arthroplasty (II). Therefore, the two groups and potential impact of bone grafts and bone graft substitutes on the procedures will be discussed separately. There is a complete lack of randomized controlled clinical trials on different treatment options combined with the use of bone grafts and bone graft substitutes in the presence of an infected arthroplasty; thus, only an overview over the current literature is given.

24.2 Two-Stage Exchange

Regarding the use of bone grafts and bone graft substitutes, the two-stage exchange has to be analyzed as two separate procedures: (1) explantation of the infected arthroplasty and management of the dead space and (2) replantation of the arthroplasty.

The first step of a two-stage exchange of infected arthroplasties is usually the complex implant removal including cement bone graft (substitutes) and soft tissue debridement and is performed with a spacer formed out of PMMA and loaded with antibiotics. These spacers are either preformed and industrially loaded with antibiotics or custom-made with an individualized antibiotic loading. The use of antibiotic-loaded PMMA is well established from the treatment of osteomyelitis [29, 30]. The creation of a so-called bead pouch is a variation to fill cavities in the first interval of a two-stage exchange. This would increase the surface area/volume of the bone graft substitute

[31] but will not allow weight bearing of the joint. Thus, this might be an option in the exchange of, e.g., infected shoulder and elbow arthroplasties where weight bearing is not needed. We found only one study [2] dealing with infected total hip arthroplasties using a bead pouch in the first step and impaction grafting in the second step but without the use of any IV antibiotics. The authors were able to show a success rate of 86 % to cure the infection but reported various limitations of the study.

Another option to fill the cavity after explantation of the infected artificial joint might be the use of antibiotic-loaded collagen fleeces [31] or antibiotic-loaded calcium sulfate [28] which is currently used in the treatment of osteomyelitis. There are various other synthetic materials which are currently tested in vitro and in vivo but are currently lacking clinical data.

The concept of generating a bead pouch is as mentioned well established in the treatment of chronic osteomyelitis, but we are not aware of any clinical study dealing with other materials than PMMA in the context of infected arthroplasties.

During replantation (step two), the infection is expected to be cured; thus, the use of local antibiotics is not mandatory. The use of bone grafts and bone graft substitutes in this step therefore depends on the need to reconstruct bony defects and/or to create a stable bone bed for anchoring the implants [3, 5, 20, 22, 23, 40]. Fresh, fresh-frozen, and artificial bone grafts and bone graft substitutes can facultatively be mixed or coated with antibiotics. Buttaro et al. [9] showed good infection control in two-stage exchange on infected total hip arthroplasties with meticulous debridement in the first step followed by IV antibiotics and the use of Vancocin-loaded cancellous bone grafts and impaction grafting in the second stage. We found no clinical data in favor of one or the other concerning success rates in the treatment of infected arthroplasties.

24.3 One-Stage Exchange and Retention and Debridement

Radical debridement is a prerequisite to cure an implant-associated infection. The exchange (one step) or retention of the implant is linked to special prerequisites. Independent from exchange or retention of the implant, an infected operative site cannot be sterilized during surgery by debridement alone. The debridement shall reduce the predominant amount of bioburden, but even the most careful cleaning cannot prevent residual bacterial colonies to remain in niches of the debrided site. Therefore, systemic and/or local antibiotics are mandatory to cure the infection. Buchholz et al. were the first who proved that one-stage revision with the use of antibiotic-loaded PMMA showed reasonable results [8]. Anyhow, one-stage revision using antibiotic-loaded cement has not gained widespread use, although it shows obvious clinical and economic advantages [32].

The antibiotic release from PMMA is low concerning the whole amount of antibiotics added; thus, other carrier materials might be superior to deliver local antibiotics. In one-stage exchange, PMMA has, despite delivering antibiotics, another even more important function, namely, fixation of the implant. Thus, all other potential carrier materials must additionally be able to fix the new implant, too. To our knowledge, there is no clinical nor laboratory data on any other materials except cancellous bone loaded with antibiotics that showed the ability to substitute PMMA.

Winkler et al. developed a method to impregnate allograft bone with high levels of antibiotics and used the prepared material for impaction grafting. They performed 37 one-stage revisions of infected THRs [33] and showed a 92 % success rate curing the infection. They additionally noted that the incorporation of bone graft was comparable with non-impregnated grafts.

We found no clinical data on the additional use of bone grafts or bone graft substitutes as local antibiotic carriers in the context of debridement and retention alone. There might be a potential benefit from high local antibiotic levels in this procedure, too. Anyhow, this advantage might be dearly bought by potential third particle were from loose material finding their way into the bearing surfaces.

24.4 Outlook and Future Development

Current research in material science has developed various materials with increased resistance against infection superior to PMMA [10]. Common shortcoming of all new synthetic materials is that they are not able to withstand the load after implantation of an artificial joint without additional reinforcement [21].

From our point of view, in case of (infected) revision arthroplasty, orthopedic surgeons should rely on proven concepts like antibiotic-loaded PMMA or cancellous bone chips (with/without antibiotics) for impaction grafting at least until the promising new materials are also able to show at least equal mechanical properties.

References

1. Achermann Y, Vogt M, et al. Characteristics and outcome of 27 elbow periprosthetic joint infection: results from a 14-year cohort study of 358 elbow prostheses. Clin Microbiol Infect. 2011;17(3):432–8.
2. Ammon P, Stockley I. Allograft bone in two-stage revision of the hip for infection. Is it safe? J Bone Joint Surg Br. 2004;86(7):962–5.
3. Aulakh TS, Jayasekera N, et al. Long-term clinical outcomes following the use of synthetic hydroxyapatite and bone graft in impaction in revision hip arthroplasty. Biomaterials. 2009; 30(9):1732–8.
4. Baldoni D, Haschke M, et al. Linezolid alone or combined with rifampin against methicillin-resistant *Staphylococcus aureus* in experimental foreign-body infection. Antimicrob Agents Chemother. 2009;53(3):1142–8.
5. Blom AW, Wylde V, et al. Impaction bone grafting of the acetabulum at hip revision using a mix of bone chips and a biphasic porous ceramic bone graft substitute. Acta Orthop. 2009;80(2):150–4.
6. Bohner M. Design of ceramic-based cements and putties for bone graft substitution. Eur Cell Mater. 2010;20:1–12.
7. Brandt CM, Sistrunk WW, et al. *Staphylococcus aureus* prosthetic joint infection treated with debridement and prosthesis retention. Clin Infect Dis. 1997;24(5):914–9.

8. Buchholz HW, Elson RA, et al. Antibiotic-loaded acrylic cement: current concepts. Clin Orthop Relat Res. 1984;190:96–108.

9. Buttaro MA, Pusso R, et al. Vancomycin-supplemented impacted bone allografts in infected hip arthroplasty. Two-stage revision results. J Bone Joint Surg Br. 2005;87(3):314–9.

10. Clauss M, Trampuz A, et al. Biofilm formation on bone grafts and bone graft substitutes: comparison of different materials by a standard in vitro test and microcalorimetry. Acta Biomater. 2010;6(9):3791–7.

11. Costerton JW, Montanaro L, et al. Biofilm in implant infections: its production and regulation. Int J Artif Organs. 2005;28(11):1062–8.

12. De Long Jr WG, Einhorn TA, et al. Bone grafts and bone graft substitutes in orthopaedic trauma surgery. A critical analysis. J Bone Joint Surg Am. 2007;89(3):649–58.

13. Ehrlich GD, Stoodley P, et al. Engineering approaches for the detection and control of orthopaedic biofilm infections. Clin Orthop Relat Res. 2005;437:59–66.

14. Giulieri SG, Graber P, et al. Management of infection associated with total hip arthroplasty according to a treatment algorithm. Infection. 2004;32(4):222–8.

15. Gristina AG. Biomaterial-centered infection: microbial adhesion versus tissue integration. Science. 1987;237(4822):1588.

16. Kappe T, Cakir B, et al. Infections after bone allograft surgery: a prospective study by a hospital bone bank using frozen femoral heads from living donors. Cell Tissue Bank. 2009; 11(3):253–9.

17. Karrholm J, Hourigan P, et al. Mixing bone graft with OP-1 does not improve cup or stem fixation in revision surgery of the hip: 5-year follow-up of 10 acetabular and 11 femoral study cases and 40 control cases. Acta Orthop. 2006;77(1):39–48.

18. Ketonis C, Barr S, et al. Bacterial colonization of bone allografts: establishment and effects of antibiotics. Clin Orthop Relat Res. 2010;468(8):2113–21.

19. Laffer RR, Graber P, et al. Outcome of prosthetic knee-associated infection: evaluation of 40 consecutive episodes at a single centre. Clin Microbiol Infect. 2006;12(5):433–9.

20. Lee PT, Clayton RA, et al. Structural allograft as an option for treating infected hip arthroplasty with massive bone loss. Clin Orthop Relat Res. 2011;469(4):1016–23.

21. Richards RG. Final Presidential Lecture at the 19th Annual meeting European Society of Biomaterials, Lausanne. 2009.

22. Ritter MA, Trancik TM. Lateral acetabular bone graft in total hip arthroplasty. A three- to eight-year follow-up study without internal fixation. Clin Orthop Relat Res. 1985;193:156–9.

23. Slooff TJ, Schimmel JW, et al. Cemented fixation with bone grafts. Orthop Clin North Am. 1993;24(4):667–77.

24. Trampuz A, Zimmerli W. Diagnosis and treatment of infections associated with fracture-fixation devices. Injury. 2006;37 Suppl 2:S59–66.

25. Trampuz A, Zimmerli W. Diagnosis and treatment of implant-associated septic arthritis and osteomyelitis. Curr Infect Dis Rep. 2008;10(5):394–403.

26. Trebse R, Pisot V, et al. Treatment of infected retained implants. J Bone Joint Surg Br. 2005; 87(2):249–56.

27. Van De Pol GJ, Sturm PDJ, et al. Microbiological cultures of allografts of the femoral head just before transplantation. J Bone Joint Surg Br. 2007;89(9):1225.

28. Wahl P, Livio F, et al. Systemic exposure to tobramycin after local antibiotic treatment with calcium sulphate as carrier material. Arch Orthop Trauma Surg. 2011;131(5): 657–62.

29. Walenkamp G. Small PMMA beads improve gentamicin release. Acta Orthop Scand. 1989; 60(6):668–9.

30. Walenkamp GH. Chronic osteomyelitis. Acta Orthop Scand. 1997;68(5):497–506.

31. Walenkamp GH. Self-mixed antibiotic bone cement: western countries learn from developing countries. Acta Orthop. 2009;80(5):505–7.

32. Winkler H. Rationale for one stage exchange of infected hip replacement using uncemented implants and antibiotic impregnated bone graft. Int J Med Sci. 2009;6(5): 247–52.

33. Winkler H, Stoiber A, et al. One stage uncemented revision of infected total hip replacement using cancellous allograft bone impregnated with antibiotics. J Bone Joint Surg Br. 2008; 90(12):1580–4.

34. Winter E, Piert M, et al. Allogeneic cancellous bone graft and a Burch-Schneider ring for acetabular reconstruction in revision hip arthroplasty. J Bone Joint Surg Am. 2001;83-A(6):862–7.

35. Zimmerli W, Frei R, et al. Microbiological tests to predict treatment outcome in experimental device-related infections due to *Staphylococcus aureus*. J Antimicrob Chemother. 1994;33(5): 959.

36. Zimmerli W, Lew PD, et al. Pathogenesis of foreign body infection. Evidence for a local granulocyte defect. J Clin Invest. 1984;73(4):1191–200.

37. Zimmerli W, Trampuz A, et al. Prosthetic-joint infections. N Engl J Med. 2004;351(16): 1645–54.

38. Zimmerli W, Waldvogel FA, et al. Pathogenesis of foreign body infection: description and characteristics of an animal model. J Infect Dis. 1982;146(4):487–97.

39. Zimmerli W, Widmer AF, et al. Role of rifampin for treatment of orthopedic implant-related staphylococcal infections: a randomized controlled trial. Foreign-Body Infection (FBI) Study Group. JAMA. 1998;279(19):1537–41.

40. Zofka P. Results of acetabular reconstruction with solid bone graft in primary and revision hip arthroplasty. Acta Chir Orthop Traumatol Cech. 2006;73(3):190–6.

Appendix A
Pitfalls of Antimicrobial Therapy in Prosthetic Joint Infection

Nataša Faganeli

Abstract In this chapter, the peri- and post-operative monitoring of antibiotic therapy in infected total joint arthroplasty is presented from the clinical pharmacist's point of view. Recommendations for selection, risk factors, and monitoring are given.

The provision of clinical pharmacy service in infected total joint arthroplasty can be considered under a number of sections:

- Medicines reconciliation at every transition of care
- Perioperative medication management
- Monitoring of medical therapy
- Assuring in-patient and out-patient compliance during antimicrobial therapy

Keywords Antibiotics • Adverse events • Prevention • Rifampicin

Introduction

Periprosthetic joint infections are caused by microorganisms growing in biofilms, rendering these infections very difficult to diagnose and to eradicate. The treatment modalities differ from case to case, but always include antimicrobial therapy (Chap. 23). The current recommendations include 2 weeks of parenteral antibiotic treatment, followed by peroral antibiotics for overall duration of 3 months (6 months for knee prosthesis) [1, 2]. Most of the selected antimicrobial agents, especially

N. Faganeli, Pharm.D.
Department of Pharmacy, Orthopedic Hospital Valdoltra,
Jadranska cesta 31, Ankaran SI-6280, Slovenia
e-mail: natasa.faganeli@ob-valdotra.si

R. Trebše (ed.), *Infected Total Joint Arthroplasty*,
DOI 10.1007/978-1-4471-2482-5, © Springer-Verlag London 2012

rifampicin[1]-combination regimens, for treatment of periprosthetic joint infections are related with high incidence of adverse events. Especially the elderly patients are prone to hard-to-bear adverse drug events, which can lead to treatment failure. In this population, the adverse event rate is higher than that of younger adults due to the clinically significant changes in renal and hepatic function, and body composition associated with aging. Another important factor is the number of medications the elderly consume.

The optimal dosage regimen is also of clinical importance for effective antimicrobial therapy. High dosing is needed to achieve sufficient concentration in bone and surrounding tissues [1]. Taking into account the duration of antibiotic treatment, the adverse events are even more likely to occur.

Orthopedic surgeons frequently underestimate the impact of drug–drug and drug–disease interactions on negative results of antimicrobial treatment in these cases. It must be emphasized that most of the potential adverse drug events can be avoided with appropriate strategy, which includes medications reconciliation, drug therapy monitoring, and patient compliance assurance.

Polypharmacy in Orthopedic Surgical Patients

The majority of orthopedic patients undergoing primary total joint arthroplasty (TJA) are of age above 65, one-half of them older than 75, while revision total hip arthroplasty procedures were most commonly reported in the age group 75–84 [3–5]. Polypharmacy in the elderly is a common phenomenon secondary to the amount of medications required to treat the conditions that become more prevalent with age, such as heart disease, lung disease, metabolism problems, and diabetes. The presence of malignancy or systemic autoimmune disease such as rheumatoid arthritis also increases the incidence of polypharmacy [6]. In case of infected total joint arthroplasty, the introduction of antibiotic therapy, usually highly aggressive, can result in unexpected interactions with routinely used medications and lead to poor or negative outcomes. Patients with multiple medications, especially elderly, are at increased risk.

The potential interactions of routinely used medications with newly introduced antibiotic therapy can lead to two opposite situations: treatment failure because of decreased efficacy of antibiotic or, on the other hand, co-existing disease progression because of decreased efficacy of routinely used medications. Nevertheless, adverse drug events can significantly impact patient morbidity and mortality.

Dosing Regimen Impact

According to current concepts, long-term antibiotic treatment with high dose is needed to achieve treatment goals because of the biofilm resistance pattern. Generally the recommended antibiotics for treatment of infected total joint arthroplasty are not

---

[1] Rifampicin (INN) or rifampin (USAN) – vstaviti na dnu strani kot opombo!

officially approved for these indication, which is why the optimal dosing regimen in these cases is not established too. In most cases, the highest labeled dose of selected antibiotic (parenteral and peroral) approved for the most similar indication available is used for the treatment of prosthetic joint infections (PJI) (Chapter 23). However, the study results showed low cure rate when labeled dosing regimen was used for some antibiotics, especially rifampicin and co-trimoxazole [7–12]. Higher doses are needed. Current dosing regimens in contemporary clinical praxis are more or less empirical, without human pharmacokinetic/pharmacodynamics studies support. It must be emphasized that optimal dosing regimen, i.e., route of administration, dose and dosing interval of selected drug, is directly correlated to pharmacokinetic profile of a drug. In drugs with complex, nonlinear pharmacokinetic profile, narrow therapeutic index and significant intra-individual variability due to genetic polymorphisms of metabolizing enzymes, even slight changes in dosage regimen can result in decrease or loss of pharmacological effect and/or adverse events occurrence. Rifampicin has the most complex pharmacokinetic profile among antibiotics used in antimicrobial treatment of infected total joint arthroplasty.

The enormous inconsistency in dosing regimen is present for rifampicin, which has become the cornerstone for the treatment of infected PJI caused by *staphylococci*. According to published studies, the applied daily doses varied from 300 to 1,200 mg, as a single or subdivided doses [13–16]. On the other hand, the published evidence support only rifampicin doses of 450 mg twice daily to achieve high cure rate in combined antibiotic therapy [17]. It must be stressed that selected dosage regimen and duration of treatment strongly impacts on pharmacokinetics of rifampicin. A series of human studies indicate that daily dosages higher than 300–450 mg result in a more-than-proportional increase in both the peak concentrations of the drug and the area under the curve (AUC) in blood because of the saturation of efflux transport system through small intestine wall. The features of this effect differ if the same daily dose is administered as single dose or in subdivides doses. The daily fluctuation in serum concentration is more marked if higher doses are administered as single dose [18, 19]. It is of concern that during prolonged treatment rifampicin's bioavailability decreases from the excellent 93 % to only 68 % due to auto-induction of its own metabolism. Rifampicin's maximal auto-induction is reached in about 4 weeks [20, 21]. In the author's opinion, different dosage regimes can induce such fluctuations of serum concentration of rifampicin that therapeutic levels above MIC are not guaranteed for the entire 24-h time interval. It is very likely that this variability of serum concentrations is strongly dependent on rifampicin auto-induction mechanisms. Further studies are necessary to investigate dosage regimen impact on cure rate in these cases. Until clarification of this topic, the author endorses the use of rifampicin dosage regimen of 450 mg twice daily, supported by the only published randomized control trial (RCT), for combined antimicrobial treatment of PJI caused by *staphylococci*.

Note

- Caution is needed when using *off-label* dosing regimen especially in antibiotics with complex pharmacokinetic profile; the impact on kinetic pattern can lead to an unexpected decrease in efficacy of antibiotic treatment and increase of adverse event incidence.

The Role of Adverse Drug Interactions

In the broadest sense, a drug interaction occurs whenever one drug affects the pharmacokinetics, pharmacodynamics, efficacy, or toxicity of another drug. When the drug combination results in an undesired effect, the drug interaction becomes an adverse drug interaction.

Patients on antibiotic treatment of infected total joint arthroplasty, especially elderly, are highly exposed to adverse drug interactions because of their comorbidities and polypharmacy present. When high doses for prolong time are used, the incidence of adverse drug interactions is even higher. The question is which of them are clinically important? Readers should agree that clinically important adverse drug interactions which lead to adverse events that need treatment can negatively impact on patient compliance and contribute to poor treatment results.

With some simple calculations based on the reported magnitude of an interaction, it is possible to estimate the potential risk to a patient. Based on the degree of risk and the benefit of administering the drugs, the appropriate management options can then be selected [31].

Drug interactions of major clinical significance for antibiotics for infected PJI are listed in Table A.1 [22–30]. Of note is the fact that the beta-lactams rarely cause clinically significant drug–drug interactions.

Rifampicin

Among all antibiotics used for the treatment of infected joint replacements, rifampicin is the most problematic from the drug interaction point of view. Rifampicin is one of the strongest inducers of a number of drug-metabolizing enzymes, having the greatest effect on the expression of cytochrome P450 (CYP) in the liver and in the small intestine, among all drugs currently used. In addition, rifampicin induces some drug transporter proteins, such as intestinal and hepatic P-glycoprotein and MRP (multidrug-resistance protein). Full induction of drug-metabolizing enzymes is reached in about 1 week after starting rifampicin treatment and the induction dissipates in roughly 2 weeks after discontinuing rifampicin. Rifampicin has its greatest effects on the pharmacokinetics of orally administered drugs that are metabolized by CYP3A4, CYP2C9, and CYP2C19 and/or are transported by P-glycoprotein and MRP [32, 33].

Thus, for example, oral midazolam, triazolam, simvastatin, verapamil, and most dihydropyridine calcium channel antagonists are ineffective during rifampicin treatment. The plasma concentrations of several anti-infectives, such as the antimycotics itraconazole and ketoconazole and the HIV protease inhibitors indinavir, nelfinavir, and saquinavir, are also greatly reduced by rifampicin. The use of rifampicin with these HIV protease inhibitors is contraindicated to avoid treatment failures. Rifampicin can cause acute transplant rejection in patients treated with immunosuppressive drugs, such as cyclosporin. In addition, rifampicin reduces the plasma concentrations of methadone, leading to symptoms of opioid withdrawal in most patients. Rifampicin also induces CYP2C-mediated metabolism and thus reduces the plasma concentrations of, for example, the substrate (S)-warfarin and the sulfonylurea antidiabetic drugs. In addition, rifampicin can reduce the plasma concentrations of drugs that are not metabolized (e.g., digoxin) by inducing drug transporters such as P-glycoprotein. Thus, the effects of rifampicin on drug metabolism and transport are broad and of established clinical significance [34, 35].

The main concern is caused by substantial intra- and inter-individual pharmacokinetic variability due to the presence of gene polymorphism of drug influx and efflux transporter genes. These polymorphisms result in significant reduction in rifampicin AUC0-24. The presence of transporter gene polymorphisms is highly unpredictable and probably the reason of unexpected adverse drug interaction or treatment failure [36].

Potential drug interactions should be considered whenever beginning or discontinuing rifampicin treatment. It is particularly important to remember that the concentrations of many of the other drugs used by the patients will increase when rifampicin is discontinued as the induction starts to decrease!

Complementary and Alternative Medicines

Patients on antibiotic therapy are very likely to use complementary and alternative medicines (CAMs) in good faith of avoiding adverse event due to antibiotics and contribute to better treatment outcome. However, CAMs, i.e., glucosamine, chitosan, St. John's Worth, vitamins and minerals, CoQ10, therapeutic nutrition shakes, are related with potentially or confirmed serious interactions with prescription medicines concurrently taken [37]. We must take into account the unregulated nature of many CAM products and that the suspected mechanism of an interaction may not be what it appears. During antibiotic treatment, especially rifampicin-based, all CAMs should be avoided. Caution is also needed in the enterally fed patients because of increased incidence of diarrhea due to concomitant therapy with antibiotics [38]. Enteral feeding products also significantly decrease the absorption of quinolones, thus a particular attention must be put on correct dosing time between both [39].

Note

- The majority of adverse drug–drug and drug–disease interactions can be predicted.
- Half-lives of two interacting drugs are not good indicators to estimate the time required for induction onset and offset.
- Adverse drug interaction could result not only after drug introduction, but also after drug discontinuation.
- Drug interaction classification systems should be used only for general guidance! The individual patient risk factors and variables evaluation should always be the platform for decision on suitable course of action.

Table A.1 Antibiotics, used in infected TJA, drug interaction of major clinical significance

Antibiotic	Drug	Interaction type	Action
Rifampicin	Warfarin	Increased warfarin metabolism	Switch to LMWH[a]
	Dabigatran	Increased dabigatran efflux transport	Switch to LMWH
	Rivaroxaban	Increased rivaroxaban efflux transport and metabolism	Switch to LMWH
	Clopidrogel	Increased clopidrogel active metabolite production	Therapy monitoring or change therapy
	PPI[b]	Dose dependent induction of PPI metabolism (no clinical sign of pantoprazole metabolism induction)	Switch to pantoprazole
	Tamoxifen	Increased tamoxifen metabolism	Change therapy
	Cyclosporine	Increased cyclosporine metabolism	Change therapy
	Antiarrhytmics[c]	Increased antiarrhytmic metabolism	Change therapy; in case of amiodarone, increase dose and monitor efficacy
	Calcium channel blockers	Increased metabolism	Change therapy
	Azole antifungal agents[d]	Decrease concentration of azole antifungal agents	Avoid combination, change therapy
	Leflunomide	Increased serum concentrations of the active metabolite of leflunomide	Therapy monitoring or change therapy
	Benzodiazepines (metabolized by oxidation)	Increase the metabolism	Therapy monitoring or change therapy to lorazepam, oxazepam
	Boosted saquinavir	Significant hepatocellular toxicity	Avoid combination, change therapy
	Atazanavir	Decrease the serum concentration of atazanavir	Avoid combination, change therapy
	Oral contraceptives	Decreased contraceptive efficacy	Change to alternative method of contraception
	Food	Significantly decrease absorbtion	Only on empty stomach

Ciprofloxacin	Warfarin	Enhance the anticoagulant effect of warfarin	Therapy monitoring
	Antacides	Decrease the absorption	Correct dosing time or change therapy
	BCG	Diminish the therapeutic effect of BCG	Avoid combination
	Didanosine	Decrease the serum concentration	Use systemic route of administration of ciprofloxacin or change therapy
	Tizanidine	Increased concentration of tizanidine	Avoid combination
	Theophylline derivatives	Decrease the metabolism of theophylline derivatives	Therapy monitoring
Minocyclin	Cyclosporine	Increased concentration of cyclosporine	Therapy monitoring
	Phenitoin	Decrease concentration of phenitoin	Therapy monitoring
	Retinoic acid derivatives	Enhance the adverse/toxic effect of retinoic acid derivatives	Avoid combination
	Divalent or trivalent cation	Decrease the absorption	Correct dosing time or change therapy
Fusidic acid	Protease inhibitors	Decrease the metabolism of fusidic acid	Change therapy
Cotrimoxazole	Methotrexate	Enhance the adverse/toxic effect of methotrexate	Change therapy
	Warfarin	Enhance the anticoagulant effect of warfarin	Avoid combination
Gentamicin	Agalsidase alfa	Diminish the therapeutic effect of agalsidase alfa	Avoid combination
Imipenem/cilastatin	Ganciclovir	Increase risk of seizures	Avoid combination
Penicillin G	Probenecid	Increase the serum concentration	Therapy monitoring
Cephalosporins	Probenecid	increase the serum concentration	Therapy monitoring
Daptomycin	HMG-CoA reductase inhibitors (statins)	Increase skeletal muscle toxicity	Avoid combination

[a] *LMWH* low molecular weight heparins
[b] *PPI* proton pump inhibitors
[c] Antiarrhymics – propafenone, dronedarone
[d] Azole antifungal agents – fluconazole, itraconazole, ketoconazole

Adverse Events Impact

Among orthopedic surgeons, there is a common belief that side effects of prolong antibiotic treatment are mild and there is no need of treatment interruption [1, 2, 15]. In fact, none of the published studies on treatment of PJI have discussed this issue. Antibiotics commonly used in PJI treatment are very likely to cause adverse events. The incidence and severity of antibiotic adverse event is increased especially in elderly patients due to their altered pharmacokinetic and pharmacodynamics patterns, comorbidities, and the presence of polypharmacy. High dosing regimen and prolonged duration of antibiotic therapy are additional factors. Severe adverse event leads to discontinuation of treatment with selected antibiotic and transition to, in most cases, suboptimal antibiotics. Additionally interruption of treatment or noncompliance with treatment regimen is highly present in case of hard-to-bear adverse events among outpatients on prolonged antibiotic treatment. All these facts have strong negative impact on the cure rate of infected total joint arthroplasty.

These adverse events are in most cases preventable or at least ameliorable if the strict and continuous therapy monitoring is implemented during hospital stay and after discharge [6, 40].

Hypersensitivity

Among all antibiotics used in the treatment of infected TJA, beta-lactams have the greatest potential to induce hypersensitivity reactions. Immunoglobulin E (IgE)-mediated hypersensitivity reactions to penicillins occur in between 1 and 10 % of exposed patients, but true anaphylactic reactions occur in less than 0.05 % of treated patients. There is an association with increased incidence when beta-blockers are used concomitantly with penicillins. Delayed hypersensitivity reactions include drug fever, erythema nodosum, and a serum-sickness-like syndrome, hypersensitivity rashes are particularly common with semisynthetic penicillins such as ampicillin, cotrimoxazol, and clindamycin. Cephalosporins, fluoroquinolones, and vancomycin are implicated as well, but to a lesser degree [39]. The use of minocycline is associated with serum-sickness-like reactions [41]. Daptomycin is associated with rare but life-threatening eosinophilic pneumonia in cases of treatment that last >2 weeks [42]. Predicting hypersensitivity is difficult. Skin testing is only helpful in predicting reactions caused by IgE antibodies. Most nonpruritic maculopapular rashes are not predictable by skin testing. Very useful in detecting the sensitization in progress is the monitoring the eosinophil count during the antibiotic therapy, especially with penicillins, vancomycin, and daptomycin. Although significant allergic disease can occur in the absence of eosinophilia, allergic disorder remains the most common cause of significant increase of eosinophil count [43].

Note

- Most allergic reactions occur within hours to 2 weeks after taking the medication. However, rashes may develop up to 6 weeks after starting certain types of medications.

- Fever, nausea, vomiting, diarrhea, abdominal pain or cramps are uncommon symptoms of a drug allergy, often unrecognizable as such.
- Eosinophil count especially during parenteral antibiotic therapy should be monitored.

Nephrotoxicity

In PJI antibiotic treatment, nephrotoxicity is relatively frequent because it is mostly dose related. Age depending changes in renal function and nephrotoxic concomitant drugs are additional factors. It must be emphasized that nephrotoxicity means toxic effect of the drug on kidneys and should not be confused with dose adjustment needed in antibiotics with predominately renal excretion because of decreased renal function. Aminoglycosides, sulfonamides (cotrimoxazole), and minocyclin may affect renal function by directly effecting tubules, while rifampicin and vancomycin are associated with acute interstitial nephritis.

Note

- Nephrotoxicity should not be confused with the fact that some medications have a predominantly renal excretion and need their dose adjusted for the decreased renal function.

Gastrointestinal Toxicity

Nausea, vomiting, and increased bowel peristalsis, sometimes amounting to diarrhea, are common, but are generally of minor inconvenience during the majority of oral antibiotic treatment regimens. Oral treatment for PJI is mostly based on rifampicin, ciprofloxacin, minocyclin, clindamycin, fusidic acid, cotrimoxazole, and amoxicillin, depending on the causing microorganism. Gastrointestinal side effects in this cases are very common and hard-to-bear because large doses are applied for a long time mainly in elderly patients with polypharmacy as a rule. Rifampicin, fusidic acid, clindamycin, and minocycline are associated with high incidence of epigastric distress, flatulence, heartburn, nausea, and vomiting. The author recommends to introduce proton pump inhibitors (PPI) until the end of the antibiotic treatment. Pantoprazole should be the therapy of choice because of the smallest impact on CYP-mediated metabolism of concomitant antibiotics. Nausea and vomiting, if present, occur mostly in 3–5 days after introduction of oral antibiotic treatment and in most cases disappears after a few days. Short-term therapy with an antiemetic is reasonable in these cases, especially considering the potential patient rejection and omission of antibiotic treatment. Diarrhea occurs in 2 % of patients on ciprofloxacin and in about 5–10 % of patients taking oral ampicillin or clindamycin [23]. The most notorious complication is *Clostridium difficile*-related colitis with high mortality rate among elderly patients. To avoid the development of pseudomembranous colitis, the author recommends to interrupt the antibiotic treatment in elderly patients as soon diarrhea occurs and to switch to another antibiotic, if possible.

Hepatotoxicity

Several antibiotics used for treatment of PJI, including clindamycin and fusidic acid, can produce minor elevation in liver enzymes. However, rifampicin, amoxicillin-clavunate, and cotrimoxazole are associated with acute cholestatic injury. Elderly patients receiving >2 weeks of treatment appear at significantly increased risk of flucloxacillin-associated jaundice. Prolonged treatment with linezolid has been associated with severe liver failure and lactic acidosis [44]. Rifampicin has the highest rate of hepatotoxic adverse events due to prolong treatment with high doses. Hepatitis and jaundice have occurred mainly in patients with underlying liver disease and in combination with other hepatotoxic agents [45]. Serum transaminases and bilirubin should be measured at baseline and every 2–4 weeks during therapy. Elevated liver function tests per se are not a contraindication to the use of rifampicin unless they indicate worsening or acute liver disease. Strict monitoring of these patients, however, is crucial. In cases when high levels persist, rifampicin should be discontinued at once.

Note

- Elevated levels often occur transiently in 10–15 % of patients, usually during first 3–5 days of treatment with rifampicin. Rifampicin should be promptly discontinued when high levels persist.

Administration Type Impact

Due to high dosing of antibiotics used in treatment of PJI, the occurrence of peripheral vein thrombophlebitis during intravenous therapy is very likely, especially with antimicrobial agents available in powder. The incidence of adverse events due to intravenous administration depends directly on reconstruction technic (filters should be routinely used to minimize particle contamination), diluent used, concentration of the reconstructed solution and flowrate. Clinical signs of peripheral vein thrombophlebitis (i.e., increased CRP level, fever) are too often underestimated and wrongly interpreted as symptoms of the current infection rather than side effects of the intravenous therapy. The highest rate of complications related to intravenous administration is present with strongly acidic drugs such as vancomycin, penicillin G, and ceftazidime.

The rate and clinical importance of these complications can be highly reduced or prevented by following precise reconstruction and administration instructions provided by pharmacy service and adapted to each case separately.

Fluid and electrolyte overload is another possible, but in clinical praxis often overlooked adverse event after administration of large parenteral doses of certain antibiotics, available as sodium or potassium salts. Ampicillin, piperacillin and ticarcillin, imipenem/cilastatin and ceftazidime contain high quantity of sodium. Large doses for prolonged time can result in sodium overloading and congestive cardiac failure, particularly in patients with impaired renal function. Thus, sodium-containing agents should be avoided in patients who are edematous or hypervolemic. Penicillin G is available as sodium or potassium salt. Alternating both types of salts when large doses are needed is advantageous in patient with impaired renal function.

How to Avoid Pitfalls?

Medicine Reconciliation

Medicine reconciliation is the process of comparing a patient's medicine orders to all of the medicines that the patient has already been taking. This reconciliation is done to avoid medication errors such as omissions, duplications, and dosing errors at every transition of care [46]. Interventions by clinical pharmacists also address and correct some of recognized weaknesses in prescribing arrangements due to drug interactions. In this way, the negative impact of drug–drug and drug–disease interactions on efficacy of antimicrobial treatment can be avoided or minimized.

Perioperative Medication Management

In the case of surgical intervention in PJI surgery-specific drugs and typical medications used for the treatment of intra- and early post-operative complications can interact with concomitant antimicrobial agents, leading to significant adverse events. On the other hand, parenteral antibiotic treatment as a rule in early postoperative period can result in high increase of surgery-related complication rate. Elderly patients with significant renal failure, presence of pulmonary embolism, significant electrolyte imbalance, excessive blood loss are the most frequently exposed to this danger. The selection of antibiotic agent and its dosage regimen should be promptly adjusted on patient current status.

Therapeutic Drug Monitoring

Therapeutic drug monitoring (TDM) is defined as a strategy by which the dosing regimen for a patient is guided by repeated measurements of plasma drug concentrations [47]. TDM is used to avoid drug toxicity and to improve therapeutic efficacy. In PJI it is reasonable to undertake TDM during treatment with vancomycin and aminoglycosides (gentamycin), especially in elderly patients, receiving >2 weeks of treatment, significant blood loss (hemoglobin < 100 g/L) and renal impairment. It must be emphasized that the inappropriate timing of blood sampling leads to misleading results!

Drug Therapy Monitoring

Monitoring drug treatment allows for assessing the degree of therapeutic response and detecting the adverse events. Through targeted routine lab testing it is possible to detect declinations prior the adverse events occurrence. Laboratory tests include monitoring parameters for liver and kidney functions, complete blood count and all other relevant laboratory data, depending on pharmacokinetic and pharmacodynamic profile of the target drug. The frequency of these tests should be based on clinical judgment of the patient's status and the anticipated frequency of the incidence of the potential singular adverse event.

Patient Compliance

In prolonged antibiotic treatment, patient adherence to therapeutic regimen is of great importance for good clinical outcome. Patient compliance influence on treatment failure is underestimated. In published studies on the treatment of PJI, this issue is regularly missing. Duration of antibiotic treatment and hard-to-bear side effects are the main reasons for poor compliance, increased by older age, lower educational levels and lower socioeconomic status. Strategies for improving patient compliance include better patient education, clear and simple instructions, tailoring the treatment to the patient's life-style, encouragement of family support, informing patients about side-effects, monitoring of adherence and provision of feedback to the patient in case of problems.

Conclusion

Current recommendations for the treatment of PJI include prolonged antibiotic treatment with application of high doses because of biofilm resistance pattern. Rifampicin-based combination regimen is the most common due to high incidence of staphylococcal infections. Although drug-related complications in patients with PJI are common and severe, orthopedic surgeons still underestimate their impact on the treatment failure.

The majority of patients with PJI are elderly and are prone to hard-to-bear adverse drug events which can lead to treatment failure. In this population, the adverse event rate is higher than in younger adults due to clinically significant changes in renal and hepatic function, and body composition associated with aging. Polypharmacy is another important issue which must be taken into account when introducing antibiotic therapy. Unexpected drug–drug or drug–disease interaction can result in high incidence of adverse events, leading to antibiotic treatment discontinuation and significant increase in patient morbidity and mortality rate.

Another important issue is patient adherence to antibiotic treatment. Especially out-patient compliance can be very poor due to duration of therapy and high rate of adverse events.

There are therefore different approaches from clinical pharmacy service for the prevention of drug-related complications impact on treatment failure:

- Medicines reconciliation of newly introduce antibiotic agent with already taken drugs
- Perioperative medication management in surgery patients
- Monitoring of medicine therapy
- Assuring in-patient and out-patient compliance during antimicrobial therapy

In this way the majority of drug-related complications can be avoided.

Take Home Messages

- Medicines reconciliation, perioperative medication management, monitoring of medicine therapy and assuring in-patient and out-patient compliance during antimicrobial therapy are essential tools for avoiding drug-related complications during antibiotic treatment of infected TJA.
- The dosing regimen of parenteral antibiotic should be always adjusted to individual patients before its introduction.
- When a change/adjustment in concurrently medication therapy with introduction of antibiotic treatment is needed, the readjustment should be done after the discontinuation of antibiotic treatment.
- Routine out-patient clinical pharmacy services should be adopted for patient on prolong antibiotic treatment.

References

1. Trampuz A, Zimmerli W. Persistence of infection in device-associated infection. J Bone Joint Surg Br. 2011;93-B:320–1.
2. Trampuz A, Zimmerli W. Diagnosis and treatment of implant-associated septic arthritis and osteomyelitis. Curr Infect Dis Rep. 2008;10(5):394–403.
3. DeFrances CJ, Podgornik MN. National Hospital Discharge Survey. Adv Data. 2006;371:1–19.

4. Mahomed NN, Barrett J, Katz JN, Baron JA, Wright J, Losina E. Epidemiology of total knee replacement in the United States Medicare population. J Bone Joint Surg Am. 2005;87(6):1222–8.

5. Bozic KJ, Kurtz SM, Lau E, Ong K, Vail TP, Berry DJ. The epidemiology of revision total hip arthroplasty in the United States. J Bone Joint Surg Am. 2009;91:128–33.

6. Wooten J, Galavis J. Polypharmacy. Keeping the elderly safe. RN. 2005;68(8):44–50.

7. Blaser J, Vergères P, Widmer AF, Zimmerli W. In vivo verification of in vitro model of antibiotic treatment of device-related infection. Antimicrob Agents Chemother. 1995;39(5):1134–9.

8. Zimmerli W, Frei R, Widmer AF, Rajacic Z. Microbiological tests to predict treatment outcome in experimental device-related infections due to *Staphylococcus aureus*. J Antimicrob Chemother. 1994;33:959–67.

9. Stein A, Bataille JF, Drancourt M, Curvale G, Argenson JN, Groulier P, Raoult D. Ambulatory treatment of multidrug-resistant Staphylococcus-infected orthopedic implants with high-dose oral co-trimoxazole (trimethoprim-sulfamethoxazole). Antimicrob Agents Chemother. 1998;42(12):3086–91.

10. Sánchez C, Matamala A, Salavert M, Cuchí E, Pons M, Anglés F, Garau J. Cotrimoxazole plus rifampicin in the treatment of staphylococcal osteoarticular infection. Enferm Infecc Microbiol Clin. 1997;15(1):10–3.

11. Norden CW, Keleti E. Treatment of experimental staphylococcal osteomyelitis with rifampin and trimethoprim, alone and in combination. Antimicrob Agents Chemother. 1980;17:591–4.

12. Stein A, et al. Ambulatory treatment of Staphylococcus-infected orthopedic implants. In: Waldvogel FA, Bisno AL, editors. Infections associated with indwelling medical devices. 3rd ed. Washington, DC: ASM Press; 2000.

13. Moran E, Byren I, Atkins BL. The diagnosis and management of prosthetic joint infections. Antimicrob Chemother. 2010;65 Suppl 3:iii45–54.

14. Barberán J. Management of infections of osteoarticular prosthesis. Clin Microbiol Infect. 2006;12 Suppl 3:93–101.

15. Bliziotis IA, Ntziora F, Lawrence KR, Falagas ME. Rifampin as adjuvant treatment of Gram-positive bacterial infections: a systematic review of comparative clinical trials. Eur J Clin Microbiol Infect Dis. 2007;26(12):849–56.

16. Gómez J, Rodríguez M, Baños V, et al. Orthopedic implant infection: prognostic factors and influence of long-term antibiotic treatment on evolution. Prospective study, 1992–1999. Enferm Infecc Microbiol Clin. 2003;21(5):232–6.

17. Zimmerli W, Widmer AF, Blatter M, Frei R, Ochsner PE. Role of rifampin for treatment of orthopedic implant-related staphylococcal infections. JAMA. 1998;279:1537–41.

18. Acocella G. Clinical pharmacokinetics of rifampicin. Clin Pharmacokinet. 1978;3:108–27.

19. Acocella G. Pharmacokinetics and metabolism of rifampin in humans. Clin Infect Dis. 1983;5 Suppl 3:S428–32.

20. Denti P, et al. A population pharmacokinetic model for rifampicin auto-induction. In: 3rd International Workshop on Clinical Pharmacology of TB Drugs, Boston. September 2010.

21. Loos U, Musch E, Jensen JC, Mikus G, Schwabe HK, Eichelbaum M. Pharmacokinetics of oral and intravenous rifampicin during chronic administration. Klin Wochenschr. 1985;63(23):1205–11.

22. Baxter K, editor. Stockley's drug interactions 9. [CD-ROM]. London: Pharmaceutical Press; 2010.

23. Lexi-Comp, Inc. (Lexi-Drugs™). Hudson: Lexi-Comp, Inc.; 29 January 2011.

24. Bound BL, Johnstone L, McKay GA. Long term treatment with rifampicin for pruritis has implications for warfarin use. SMJ. 2009;54(1):58.

25. Krajewski KC. Inability to achieve a therapeutic INR value while on concurrent warfarin and rifampin. J Clin Pharmacol. 2010;50(6):710–3.

26. Craig RL, Kimberly AT. Difficulties in anticoagulation management during coadministration of warfarin and rifampin. Pharmacotherapy. 2001;21:1240–6.

27. Prescribing information. Pradaxa (dabigatran etexilate). Ridgefield: Boehringer Ingelheim Pharmaceuticals, Inc.; October 2010.

28. Ogilvie BW, et al. The proton pump inhibitor, omeprazole, but not lansoprazole or pantoprazole, is a metabolism-dependent inhibitor of CYP2C19: implications for coadministration with clopidogrel. Drug Metab Dispos. 2011;39(11):2020–33.
29. Judge HM, Patil SB, Buckland RJ, Jakubowski JA, Storey RF. Potentiation of clopidogrel active metabolite formation by rifampicin leads to greater P2Y12 receptor blockade and inhibition of platelet aggregation after clopidogrel. J Thromb Haemost. 2010;8(8):1820–7.
30. Kivisto KT, Billikka K, Nyman L, et al. Tamoxifen and toremifene concentrations in plasma are greatly decreased by rifampin. Clin Pharmacol Ther. 1998;64:648–54.
31. Horn JR, Hansten PD. Ignoring drug interactions for the right reasons. Available on: http://www.pharmacytimes.com/publications/issue/2009/november2009/DrugInteractions-1109/. Accessed on Sept 2011.
32. Rae JM, Johnson MD, Lippman ME, Flockhart DA. Rifampin is a selective, pleiotropic inducer of drug metabolism genes in human hepatocytes: studies with cDNA and oligonucleotide expression arrays. J Pharmacol Exp Ther. 2001;299(3):849–57.
33. Niemi M, Backman JT, Fromm MF, Neuvonen PJ, Kivistö KT. Pharmacokinetic interactions with rifampicin: clinical relevance. Clin Pharmacokinet. 2003;42(9):819–50.
34. Horn JR, Hansten PD. Drug interactions: insights and observations time course for enzyme induction and de-induction. Available on: http://www.hanstenandhorn.com/hh-article04-11.pdf. Accessed on 29 Aug 2011.
35. Finch CK, Chrisman CR, Baciewicz AM, Self TH. Rifampin and rifabutin drug interactions: an update. Arch Intern Med. 2002;162(9):985–92.
36. Weiner M, et al. Effects of tuberculosis, race, and human gene SLCO1B1 polymorphisms on rifampin concentrations. Antimicrob Agents Chemother. 2010;54(10):4192–200.
37. Dietary supplements – balancing consumer choice and safety. Task force on life and the law, New York State Department of Health. Available on: http://www.health.state.ny.us/regulations/task_force/docs/dietary_supplement_safety.pdf. Accessed on Sept 2011.
38. Bowling TE. Clinical quality. Diarrhoea in the enterally fed patient. Frontline Gastroenterol. 2010;1:140–3.
39. Gleckman RA, Czachor JS. Antibiotic side effects. Semin Respir Crit Care Med. 2000;21(1):53–60.
40. Pirmohamed M, James S, Meakin S, Green C, Scott AK, Walley TJ, Farrar K, Park BK, Breckenridge AM. Adverse drug reactions as cause of admission to hospital: prospective analysis of 18 820 patients. BMJ. 2004;329(7456):15–9.
41. Bettge AM, Gross GN. A serum sickness-like reaction to a commonly used acne drug. JAAPA. 2008;21(3):33–4.
42. Medicines and Healthcare products Regulatory Agency. Drug Safety Update. February 2011;4(7):S1.
43. ASCIA Education Resources. Laboratory tests in the diagnosis of allergic diseases. Last Updated November 2010. Available on http://www.allergy.org.au/aer/infobulletins/Laboratory_Tests.htm. Accessed on Sept 2011.
44. Andrade RJ, Tulkens PM. Hepatic safety of antibiotics used in primary care. J Antimicrob Chemother. 2011;66(7):1431–46.
45. Prince MI, Burt AD, Jones DE. Hepatitis and liver dysfunction with rifampicin therapy for pruritus in primary biliary cirrhosis. Gut. 2002;50(3):436–9.
46. The Joint Commission. Issue 35: using medication reconciliation to prevent errors. Sentinel Event Alert. 2006. Accessed on July 2011.
47. Jones D. Therapeutic drug monitoring – a vital pharmacy role. Br J Clin Pharmacol. 2009;1:171.

Index

A

Agency of Healthcare Quality and Research (AHRQ), 38

American academy of orthopedic surgeons (AAOS), 64, 275

Amputation, 216

Antibiotic-loaded bone cement (ALBC), 68

Antimicrobial susceptibility testing, 187–188

Antimicrobial therapy
administration type impact, 306–307
adverse drug interactions
clinical significance, 302–303
complementary and alternative medicines, 300–301
P-glycoprotein, 301
rifampicin, 300–301
antibiotic adverse event, 304
dosing regimen impact, 298–299
drug–disease interactions, 298
drug-related complications, 308, 309
drug therapy monitoring, 308
gastrointestinal toxicity, 305–306
hepatotoxicity, 306
hypersensitivity, 304–305
medicine reconciliation, 307
nephrotoxicity, 305
optimal dosage regimen, 298
patient compliance, 308
perioperative medication management, 307
polypharmacy, 298
therapeutic drug monitoring, 307–308

Arthrodesis
ankle fusion, 216, 217
disadvantage, 218
dorsal and plantar flexion, 216, 218
external fixator, 218, 219
indications, 216

intramedullary nail, 218, 220
plates and screws, 218, 221
two-stage revision, 217

Artificial bone grafts, 291

B

Bacteria–biomaterial interactions. *See* Biomaterial-associated infection (BAI)

Bacterial adhesion, PJI
cellular second phase, 97–98
clinical infection, 96, 97
matrix proteins, 96
physical reversible first phase, 97

Biofilm
bacterial biomass, 98
bone grafts, 292
Candida albicans, 99
PIA, 198–199
planktonic form, 100
Propionibacterium acnes, 99
septic loosening, 122
sonication, 174
synovial fluid cytology, 153

Biomaterial-associated infection (BAI)
biofilm, 105
Candida interactions, 110
microbial interactions
quaternary ammonium compounds, 110–111
silver and copper, 111–112
mycobacterial interactions
biofilm formation, 108
COPD, 109
human infections, 108
tuberculous arthritis, 109–110

R. Trebše (ed.), *Infected Total Joint Arthroplasty*,
DOI 10.1007/978-1-4471-2482-5, © Springer-Verlag London 2012

Printed by Publishers' Graphics LLC